SHAMELESS

SHAMELESS

THE VISIONARY LIFE

of

MARY GOVE NICHOLS

ॐ   ॐ   ॐ

JEAN L. SILVER-ISENSTADT

The Johns Hopkins University Press • Baltimore & London

© 2002 The Johns Hopkins University Press
All rights reserved. Published 2002
Printed in the United States of America on acid-free paper

9 8 7 6 5 4 3 2 1

The Johns Hopkins University Press
2715 North Charles Street
Baltimore, Maryland 21218-4363
www.press.jhu.edu

Library of Congress Cataloging-in-Publication Data
Silver-Isenstadt, Jean L.
Shameless : The visionary life of Mary Gove Nichols / Jean L. Silver-Isenstadt.
p.   cm.
Includes bibliographical references and index.
ISBN 0-8018-6848-3
1. Nichols, Mary Sargeant Gove, 1810–1884.   2. Women social reformers—United
States—Biography—19th century.   3. Women health reformers—United States—
Biography.   4. Nichols, Thomas Low, 1815–1901.   5. Hydrotherapy.   6. Physicians—
United States—Biography.   I. Title.
HQ1413.N53 S55 2002
303.484′092—dc21

2001002226

A catalog record for this book is available from the British Library.

Dedicated to Sophie, Maya, and Ezra,
the coming tide,
and to Ari,
for refusing separate spheres

A new thought has dawned upon the world—
that of fidelity to one's self.
MARY GOVE NICHOLS, *Marriage, 1854*

CONTENTS

ILLUSTRATIONS

FOLLOW P. 128

Advertisement for Mary Gove's Graham Boarding School

Lynn Lyceum

"The Wrong and the Right Way" to Heal a Child

Advertisement for the Brattleboro Water Cure

Various Water-Cure Techniques,
Joel Shew's *Hand-Book of Hydropathy*, 1845

Sitz Bath

Vaginal Syringe Kit

Indictment of the Corset in the *Water-Cure Journal*

Bloomer Costume

Advertisement for *Mary Lyndon*

Yellow Springs Water Cure, 1853

Advertisements for the Inventions and Supplies of
Thomas L. Nichols

Letter from Mary Gove Nichols to Paulina Wright Davis

Engraving of Mary Gove Nichols

———— A C K N O W L E D G M E N T S ————

I AM GRATEFUL for the financial support provided by the American
Antiquarian Society's Kate B. and Hall J. Peterson Fellowship, by a Research Fellowship from the College of Physicians of Philadelphia's Wood
Institute, and by a Dissertation Fellowship from the University of Pennsylvania's School of Arts and Sciences. Many generous individuals provided me with research assistance as well. I would particularly like to
thank Joane Chaison, Laura Wasowicz, Thomas Horrocks, Scott Sanders,
Patricia Cline Cohen, and Ronald Walters for their warmth and assistance.

I am also indebted to the following people for their knowledgeable
hunting of sources: Patricia Albright, Mt. Holyoke College Archives; Eve-
lyn Bechtel, New Hampshire Historical Society; Kathryn Black, New
England Historic Genealogical Society; Kevin Cawley, University of Notre
Dame Archives; Victoria Douglas, Columbia Readers' Guild; Kelly R. Fal-
cone, Western Reserve Historical Society; David Gross, College of William
and Mary; Karl Kabelac, University of Rochester Library; Martha Lan-
dis, University of Illinois Library; Charles Longley, Boston Public Library;
Nancy MacKechnie and Dean Rogers, Vassar College Library; Leslie Morris, Harvard University Library; Nina D. Myatt, Antioch University
Archives; Maureen O'Shea and Sister Janice McQuade of St. John the
Evangelist Roman Catholic Community of Columbia, Maryland; Anne-
Marie Perrault, American-Canadian Genealogical Society; Michael Plun-
kett, University of Virginia Library; Debbie Randorf, New York Histori-
cal Society; Jennie Rathbun, Harvard University Library; Diane Roden,
St. Xavier Church, Cincinnati, Ohio; Diane Shephard, Lynn Historical So-
ciety; Janice Simon, University of Georgia Department of Art History;
Mariam Touba, New York Historical Society; William Vann, the New York

State Newspaper Project; Cynthia Van Ness, Buffalo and Erie County Public Library; Virginia Weygandt, Clark County Historical Society; and Don Wilcox, University of Michigan Library. I would also like to thank Janet Noever, whose well-researched dissertation on Mary Gove Nichols inspired my own work and guided me to many primary sources. To any whose names I have missed, my apologies and sincere appreciation.

Insightful feedback on my manuscript was provided by historians Charles E. Rosenberg, Regina Morantz-Sanchez, Robert Richardson Jr., Judith McGaw, Elizabeth Hunt, and Andrew Rapoza. I consider myself very fortunate to have been able to work closely with these outstanding scholars. I also want to thank Annie Dillard—a sequoia among mentors; the immediacy of her influence astounds me still. This work also owes much to my wonderfully patient, direct, and encouraging editor, Jacqueline Wehmueller, who made the process a pleasure; to Elizabeth Yoder, whose careful copyediting smoothed and strengthened every page; and to Carol Zimmerman and the Press staff, who vitalized the home stretch.

Lastly, I would like to acknowledge the enormous family support I have received for this project. Meralda Velazquez has provided my daughters a wealth of loving care; without her this book would not exist. My brothers, Ted and Dan Silver; my sister-in-law, Ellen Rose Silver; and the extended Isenstadt family have all encouraged both my writing and my happiness. Likewise my diligent grandmother, Lillian Leopold, has never let me lose sight of the finish line. My parents, Ann-Louise and Stuart Silver, have critiqued my drafts; bestowed a rare-book budget; and fueled my stamina. Most important, my husband Ari has inspired, motivated, calmed, energized, provoked, and nurtured me through every phase of this project. He even *proofread the notes*. There is no deeper love. I am inordinately grateful to my entire family.

INTRODUCTION

THIS BOOK TELLS the story of Mary S. Gove Nichols (1810–84), an advocate of happiness whose work continues to influence how we live and how we think about our lives. Her first husband considered her deranged; her second considered her a genius. The *New York Morning Herald* called her an "extraordinary woman, saint, *savante*, serpent, or whatever else she may be."[1] When this leader of the free-love and water-cure movements published her autobiography in 1855, the *New York Daily Times* devoted four vituperative columns to denouncing the work and its infamous author. Mary's personal journey alarmed mainstream sensibilities. While outraged moralists ardently savaged her book, others ordered advance copies.

Mary's life brought her into remarkable company and circumstance. She was a national figure in the 1840s and 50s. Thousands came to hear the scandalous anatomy lectures of this young, dark-eyed educator, who dared—with all possible propriety—to discuss the healthy, undressed female body. She addressed not only its tangible parts but also its longings, capacities, and political relevance. A social reformer and able writer, Mary socialized with Edgar Allan Poe, Albert Brisbane, Horace Greeley, John Neal, and Charles Dickens (though she did antagonize Horace Mann). A radical thinker, she also led the way for Paulina Wright Davis, Elizabeth Cady Stanton, Margaret Sanger, Emma Goldman, Gloria Steinem, and Dr. Ruth Westheimer, to name but a few.

Mary's life story reflects the complexity and energy of nineteenth-century social reform—for there were many forces driving Mary and much that she sought to improve. In this, Mary Gove Nichols was typical. Her odyssey, on the other hand, was not. Like many dutiful wives of her day,

she had submitted to the unwanted sexual clutches of a husband she detested, while silently questioning whether God intended such suffering. Like
so many others, she prayed, she endured, and she gave birth to stillborn
children. But then, unlike most women, she said *Enough*. The form of this
"enough," the sequelae of this "enough," are part of a unique story whose
cultural context was shared by thousands. Because Mary Gove Nichols
publicly struggled with issues that engaged everyone, she acquired fame
and influence in her lifetime. Yet because her epiphanies and methods do
not fit neatly into established story lines of progressivism, she has been
largely neglected by historians. Mary vigorously and self-consciously confronted issues that remain central to identity and conduct: sex roles, intimacy, parenthood, marriage, the question of human equality, the role of
religion, the dangers of isolation, the management of illness, the nature
of sex, the pleasure of work, and the route to political and social progress.

"THE THING CALLED A WIFE"

Mary's first question was simple: to whom did her body belong? From this
painful beginning evolved a life's work. She struggled with her relationship to both men and God, who were conflated in many ways. The civil
laws of nineteenth-century marriage derived from biblical teachings: the
nature and intentions of God were ostensibly manifest in a legal system
that deemed wives akin to property, that denied them the right to negotiate contracts or to maintain control of their own earnings, and that refused to recognize mothers' custody rights as equal to those of fathers. All
women, whether married or single, were vehemently discouraged from
any form of public speaking. Few had access to substantive education. And
of course no woman had the right to sit on a jury or to vote.

Mary Gove Nichols helped initiate a wave of resistance to this version
of "God's will." Hers was among the new voices of medical expertise that
effectively competed with the church as arbiter of morality. The health
reform movement was not merely medical; it was political. It offered an
authoritative endorsement of women's strength. As one of Mary's water-
cure colleagues wrote in 1852, women should make it "absolutely impossible for man to philosophize correctly, to exhort edifyingly, to enter into
society properly, to legislate with permanency, unless he proceeds on the
recognition that woman, as well as man, has a soul, an organization, an

entity not to be buried up in him, or in arrangements solely contemplating him."[2] These were fighting words. As Mary wrote, "I have been 'the thing called a wife,' having no individuality, no spontaneity. I have suffered a degradation that the Church and the world call purity and virtue."[3] Seeing little alternative, she wrought a new ideal.

That sex shaped Mary's search for women's rightful place with regard to men and God has a logic easier to appreciate today than it was in antebellum America. Discussions of sexual politics now saturate our culture. But in the agony of her first marriage bed, Mary lacked such language. Gradually, through the lenses of the health-reform movement and the social experiments of utopian communalists, Mary began to view women's health and happiness as dependent upon personal freedom. Her growing commitment to women's self-knowledge and self-ownership drew her into the public domain. She lectured to the newly founded "physiological societies," at urban lyceums, and in parlor classes. She began writing for national journals (sometimes under pseudonyms). And she, like thousands of other women denied the legal right to divorce, still managed to separate from her first husband and to find a truer match. Few remarried women, however, found themselves in the empowering company of men as progressive as Thomas Low Nichols.

In many ways this book constitutes a dual biography, for Mary's story is wonderfully intertwined with that of her second husband, a journalist-turned-physician who, with his wife's partnership, became an outspoken feminist in his own right. Passionate, articulate, resilient, and unabashed, Thomas Low Nichols produced one of the most popular and sexually explicit medical textbooks of his day. Likewise slandered for his endorsement of "free love," Thomas agreed with Mary and others in the movement that God intended balanced expression of all physiologic passions, including sexual passion, and that traditional social institutions such as indissoluble marriage led to widespread misery and consequent disease. Most nineteenth-century readers viewed "free lovers" as defenders of promiscuity, yet the Nicholses advocated—and seem to have practiced—extreme restraint when it came to sex. Nonetheless, many who read their work looked at the world's pervasive selfishness, lust, and indulgence and concluded that instinct and purity could not reinforce one another. The Nicholses had greater faith in humanity.

Mary and Thomas worked synergistically for the cause of universal health, which they believed prerequisite to all other social improvements. Theirs was an intellectually and professionally collaborative marriage. Together they established journals, wrote books, founded a medical school, treated patients, parented children, earned money, faced critics, and sustained love. At one point Thomas wrote of his life with Mary, "Alike, almost to identity, in thought and work, we have been united, as few persons have ever been, in what we conceived to be our sacred mission."[4]

The Nicholses' success in work and matrimony constituted a great irony in their attack on the institution of marriage. That they willingly adopted one another as husband and wife at all speaks to the power of this cultural expectation, for neither entered their union naïve as to its risks. Everything Mary wrote blatantly contradicted Alexis de Tocqueville's perception that American wives "take pride in the free relinquishment of their will" and refuse to regard "conjugal authority as a blessed usurpation of their rights."[5] But she had a professional reputation to maintain and a child from her first marriage to support. The reality was that whether one chose to live within the social code or to seek its absolute limits, everyone had to make some sort of peace with convention. There were stark consequences to a life of radicalism, just as there were great costs to compliance.

THE WATER CURE

With the advent of indoor plumbing, bathing has become commonplace. But in the mid-nineteenth century, before the discovery of bacteria, professional health reformers earnestly taught people how and why to wash themselves because almost no one was doing it. Mary and Thomas advocated a specific medical system called the water cure, also known as hydropathy or hydrotherapy. The cure relied on pure, cold water to both prevent and treat disease, which was thought to result from mistakes made in diet, dress, medicine, and daily self-management. Mary put it strongly: "Believing all sickness to be the ultimation of sin in the individual, or the inherited consequence of the sins of our progenitors, I am of necessity a religious teacher. If there were no sin, there would be no sickness."[6] The pursuit of health had become a new form of worship—a demonstrated respect for God's "laws of life."

Founded by the Austrian Vincent Priessnitz in 1826, the water cure attracted many followers in antebellum America. It reached its peak of popularity in the 1850s amidst an explosion of alternative medical theories in the United States. Diverse practitioners condemned regular physicians as destructive and profiteering. The regular physicians (also termed allopathic or orthodox physicians) replied in kind. Dire warnings about one's competitors filled the many medical journals. Choosing among self-proclaimed medical experts must have felt something like playing Russian roulette. Regular medicine felt itself utterly besieged. Mary joined in this critique, but she preferred to attack "ignorance" rather than physicians per se, many of whom had helped her acquire medical education and had supported her professional lecturing. For general health and equilibrium, Mary taught her patients to pursue eight hours of work, eight hours of sleep, and eight hours of "devotion, recreation, and sustentation" each day.[7]

Those like Mary who adopted the water-cure system ate a vegetarian diet, exercised regularly, shunned corsets, bathed daily, drank many glasses of cold water, slept in well-ventilated rooms, and avoided alcohol, tobacco, and excessive "carnality." In times of illness, they preferred to consult hydropathic medical practitioners rather than regular doctors. Hydrotherapists rejected drugs. They relied instead on elaborate bathing regimens to free the body of disease, whereas allopaths favored blistering, bloodletting, opiates, cathartics, and mercury-based medications. The two systems also differed dramatically in the management of pregnancy and childbirth. Hydrotherapists believed that nature rarely required medical assistance in producing healthy children. They therefore sought to avoid the use of instruments or surgical interventions, which in difficult births were becoming standard practice for their allopathic competitors.

For other reasons as well, the water-cure movement had special appeal for women.[8] Although both sexes believed in and practiced the cure, women stood to gain in new ways by adopting its methods. Retreat to bucolic hydropathic resorts released female patients from the isolation of their daily household responsibilities and provided the company of other women. Whether under supervision at a water-cure establishment or simply by reading a water-cure journal at home, women learned how to prevent and treat disease themselves. This saved the cost and often the embarrassment of calling on private physicians, especially for the treatment of "female complaints."

Even more important, however, was hydrotherapy's refusal to pathologize natural processes such as menstruation and childbirth. Hydropathic practitioners believed that women's bodies were inherently well and strong. At a time when regular medicine portrayed women's bodies as perpetually at risk—with menarche and menopause understood as veritable crises of vulnerability—hydrotherapy rejected notions of female fragility. God, they believed, did not intend women for sickly lives of domestic caution. And rather than view a woman's mind as the hostile competitor of her reproductive organs, hydrotherapists taught that health demanded the equilibrium and generalized tone of all systems, including the intellect. The political implications of this new perspective were liberating and significant.[9] By the early 1850s, the editor of the *Water-Cure Journal, and Herald of Reforms* celebrated women's progress: "We believe there are now in the United States one hundred well-qualified female lecturers, and they can wield an influence more potent for human good, in the capacity of reform lecturers, than that of any five hundred men now existing on the face of the earth. Woman's first right is the right to herself; and her proper sphere is wherever she can be most useful to the human race."[10] Mary Gove Nichols had been the first woman to give such public health lectures to female audiences. Her labor had convinced many besides Thomas Low Nichols that the "reform of health must be the pivot of all other reforms."[11]

AN OBSESSION WITH SEX

Although her role as a leader of the health-reform movement has been recognized by historians, Mary's perspectives on sexual self-direction have been largely overlooked by scholars. The old myth of Victorian prudery has been replaced by sophisticated analyses of the tensions between prescriptive (often proscriptive) medical writing and the actual sexy content of nineteenth-century love letters and diaries. Historians have identified a virtual "obsession" with sex in Victorian America. Yet once again, Mary Gove Nichols does not fit easily into any of the dominant schools of thought. Nor does her thinking follow the evolution generally associated with her century's framing of sex.

While many viewed sexual intimacy as sanctified only by marriage and believed matrimony to protect against moral degradation, Mary saw the dangers reversed. But despite her antimarriage stance, she idealized romantic love and saw harm in mere sensualism. At the same time, she defended the theoretical right of a woman to pursue multiple partners. As a water-cure physician, she recommended extreme sexual moderation, but she also wrote with a modern voice about women's healthy libidos. Mary rebelled against the notion that discussion of passion should be privatized. She knew too well the dangers of unsupervised spaces, of isolation, and of silent "respectability." Her experience offers a new angle from which to consider nineteenth-century anxiety about distinctions between public and private conduct. Though she was viewed by many as the perfect example of moral degradation in a loosening society, she was, ironically, motivated by similar concerns about social morality.

Mary also played a significant role in the women's rights movement, though she did not focus on the cause of women's suffrage. Without the reform of marital law, Mary and Thomas considered suffrage an empty demand: "To allow married women the right of suffrage would be simply giving every married man two votes, which would be an unfair advantage over bachelors." They continued:

As long as women promise to "serve" and "obey" their husbands, they can never be independent electors. . . . The social and domestic relations of husband and wife, as defined by the laws, and according to the formulas of religion, are inconsistent with their separate political action. A wife has no civil existence, separate from that of her husband. She acts but by his permission. If she disobeys him, she violates the marriage contract. . . . There must be a new code of marriage, and new ideas of marital rights, before any important change can be effected in the relative positions of the sexes.[12]

As we understand more about the political implications of health reform, lyceum teaching, and women's public outreach, the traditionally held construct of starkly separate spheres of male and female industry in the nineteenth century has been thrown into question, and the definition of political action has expanded.[13] Clearly Mary and Thomas Nichols provide one example of a politically active couple who shared professional and personal realms. Referring to Lucy Stone, the Rev. Antoinette Brown, Ernestine Rose, and other leaders of the 1853 Woman's Rights Convention in New York City, Mary wrote with all due respect: "These women know not what they ask." For as she and Thomas elaborated in their *Journal,*

Until there are great and radical changes in social institutions, there can be no such recognition of women's rights, as these ladies demand. Until then, all that can be granted is amelioration, more scope to labor, a better education, less offensive laws—but freedom and equality with man, social, religious, and political? . . . It would be a revolution, before which all others sink into insignificance. . . . The blindness of so many reformers may be very well for reform, for if they saw what they were doing, they would stop in terror at their work, and at its consequences.[14]

FROM FAME TO OBSCURITY

The story of how a young, abused, and isolated small-town wife resituated herself as a strong public presence illuminates the boundaries facing American women during the 1800s. These confines were legal, spiritual, physical, and *negotiable*. Over time, role expectations changed because neither women nor men simply conformed to expectation. As individuals, they navigated, they chose, and sometimes they rebelled. Mary's journey traverses nineteenth-century divorce law; the anxious search for moral authority in a secularizing world; and the nature of privacy, freedom, sickness, love, sex, and ambition. Such powerful themes are best appreciated when magnified through specific experience.

It is worth considering why many people know nothing about Mary Gove Nichols. Her writings foreshadowed those of Elizabeth Cady Stanton, Emma Goldman, and Margaret Sanger; she was included in Sarah Josepha Hale's famous *Woman's Record* of 1855; and Edgar Allan Poe included her among his "literati of New York." Her lectures were front-page news, and she published widely. But today she is virtually unknown. One reason for Mary's relative obscurity in historical accounts is surely her geographical rootlessness and eventual emigration. Rather than remain in New York City where they had established a successful medical practice and hydropathic training institute, Mary and Thomas bounced from one location to another, and in 1861 they finally emigrated to England. Though they continued to publish, the Nicholses repeatedly removed themselves from networks of friends and colleagues, always seeking richer soil for their utopian visions. Thus, they appear as transient visitors in a variety of nineteenth-century causes and never as central characters in the stories of social reform. In fact, when writing their own history, leaders of the suffrage movement never credited Mary for her enormous influence on women's sense of political entitlement. Because she had endorsed free love—a cause that seemed to threaten family unity—Mary was perceived as a liability to the movement. Political expediency required suffragists not to stray too far from traditional American values. But Mary had not prized the mere vote enough to temper her broad demands. By this, she sacrificed later recognition.[15]

The Nicholses' radicalism alienated fellow reformers to the point that some attempted to marginalize the couple even at the peak of their influence. Longtime colleagues turned on them. Callously broadcast slander made new friendships difficult to establish. As novelist John Neal put it in 1843: "All reformers have gone too far—else were they no reformers. If you mean to clear a ditch, you must try to jump *over* it, and therefore *beyond* it." And as Mary herself acknowledged, "It has often been my lot to stand among those who were foremost, and consequently to bear the blame of 'going too far.'" With this came the price of historical submersion.[16]

It is also significant that Mary and Thomas retreated from some of the most powerful of their own initiatives, confusing peers and historians alike. Their recantation of free-love doctrine—combined with their ultimate conversion to Catholicism, the most traditional of Christian denominations—have left the two very difficult to classify. To those for whom the integration of traditional religion and undiluted feminism seems fundamentally impossible—a core contradiction—Mary may invite quick dismissal as a flawed revolutionary whose religious conversion is not only intellectually indefensible but also profoundly disappointing. Such an unforeseen transition by this champion of personal freedom is extremely provocative: *What was she thinking?* This, in fact, is the central question to anyone interested in the history of women. It is the drive to biography.

We have a spectacular gold mine in the prolific writings of Mary Gove Nichols, who deserves serious attention not only from scholars of social history but also from anyone interested in how our own paths were worn for us, and against what thorny obstacles. Without question, Mary Gove Nichols was one of the most articulate and clear-headed leaders of the early feminist movement, broadly defined. She launched our unembar-

rassed expectation of sexual education. She proved that traditionally se-
questered topics (and naked French mannequins) could withstand the
heat of the public lecture hall. She enabled women to see connections between their bodies, their laws, their health, and their happiness.

I can remember first discovering "feminism" in college. I came home that
first summer horrified to discover that my physician-mother was not a
member of NOW. *Didn't she care?* She had once been a member, she said
in her own defense, and would join again with me; but my disillusionment
was not easy to counter. "I try to express my feminism in my daily work,"
she explained—weakly, I thought. At the time, I just didn't get it. Sure,
she had been the first half-time psychiatric resident at Johns Hopkins,
staying home to be involved with her three children. Sure, she later
treated patients sixty hours per week. Sure, she gave academic talks on her
professional foremothers. Sure, she would be president of the American
Academy of Psychoanalysis. Sure, she baked and gardened and sewed and
traveled and published and voted. *But what about that membership in
NOW?* It has taken me years to understand what my mother was then trying to say: Look at the life.

Like my mother, Mary Gove Nichols raised children, treated patients,
published writings, and sought to live what she believed. She also, in the
eyes of her contemporaries, dropped the ball a lot. Contradicted herself.
Didn't show up where she should have. Appeared where she shouldn't
have. Spoke too bluntly. Pursued the unexpected. Because Mary's trek was
real and not rhetorical, it was rutted, steep, and circuitous. Her strivings
not only shed light on the nineteenth century, but they also give resonance
to *our* choosings from moment to moment. They reveal the inevitable
difficulty of swirling in the social current, and they perhaps enable some
self-forgiveness as well. Most importantly, an understanding of Mary's
quest can help us resist the urge for simple delineations of historical
progress or for simple, implausible heroes.

ONE

The Formative Years

TWO THOUSAND PEOPLE, a third of them children under ten, occupied Goffstown, New Hampshire, in 1810, the year of Mary Neal's birth. Goffstown had been founded in 1733, when traces of primeval forest still remained. Town lore held that a pine mast taken from the farm of George Bell had left a stump wide enough to accommodate a turning team of oxen. Located just west of Manchester near the southern border of the state, Goffstown welcomed the early sawmills that turned trees into ship planks and opened the land. In 1810 the town's residents still listened to screech owls and mourning doves, warblers and woodpeckers. Often they heard wolves. Fishing in the local Piscataquog River, they scooped up alewives, lamper-eels, shad, and salmon. Along the shores, they hunted quail and grouse.

In 1810, Goffstown farmers tilled the productive soil along the river's edge and paid taxes to support the new district schools where their children sat on simple benches and studied from Pike's *Arithmetic, The New English Primer,* the Bible, Lindley Murray's *Grammar,* and Pope's *Essay on Man.* An 1808 town statute required: "No person shall be deemed qualified to teach . . . unless they can procure a certificate from some reputable English grammar schoolmaster, learned minister of the gospel, president or professor of some college of their ability, and likewise a certificate . . . that they sustain a good moral character." Everyone knew one another; character mattered. Three local inspectors visited the schools regularly to help secure high literary, moral, and religious standards.

The Uncanoonuc Mountains, wholly encompassed in the town's 29,000 acres, sheltered deer, bears, catamount, and lynx. In the spring, pink and white laurel—called spoonhunch—bloomed thickly along the Piscataquog's southern shore. From the summit of Uncanoonuc Mountain, one could identify peaks of the distant White Mountains and Franconia Range to the north—Mt. Washington and Lafayette; to the south loomed Wachusett and the Blue Hills near Boston. One could even spot Bunker Hill. The Kuncanowet Hills separated Goffstown from Weare, to the west, and from those hills, looking east over Goffstown, one could see the wide waters of Massabesic Lake, the winding course of the Merrimack River, and the town of Amoskeag, soon to be operating the world's largest cotton mill and later known as Manchester.[1]

Mary Sargeant Neal embarked on life in 1810—the same year as did Phineas T. Barnum, Theodore Parker, and Margaret Fuller, all following close on the heels of Edgar Allan Poe and Ralph Waldo Emerson. In Europe, Frederic Chopin and Robert Schumann were born. It was the year that Samuel Hahnemann published his *Organon of Therapeutics,* describing the principles of homeopathic medicine, and the year that New York City surpassed Philadelphia in population. Harriet Beecher Stowe, Elizabeth Cady Stanton, Frederick Douglass, and Henry David Thoreau would be born before the decade ended.

But Mary Neal's birth must not have felt auspicious at all to her mother, Rebecca Neal, herself the oldest of seventeen children. Rebecca was suffering with typhus when she delivered her first daughter. Many in Goffstown had already succumbed to the disease. From that first agonizing July day forward, a lack of affinity characterized the relationship between Rebecca and her child. Mary proved to be sickly, clumsy, somnambulant, unattractive, and shy—yet full of ambition. Her mother would have preferred an efficient, robust daughter who could make a good loaf of brown bread. Mary, instead, loved to read and tended to adopt odd pets, like crows. Often weak with illness and harshly medicated by the town doctor, she took little interest in mastering household chores. She frequently burned what she put in the oven. In her sleep, she once wandered out of the house into deep snow.[2] Worst of all, Mary was developing a strong will, like her father.

Throughout Goffstown, New Hampshire, William Neal had a reputation as an infidel. He preferred to call himself a freethinker. While Rebecca discouraged Mary's ambitions and ceaselessly reiterated the need for "usefulness," William prodded his daughter to question authority. Not surprisingly, Mary grew to worship her father and resent her mother. "My mother, so conscientious and devout," Mary later wrote, "still made the misery of my young life. She had a theory that no child should have a will or way of his, or her, own. She crushed individuality as her most imperative duty." Chronic activity characterized the Neal home. In the living room, Mary recalled typically "a half-dozen kinds of industry going on at the same time." The whirl of four spinning wheels often filled the house as girls simultaneously worked linen, tow, cotton, and wool. Amidst this production, one schoolteacher who always boarded with the family stole a corner of the table for study. Mary envied him.[3]

For a woman who would later write moving, powerful descriptions of maternal love, Mary Neal only grudgingly recognized the sentiment in her own mother. Rebecca Neal stood accused of having a "false conscience" when it came to her daughter. "I wished to learn what she thought of 'no use,'" wrote Mary. "These two words were always potent with her, and her ideas of use were very limited. She could not understand me in the least." But resist it as they will, children tend to become their parents. Everything that is known about William and Rebecca Neal— whom Mary remembered as reasonable, unsuperstitious, and brave— found expansion in the life of their daughter.[4]

Both William and Rebecca Neal held extreme views. "Free thinking as to religion, and republicanism in politics, were royal roads to my father's favour," recalled Mary, who often read out loud to him from his favorite writers: Pope, Voltaire, Volney, Paine, and Cobbett.[5] One of Mary's earliest memories was of saying goodbye to her father when he left home temporarily in 1812 to lead a company of volunteers in defense of Canada. Rebecca, more religious than William, adopted Universalism and its belief that a loving God had destined all human beings for heaven. Evangelicals and Congregationalists considered Universalism an enormous threat to traditional religion because it eliminated the motivating fear of damnation. Thus, Rebecca Neal would be seen by most of her neighbors as heretical. Yet she was devout compared to her husband, who challenged "God" to persuade the family of his existence. In conversation, William provoked Mary to defend her faith:

"Little one, your Christianity commands the impossible, and does not achieve the possible. Tell me who is a Christian."
"The being who acts from love."

"Every one acts from love, but the little word self comes before it. There are a great many kinds of love."

"I only mean Divine love, father. . . . The true spirit of religion is love, and whether its professors have much or little of this spirit, it remains the same."

"That is a droll center that has no circumference."

"Oh father! . . . It is folly to talk with you. . . . You do not wish to convince—you argue to triumph and to silence."

"Pretty near the truth. Most people have no analysis, or understanding. You are quite out of the common highway for women. You are better than the best of them, and *you* always end an argument with an inundation."[6]

Such intellectual sparring fostered an assertiveness in Mary and introduced her to the world of radical ideas. "It were an easy task to find 'thirty-nine articles' in which he had no faith," Mary wrote, "but very difficult to find half a dozen to which he would give his hearty, unqualified credence." Her father, who headed the Goffstown school board and selected and boarded the schoolteachers, admitted to Mary that he enjoyed the art of persuasion and that rhetorical debate amused him. Most people, in his view, thought like sheep. As an adult, Mary came to the painful realization that her "noble father was a sophist." Still, she attributed much of her own character strength to her father. He had encouraged her to think and to argue. He had praised her mind.[7]

Strangely, though, William discouraged Mary from learning how to write. Though he brought her books and often asked her opinion of them, William did not provide his daughter with paper and pencil. Even as an adult, Mary could not understand this inconsistency. Perhaps her mother had something to do with it. Though Rebecca expected her daughter to learn "reading, writing, and arithmetic" in school, she also worried about Mary's excessive love of stories. Novels were just coming into vogue in the early nineteenth century, and many considered them dangerous—and useless. Novels rejected the traditional literary structures of sermons and psalms; they encouraged female literacy; they gave voice to the experiences of women and minorities; they even incited desire. Mary wanted to write one. As a young child she secretly taught herself how to form letters, but throughout her long life, Mary never developed polished handwriting.[8]

Like many early New England families, the Neal family was large and complex. William's family was of Scottish descent. Rebecca, whose maiden name and ancestral origins are unknown, was twenty-one when she became William's second wife after his first wife died. She mothered the three children of his first marriage as well as the three she and William had together. Details have been lost, but it seems that Mary's eldest half-sister was about fifteen years her senior. Rebecca and William's first child was a boy twenty months older than Mary, who died of consumption as a young adult. Mary, their second child, also suffered with consumption throughout her life. Then a third child, whose sex is unknown, was born to them. "My father was my peer, my mother my severe ruler, and my elder sisters my critics and satirists," Mary summarized. "All loved me, no doubt, but no one gave me any expression of affection, except my maternal grandmother."[9] And we do not know who her maternal grandmother was.

Mary describes her childhood as lonely. Goffstown, New Hampshire, is still a small and quiet town, though much greener now than in Mary's youth, when villages consumed their forests for fuel. Roads were dusty and muddy by turns. The white, spired church and its cemetery marked the center of town. Gravestones of the many women who had died between the ages twenty-five and forty reminded girls of the dangers awaiting them. Graves of children and infants encircled these. Epidemic measles, scarlatina, and typhus regularly reduced the population. "Half the children born around me died in infancy," Mary recalled.[10] Goffstown grew especially desolate for the Neals when one of Mary's elder half-sisters, only twenty, died of tuberculosis. Mary was twelve years old at the time.

In her autobiography, Mary describes her variety of adopted pets with greater affection than this ill-fated sister, whom she calls "Emma." Passionately devoted to the feminine art of fashion, Emma was beautiful and entirely uninterested in intellectual pursuits. She taunted her little sister for spending too much time with books and even mocked Mary's way of walking. When the two girls looked at themselves side by side in the mirror, it seemed to Mary a painful contrast. "I did not love my sister," wrote Mary, "and Emma did not love me."[11]

In her career as a water-cure practitioner and health advocate, Mary frequently returned to the story of her sister's death, which always seemed senseless and unnecessary, brought on by slavery to fashion and an ignorant reliance on the town doctor, a traditional blood-letter. For Mary, this version of events became a morality tale; it acquired an archetypal quality, a life of its own.

It was winter. Emma had a terrible cough. Rebecca Neal had forbidden her daughter to attend a distant evening party. Yet with promises that she would return home by ten o'clock; that she would wear a dress with a high neck, a warm shawl, a cloak, and fur-lined overshoes; and that she would arrange a ride and not walk in the snow, Emma artfully won permission. Mary watched the exchange with interest. Later she recalled the scene that evening when Emma descended the stairs "dressed in sky-blue merino, her neck, shoulders and arms exposed, as if in mockery of the warm material of her dress."[12] And in retrospect, perhaps most damaging, Emma had laced her corset so tightly that her already struggling lungs suffered terrible compression. An ugly exchange ensued between Rebecca and Emma, followed by much cajoling. Ultimately, Rebecca softened. Emma stayed late at the party, missed her ride, and returned home around midnight, trudging alone through the snow in pretty party shoes. The next day she was very ill.

Emma did not last much longer. Though she recovered from that particular bad cold, another one followed, and another. Soon she was coughing up blood. Panicked, the family called a local doctor, who bled Emma profusely. Mary remembered sitting day after day by her dying sister, watching the life drain out of her. It became difficult for Emma even to tuck stray curls back under her night cap.

The weeks of Emma's slow dying heightened Mary's awareness of her mother and father as well. Rebecca's grief was boundless. Given the cool relationship Mary shared with her mother, it must have been painful to watch her mother's anguish over Emma. Though she repeatedly insists that she harbored no envy for her sister, Mary insists too often; a powerful self-pity informs Mary's accounts of her childhood. Her anger at her sister colors such judgmental statements as "The violated law of God, established in [Emma's] nature, found no atonement."[13] In other words, her sister's death was just punishment for the sin of vanity. Well before Emma became sick, Mary considered herself wholly opposite in nature; after

Emma died, Mary had a powerful justification for maintaining and widening the perceived abyss between them. As a young adult, Mary resolved never to resign her health to a corset, never to sacrifice her warmth for a strapless dress.

Naturally, William Neal suffered greatly at the loss of his daughter. Unlike his wife, William did not have God for comfort. A young Methodist minister came to the house daily at Emma's request, praying for both Emma and her faithless father. This young man made a deep impression on Mary, for his relentless efforts to "save" William seemed as devoted as his care for Emma. This minister's dogged pursuit of argument with William—which Mary well knew would prove fruitless—served to underline her father's lonely position. Believing in neither doctors nor ministers, William had called on both for Emma. "He said *No* to every one's proposition in medicine and religion, but he had no *Yes* to utter," wrote Mary. The earnest Methodist engaged in debate after debate, flustered by William Neal's repeated heresies. "He might as well have argued with a windmill in a heavy gale," thought Mary.[14]

Others exhorted William to seek faith as well. Mary recalled one neighborhood woman in particular. Hers seemed a competitive devotion to God, richer and more public than the devotion of most. William allowed her in the house only because Emma wished the visit. "She hated the enemies of Jesus Christ with a holy hatred," wrote Mary of the neighbor. "[S]he hurled her anathemas with sufficient force against my father to injure herself in the rebound." These dramatic scenes must have been both disturbing and exhilarating for twelve-year-old Mary, who revered her independent father but also feared for his want of religion and his lack of solace. When Emma finally died and William closed her eyes, Mary watched the unaccustomed sight of tears flowing down her father's cheeks. Listening to her mother wail, Mary felt numb and did not cry. At the funeral, the unsympathetic neighbor woman denounced William as "a millstone about the neck of his now sainted daughter, to sink her into the pit that is bottomless."[15] For many years, Mary would have an ambivalent relationship to Christianity.

Not long after Emma's death, the Neals moved away from Goffstown. Mary's eldest brother had left home for medical school. The Goffstown house, oppressively quiet, constantly reminded the family of Emma, and they sought distraction from their grief. As if to finalize the decision, cotton mills had polluted William's fishing grounds, and the Neals found little reason to linger. They packed their belongings.

Merely locating Craftsbury, Vermont, on a map gives one a sense of their new town's isolation. About thirty miles south of the Canadian border and right in the center of Vermont, Craftsbury offered little more than snow. Mary considered their plank home "aristocratic" when compared with the log houses of their neighbors. The family cooked their meals over an open fire in the yard—a ruggedness Mary claimed to enjoy. Nonetheless, during their two years in Craftsbury, Mary suffered with illness and depression. Before her sister's death, Mary had attended the local school six or seven months out of every year; afterward, she received only "snatches of schooling," totaling perhaps seven or eight months. At times her parents heeded a local doctor's advice that she should be forbidden to read lest the activity further weaken her. This "treatment" mortified Mary. Her daily access to books resumed after a second local physician diagnosed the depth of Mary's homesickness for Goffstown. He also endorsed a treatment favored by Mary's parents. Each morning, for a bath, her mother poured cold water over Mary, then tucked her under warm comforters for an hour of deeply restful sleep. This maternal nurture, combined with reading, soothed a profound loneliness.[16]

Mary's description of the period reveals not only an isolated longing for faith but also the desperate need to atone—for what, she could not clearly say. One late afternoon, as she watched the low sun flash through the trees behind her house, Mary experienced a profound, transient, and mystical wave of faith. It was three years after Emma's death. She felt "a sense of pardon." During the ephemeral moment, Mary felt the sunlight as "the light of God's love." She felt holy. But soon the force of this epiphany waned. She began to think about suicide, an obsession her Christian friends explained as the devil's temptation placed before those in a "state of grace." Specifically, Mary imagined walking through snow drifts, getting sick, and dying of exposure. Perhaps, struggling on with her bereaved parents, she imagined that God had taken the wrong daughter. She constantly struggled with an overwhelming sense of her own sinfulness.[17]

When her older brother at medical school sent her money for a new dress, Mary instead paid the $3 tuition at a local Presbyterian school headed by the minister's wife. She had little love for new dresses. Before long, however, Mary found herself expelled. Overly precocious (and probably a bit like her father in manner), Mary was dismissed by the minister for disrespect. The Methodists back in Goffstown had secured none of her love, and now she faced expulsion by the Presbyterians. Disillusioned and surely embarrassed, Mary still sought a theology that her father lacked.

Books led her to a fascination with Quakerism. *The Monitor*, a Quaker schoolbook she had borrowed, described the early history of the Friends and summarized many of their beliefs. Mary was drawn to the society's "temperance, frugality, self-denial, and exceeding piety." That she had never met a Quaker probably made the sect especially easy to romanticize. She had no Quaker blood on either side, but she must have given substantial weight to her father's opinion that "Christians are a poor set, but I believe the Quakers are the best of the bunch." Thus, when she was about fifteen years old, Mary formally declared herself a Quaker. William abided his daughter's decision until she would grow "wise enough not to be a Christian." Rebecca chose to remain silent.[18] Mary altered her dress and speech accordingly, seeking plainness. She pulled her dark, thick ringlets straight back into an unattractive bun. In her mind, these acts of devotion guarded her against the sins of vanity and worldliness.

Mary found herself accepted as the lone Quaker in town, though her mother criticized the unbecoming simplicity of her daughter's clothes and hair. Through this conversion, Mary had found a means to extricate herself from the Presbyterian Church, avoid the minister and his wife, and satisfy her need for a pious life. She found heroes among the Quakers in her reading and felt part of a larger community for the first time in her life. She admired Quaker values and enjoyed the structure of their rules. She enjoyed not having to go to church. Retrospectively, Mary described the religious confusion of her adolescence: "I wanted to present myself before God as one who humbly accepted the atonement made by Christ, though I did not understand it at all, and was told that it was a mystery, and therefore was not intended to be understood; yet I wanted to work out my own salvation."[19] This would prove a lifelong struggle.

Within a few years, however, Mary's spiritual uncertainty was forced to compete with more earthly concerns. Financial trouble beset the Neal family. William Neal had entered into a business partnership with a dishonest man, who, as Mary tells it, stole the company profits, burned the warehouse, and disappeared, leaving her father to pay debts he could not meet. The threat of debtors' jail time and the community service of chopping one hundred cords of wood served as William's punishment. Rebecca and Mary sold homemade socks and gloves. The debts were met, but the family was in a terrible situation. Though his name was ultimately cleared, William Neal's reputation had suffered drastically; many in town suspected him of having burned his own warehouse.[20]

Rebecca had never brooked snobbery in anyone. Being the subject of nasty gossip must have been a torment to her. Mary recalled that her mother disdained all aristocratic pretensions and had only contempt for those who thought themselves exempt from labor. "With a democracy that would forever level downward, her bitterness toward all above her in talents or position can hardly be conceived," recalled Mary.[21]

LEAVING HOME

To contribute all she could, Mary decided to become a schoolteacher. This choice was appropriate for a single young woman who enjoyed study, but it required her to jump through several intimidating hoops. First, she had to acquire a written recommendation from the minister who had expelled her from his wife's school. Though this did not prove difficult, Mary had to steel herself for the asking. Subsequently, she had to meet the requirements of the town's school committee, consisting of a merchant, a mechanic, and a lawyer. These men quizzed her knowledge of spelling, mathematics, geography, grammar, and religion. They also expected her to write her own name with a goose quill pen of her own construction. She passed these various tests and then waited for a teaching position to become available. In the meantime, she wrote stories and poems for publication in a weekly New England paper, the *Boston Traveller*. Not only did this earn her a bit of money, but the editors of the paper obligingly sent her the medical books they had been sent to review. She swapped these books with a local doctor and quietly began her private medical education.

By summer, a teaching position had opened in a neighboring town, and she had her own class of scholars. Mary was not asked to "board round," a common custom wherein a hired schoolteacher lived for several weeks in the home of each of her students so as to spare the community the cost of a separate rent while not overburdening any one family. Rather, she was offered her own room in a pleasant home. This room opened onto a flower garden. With its white floor and white bedspread, the bedroom offered a peaceful, private space for study.

Income from their daughter's teaching and writing helped the Neals. It also allowed Mary to feel the power that comes from earning one's own money and spending it as one chooses. After sending money to her family, Mary bought writing paper for herself. She set for herself two goals in teaching: "to teach my pupils what their parents wished them to learn" and "to learn as much as was possible myself." The mistress of the house had spent some time at an academy, and Mary liked her very much.[22]

Mothers of several students, however, proved to be another story. Curious about the new schoolteacher, a group of six women from the town called on Mary at her boardinghouse. Rather than graciously meeting these women, Mary sent the message that she saw no reason for a second evaluation, as she had already passed formal qualifying examinations. She refused to come out of her room. It is easy to imagine that Mary was really more terrified than insulted; her anxiety seems to have been that the women considered themselves superior and had arrived to judge her. Rebecca had fostered in her daughter a deep aversion to such people. Mary's defensive hostility in the unexpected situation did not make a tolerable impression. The women, greatly affronted, left the house imbued with strong opinions about the new schoolteacher.

It was the master of the boarding house who explained to Mary how to go about redeeming herself: she must make visits to each of the women she had snubbed. When she objected that it would be sheer hypocrisy for her to spend time visiting people she had absolutely no interest in meeting, he responded: "That's the way people excuse pleasing themselves, by considering it hypocrisy to please others."[23] Thus chastened, Mary began to reevaluate her behavior. She made the requisite visits and salvaged her reputation.

That Mary chose to recount this somewhat embarrassing story thirty years later in an autobiography reveals its significance in her life. The whole process of performing before an evaluating committee, leaving home, and taking responsibility for the education of a group of children had demanded new levels of courage and maturity, as had receiving new visitors. The defenses she brought to the situation mirrored her parents' reactions: who are these people to judge me? The immediate need to recover her lost reputation must have stung doubly, following on the heels of her father's difficulties. Even as an adult, she had not entirely gotten over the incident. Framing her account of the experience are snipes at "gossiping women." Her offense had pleased the women, she believed. "It raised them to the dignity of critics, and gave them a chance to discuss my character, and also to gratify their envy, and occupy their idleness." Later in life, when writing reflectively about her own character, Mary was able to recognize both her deep need for approbation and her pride.[24]

During this time, Mary maintained her interest in medical books. It is difficult to appreciate the depth of anatomical ignorance surrounding children in the 1820s. Remembering a house call from her Craftsbury doctor, Mary later wrote, "I [then] had no idea of the complex machinery of my body. I did not even know what he meant by my lungs."[25] Given access to the library of the house where she boarded, Mary secretly exhausted its medical collection. On a visit home, she happily discovered her older brother's medical text, Bells' *Anatomy*. Though doctors had never seemed effective to her—especially after her sister's death—their calling appealed to her. No women received medical degrees in the 1820s, and Mary did not aspire to become a physician in any formal sense. Still, she could learn from books.[26] When her brother discovered his textbook in her hands, however, he took it from her immediately. Anatomy was not a fit subject for females. In fact, he even teased his sister with the threat of getting her some books on obstetrics; it was an exchange that left her painfully embarrassed. Without her brother's books, Mary resigned herself to the study of French and Latin—languages ideally suited to the study of medicine, though she did not realize it at the time.[27]

Once she had settled into the routine of teaching and the pleasures of independent study, Mary found the work rewarding and her salary generous. She also grew attached to the students. When the community invited her to stay on to teach the winter session, she renewed her housing arrangement and accepted. Schools were not graded by age at that time, and Mary found the youngest children most difficult to manage. How they learned to read mystified her; she felt she had practically nothing to do with their progress.

While she was teaching the summer session, Mary had her first opportunity to attend a meeting of Quakers. Two men, one about sixty and the other a bit younger, arrived in the town hoping to hold a meeting.

They wore standard garb for the Society of Friends: broad-brimmed hats and plain brown suits. The first was a "Public Friend," a minister who traveled to various communities apart from his own to hold meetings and speak as the spirit moved him. He and his companion received permission to use the schoolhouse for their gathering. They posted notices about town and drew a small number of curious people, including Mary. She found herself extremely disappointed by their brief, predominantly silent meeting, punctuated only by "a sort of exhortation in a singing tone" from the minister, then more silence. After they left, Mary found herself thinking more highly of the Methodists.

Later that year, in the midst of an evening snowstorm, Mary once again received an unexpected visit from unfamiliar Friends. A young man came to the house asking after her. Behind him she saw an elaborate sleigh loaded with furs and pulled by a team of white horses. He explained that his family had been passing through the town and had decided to stay overnight at the local hotel in order to get to know the town's only Quaker. Mary returned to the hotel with the young man to discover that his father was the younger of the two Quakers who had visited the town that summer.

The family made a deep impression on her, particularly the mother. While this woman's three children did not adhere to Quaker severity of dress, their mother presented a very formal devotion to the law of plain appearance. Though attractive, she made herself look stern, with a black bonnet and drab coat. Personally, however, she exuded warmth, and Mary was drawn to her immediately. The woman clearly governed her family. Of the husband, Mary observed, "He seldom spoke, and was never guilty of uttering an idea when he did speak."[28]

Mary learned that the family lived in a town where, like her, they were the only Quakers. They held meetings in their own home with the mother serving as minister. Mary spent several weeks of the following summer with this family, observing the sheepish husband, the powerful wife, and the strikingly beautiful children. When the father returned from a gathering with evidence of sinful drink about him, "his wife divined his state at a glance, and fixing her severe gaze upon him . . . *looked* him out of the room."[29] This was Mary's only intimate view of Quaker marriage before she embarked on her own marriage. She was impressed above all with the power of that pious mother to regulate her husband and children.

Mary compared the son to a puppy for his mindless, happy devotion. Significantly, she had not met a domineering—or even assertive—man among the very few Friends she had encountered.

This would all change when Mary responded to a letter from one of her mother's younger brothers back in Goffstown, an uncle who had, like her, developed an interest in Quakerism. He had joined a meeting of Friends in the nearby town of Weare, and there he had become close friends with a good-looking, thirty-one-year-old bachelor named Hiram Gove, a hatter. Mary's uncle had described his young niece to this devout friend, who seemed very interested in meeting the twenty-year-old woman who had independently joined the Society of Friends. This uncle did not, however, specifically mention the hatter in his letter to Mary; he merely expressed his wish to provide her sympathy as a Quaker. But it is not unlikely that Mary hoped to meet some of her uncle's Quaker acquaintances. She was aware that the Society of Friends disowned any member who married outside the faith; her local prospects for marriage were therefore nonexistent. Perhaps with this difficulty in mind and accepting of their daughter's faith, Mary's parents encouraged her to make an early fall trip back to the Goffstown area and visit with her uncle.

It did not take long for introductions to take place. In describing her first impressions of the man who would become her husband, Mary granted that it "is very difficult to do justice to persons who have blessed or blasted our lives deeply, especially the last." With this qualification, she went on to describe an instant antipathy: "My first feeling, on being introduced to my uncle's friend, was one of deep and most decided aversion. There was a seeming all over and around him, which no word could express but meanness."[30] Hiram was a tall man with green eyes and a protruding chin. Though his dress was "the perfection of Quaker ugliness," Mary wrote that many women considered him beautiful. He wore a rounded hat with a broad brim. His sleeves were cut short, leaving him wristy. Mary noted that his phrenological profile indicated high firmness. Mary's uncle assured her that Hiram would surely alter his clothing somewhat to make it more appealing.

For Hiram Gove's part, he immediately fell in love with Mary. He had a nice home in a community of Quakers who all took a deep interest in Mary. He was attentive and kind during Mary's visit, though he relentlessly avoided discussion of all secular topics so far as he could manage.

Hiram had the unpleasant habit of sighing deeply and often, and though "he had nothing to recommend him but piety," Mary soon found herself pressured to accept his proposal of marriage. Neighbors, friends, and particularly her uncle beseeched Mary to accept Hiram's hand. Amid a dizzying "whirl of persuasions," Mary agreed. "My promise was given when appeals had been made to my benevolence, and I was assured that I might avert great evil if I gave this promise. Under a false excitement I gave my word, and then dared not break it. . . . I would have been considered mad, or wicked to the last degree, if I had had the courage to avow my real feeling—my detestation of the man."[31] She would learn, over the next eleven years with Hiram, never to overfear public censure again.

That night, horrified with regret, Mary cried and prayed alone in bed. After several days of agonized engagement, she told Hiram she could not go through with the marriage, that she did not love him and did not think she could ever love him. Hiram responded with "prayers and weeping, and a misery so real, apparently, that, full of the spirit of self-abnegation, I determined to be sacrificed."[32] She then commenced hoping that she would die before the wedding. Meanwhile, Hiram and her uncle together wrote to William and Rebecca, seeking their consent to the marriage, which they received.

As if this were not affliction enough, Mary proceeded to fall in love with someone else. Soon after the engagement, Hiram introduced his fiancée to an attractive young man with whom Mary began to spend many hours. When Hiram discovered the two of them reciting impassioned poetry to one another, he became enraged. Reminding her of hell's damnation that awaited sinners—sinners who broke engagements—Hiram beckoned a group of Friends into the room as witnesses and as threat. Mary cried fitfully as Hiram elaborated on the hell that to Mary was "no vague fear, but a . . . flaming reality." Hiram believed that if Mary did not go through with the marriage, she would burn in hell. In the end, the young man with whom Mary had fallen in love attended her wedding to Hiram on March 5, 1831. In private, soon after the wedding, he told Mary that he would never marry. It was during her own wedding ceremony that Mary first experienced trouble with her eyesight—a literal dimming of her vision. This incapacitating symptom would recur in her life at times of tragedy.[33]

MARRIAGE

The decade that followed Mary's wedding to Hiram proved bleak but also formative. Mary spent the first week of married life in tears, telling Hiram how much she hated and dreaded him. Thinking her more ill and overwrought than honest, he took her on a long journey, which failed to improve their relationship. The few private documents that survive from this period corroborate in tone and detail the misery described in Mary's retrospective accounts. The consistency of her narrative is impressive. Mary's 1855 autobiography, *Mary Lyndon, or Revelations of a Life,* portrays her first marriage to "Hervey" as life-sapping.

In the 1830s a woman might turn to her mother, her sister, her female friends, or perhaps her church leader for confidential support in times of marital crisis. But Mary had never felt close to her mother. The older sister with whom she had been raised had died. She was 150 long miles from her father and 10 from her childhood home, surrounded by her husband's family and friends. And it was her involvement with the Quakers that had led to her most profound problems. Isolated, Mary turned to medical books for guidance. She devoted herself to the study of the human body—its anatomy, its physiology, its relationship to the soul.

Debilitated in body and spirit, Mary desperately sought control over her situation. She knew that her mental anguish induced nervous illness and that powerlessness lay at the root. Her quest for health merged with her quest for happiness. By acquiring a man's knowledge of medicine, she tempered her overwhelming feelings of impotence. Medicine offered Mary an esoteric framework for understanding her symptoms and her life. Her pain was, in large measure, physical. Mary lacked prior sexual experience. Marriage required her to establish a new relationship with her own body, which was no longer hers alone but was available always, by law, to her husband's desires. Her physical being had become his entitlement. Mary called her years with Hiram "an abyss of evil that I can never describe."[34]

Eleven years her senior, Hiram Gove was born in Berwick, Maine, the child of Hannah Dow (of Berwick) and David Gove, of Weare, New Hampshire. Hiram was the third of five children, all of whom were born in near succession after their parents' 1796 wedding in Berwick. David Gove died in 1805 in Weare when Hiram was only five years old, probably while the family was visiting with paternal relatives. After David's death, Hannah returned to her family in Berwick, and the five children were sent to live with friends. Additional details of Hiram's childhood are unknown.[35]

Hiram's family on both sides were Quakers, and those who met Mary most likely viewed her with some measure of suspicion. After all, the daughter of an outspoken freethinker and a Universalist, she had abruptly adopted the Quaker faith based on her readings, with no firsthand knowledge of the community. Did she understand that the true Quaker life involved more than plain dress, and "thee" and "thou"? Mary, for her part, found the actual Quakers she met profoundly disappointing; they were petty and controlling—particularly her husband, who she called "a Quaker of the narrowest kind."[36] Living in Weare proved to be even more isolating to Mary than Craftsbury. The Quakers disapproved of poetry, novels, and short stories. Her beloved father had been replaced by Hiram, a lustful nonintellect who believed devoutly in a woman's obligation to obey her husband. The two did not enjoy the rich debates that Mary so cherished. As Saint Paul taught: man shall be the head of the woman.

On March 1, 1832, their first and only child, Elma Penn Gove, was born. Mary's subsequent four pregnancies during her marriage to Hiram ended in miscarriage or stillbirth. "I endured all the sufferings of maternity, without its solace," Mary later wrote. And for Mary, the suffering of maternity began in the marriage bed. Though not described anywhere, nights with Hiram must have been sheer torment for Mary, who spent most of her life arguing for (among other things) a woman's right to determine the frequency of her sexual encounters. As a wife, Mary could claim no self-dominion. Memorizing anatomical drawings may have given her some sense of ownership over her own body parts, but this could have done little to mediate her life as a married woman.[37]

Mary's accounts of Hiram leave nothing to recommend the man. She describes multiple examples of his paranoid and violent behavior, not to mention his inability to support the family financially. According to Mary, when Elma was only three months old, her father beat her. "It is only at a distance that we can describe the burning prairie with calmness," Mary wrote of her first marriage. "I believed then, and I believe now, that he had some dreadful disease of the will—a sort of spiritual paralysis, that made him unable to act for any useful purpose. . . . I do not think I blamed

. . . [Hiram] more than I would have blamed a machine, whose construction I perfectly understood, that was crushing me to death."[38] This graphic image of a wife being crushed to death by her husband may be the closest we get to a description of the Gove's sexual relationship. She compares Hiram to a machine, assembled of parts whose arrangement might be clear, but which still does not constitute a human being. Better to think of Hiram as fundamentally disordered than as evil. In her reading, Mary was seeking a medical explanation for Hiram's physical and mental abuses. And it was the study of medicine that ultimately liberated her. "Woman," she later wrote, should "be faithful to herself" and "go not shuddering and loathing to the bed of the drunkard, or any diseased monster."[39]

Between 1831 and 1837, the Goves struggled to meet their growing debts. Trained by his uncle to make hats, Hiram did not earn enough to pay their rent; in fact, he seems not to have tried very hard. Soon Mary became the only breadwinner in the family, with Hiram haunting the house and leaving his wife no solitude. She took in needlework at night, torturous labor by candlelight that cramped her body and strained her eyes. During the day she cared for the household and Elma, stealing time to write short pieces of fiction for publication. It is not clear how Hiram passed his time. Meanwhile, Mary hid her misery from her parents. Pleasure came from cuddling Elma, from writing, and from reading borrowed medical texts—books Hiram distrusted. He began to burn Mary's personal letters before she could read them, suspicious of her correspondence and intellectual activities. He also began to restrict her physical freedom. Twenty years later, Mary wrote that she had been forbidden from going anywhere outside the house without Hiram's permission, except to the Quaker Meeting or to a funeral. She was not allowed to read or to write creatively. Any letter she composed underwent his scrutiny and was subject to destruction should it contain a single sentence of which he disapproved. "He arrogated the rule over my soul and body, with the utmost confidence. I was to do his bidding," she later wrote.[40]

That Mary never became energetically committed to the growing abolitionist movement bears a relationship to her own sense of marital enslavement. The American Anti-Slavery Society had been founded in 1833, and the Female Anti-Slavery Society began recruiting members the following year. Though sympathetic to the cause, Mary remained distant. She despised all despotism. She did not support slavery, but her own chains distracted her from those of others. The oppressor in her line of vision was a very immediate husband, not the abstract southern slaveholder. In 1853 she would write, "Everywhere are fetters and chains. African slavery is the simple, external type of the more oppressive and crushing institutions of civilization. The sufferings which grow out of the Southern institution, are not to be compared, for depth and intensity, to those which come of many other civilized oppressions." In short, "there are few civilized institutions, upon which we could not write an 'Uncle Tom's Cabin,'" she added. "Modern finance is a scheme of oppression and slavery. . . . We cannot be satisfied until every yoke is broken." This global vision of social reform demanded universal health and happiness; it framed abolition and suffrage as relatively narrow pursuits. Thus, Mary considered herself an abolitionist "in rather a wider sense, than some . . . readers may have thought of being."[41] Because neither suffragists nor abolitionists apparently intended to free Mary from Hiram, they could not attract her impassioned energy. In her mid-twenties, Mary craved a reform movement that would fight for *her* personal freedom and happiness.

LYNN

In 1837 the Goves moved to Lynn, Massachusetts, a town famous for shoes. Lynn's sixty-two manufactories produced one and a half million pairs for distribution throughout the United States and abroad in 1829. They employed three thousand workers: fifteen hundred men who cut materials— satin, leather, calamanco—and fifteen hundred women who stitched them together. Nine miles northeast of Boston on the north shore of Massachusetts Bay, Lynn encompassed salt marsh and pasture, woodland and beach. The town center buzzed with industry. Many of Lynn's 7,000 inhabitants who did not make shoes instead produced glue, chocolate, printed silks, grain, spices, goatskin leather, and "lasts"—foot molds used in the repair of shoes and boots. The town supported two Congregational, two Methodist, one Baptist, and one Quaker congregation. In addition to eight schools, a savings bank, Masonic lodge, lyceum, insurance company, Temperance Society, Benevolent Society, almshouse, and circulating library, Lynn even boasted a society of Watchers for the Sick. Comparatively busy, urban, even worldly, Lynn saved Mary from Weare.[42]

The same year that the Goves moved, America fell into an economic depression initiated by inflated property prices and wild land speculation in the West. Strangely, during every month of that year, Lynn experienced a frost. Hiram, who had conceded the necessity of Mary's labor, meticulously unburdened her of every penny she earned. Needlework had proven devastating to her health, and Mary refused to join Lynn's population of lady stitchers. Instead, she wanted to open a school for girls. In this same year, Mary Lyon had established Mt. Holyoke Female Seminary in South Hadley, Massachusetts, and Horace Mann had begun agitating in the state legislature for greater emphasis on quality public education. Persuading Hiram to allow such an endeavor required more than rhetoric, however. It was only after she fell ill—most likely too ill to continue with the needlework that was sustaining the family—that Hiram grudgingly tolerated Mary's initiative.

He did not make the work easy, however. Mary could not buy books or supplies for her students without begging each cent from Hiram, who would not always part with the coins. Though the family's earnings came solely from Mary's teaching, by law she had no control of this money. Mary did find emotional support, however. By 1842 her parents, William and Rebecca Neal, had moved to Lynn. It was also in Lynn that Mary began her lifelong friendship with writer and editor Alonzo Lewis.

An ardent abolitionist known as "the Lynn Bard," Alonzo Lewis edited the *Lynn Weekly Mirror*, the *Lynn Record*, and *Freedom's Amulet*. In 1829 he also published a remarkable history of Lynn, which the *Democratic Review* called "the very best history of an American town ever written."[43] Sixteen years older than Mary, Alonzo was of medium height and well built. He kept his beard closely cropped and usually wore a cloth cap or low-crowned hat. He had remarkable physical as well as mental endurance and enjoyed attending diverse public lectures. Though rarely known to laugh with zest, Alonzo had a pleasant smile. For twelve years, before becoming a noted surveyor and architect, he had taught in Lynn's public school system and may have encouraged Mary's desire to start her own school. When Mary met Alonzo, he was married to Frances Maria Swan. Before Frances died in the spring of 1839, Alonzo had fathered six children—the first named Alonzo and the second named Frances Maria. Perhaps they attended Mary's school. For decades after she left Lynn, Mary would continue to write to Alonzo, in one letter calling him "my friend of the dark time."[44]

In September of 1837, when Elma was five years old and Lynn had become familiar territory, Mary relocated her school from Nahant Street to Front Street, continuing to teach "those branches usually taught in Academies and Common Schools." She had gained new scholars as well. Now, with an assistant, she also taught needlework. Though she despised sewing, Mary well knew its value, especially in a town whose primary industry depended on women's stitching of shoe uppers. The advertisement Mary placed in the *Lynn Record* on September 20, 1837, reassured parents that "particular attention will be paid to those children confided to their care." Tuition was $2 per quarter, fuel included. The girls exercised daily. Mary exhorted them to reject the fashion of wearing corsets, teaching in detail the anatomy of respiration and circulation so dependent on the free flow of fresh air, gallon after gallon. To emphasize her philosophy, Mary taught her students "vocal philosophy," which involved gymnastic and vocal exercises, deep breathing, and attention to erect posture.[45] Lacking brothers or sisters, Elma probably enjoyed the social life of the classroom. Moreover, school gave both Elma and her mother a refuge from Hiram's oppressive presence in the house.

When she could manage it, Mary attended lectures in town. It is unknown whether she was present on the June evening when Angelina and Sarah Grimké came to Lynn. That night one thousand women and men packed the lecture hall, while others lingered outside the windows. It was an extraordinary town event. One month earlier, the Grimké sisters had acquired fame by addressing the first meeting of the Anti-Slavery Convention of American Women in Boston. With the exception of Quaker meetings, American women simply did not address group assemblies.[46] Hiram may have kept his wife home that night, but one rainy evening that year Mary did attend a lecture by the controversial Sylvester Graham. Shopkeeper-turned-minister-turned-health advocate, Sylvester Graham preached a drastic program of self-control. Had it not been for the cholera epidemic of 1832, his extreme views might never have made it to Lynn. But his lectures on how to prevent the ravaging disease drew thousands.

Born July 4, 1794, in West Suffield, Connecticut, Sylvester Graham lived only briefly with his parents. He was the youngest of his father's seventeen children by two wives. His father, a minister and physician, died when Sylvester was two, leaving his wife with an unmanageable brood. Sylvester's mother could not handle the strain. After suffering a nervous breakdown in 1801, she found her three youngest children placed with a guardian. Thus deprived of his parents and older siblings, Sylvester grew up an unhappy, dyspeptic child.

By the time he was twenty-three, Sylvester still had not prepared himself for a career. When his mother moved to Newark, New Jersey, to live with one of her older sons, Sylvester followed her there. In New Jersey Graham spent his twenties keeping a store, writing for local newspapers, and trying to find a compatible mate. At twenty-nine he enrolled in a preparatory school, Amherst Academy, but found his tenure abruptly ended after only one semester, when he was expelled for criminal assault, a charge trumped up by younger students who resented Graham's willful personality and strong opinions. From Amherst, Graham went to Compton, Rhode Island, where he met his wife, Sarah Earl. Sarah helped him overcome his academic failure and urged him to pursue private study with Emerson Paine, the minister who had officiated at their wedding.

In the fall of 1828, when he was thirty-two, Graham received his license as an evangelist. He spent the next two years preaching in Rhode Island and developing a passion for temperance. Sometime during this period, he also stopped eating meat. In June of 1830, the Pennsylvania Society for Discouraging Use of Ardent Spirits hired Graham as a regular lecturer in Philadelphia. This move marked the beginning of a new career.

In Philadelphia Graham began a crusade for health whose foot soldiers included many of the most prominent and devoted abolitionists, preachers, writers, and social reformers of the antebellum era. By 1837, when Mary first heard Sylvester Graham speak in Lynn, he had developed so uncompromising and prescriptive a vision of health reform that many contemporaries already considered him fanatical. Graham believed that stimulation enfeebled the body. Alcohol, tobacco, meat, orgasm—all these stimulants irritated and enervated a delicate system, sensitive primarily to the alimentary tract. He developed a recipe for "Graham bread," producing loaves from unbolted, unadulterated, whole-wheat flour. His followers swore by this staple breakfast. The sad little boy with the stomach aches grew up to warn others against pleasurable indulgence. Mary thought him brilliant.[47]

By March of 1838, Mary Gove was running a Graham boarding school, located on Broad Street. Graham's rainy night lecture had exhilarated her. Hearing a doctrine of *prevention* at a time when she was obsessed with regrets over her decision to marry Hiram seems to have seared the logic of such a course in her mind. After all, she had gotten herself into a family situation seemingly impossible to remedy and yet once possible to have avoided. Graham offered Mary control—a guarantee that by following certain methods, one could prevent misery in the future. One's happiness hinged on one's health; one's inner peace therefore hinged on the freedom to live a life of strict self-control. Graham legitimized Mary's craving for autonomy and for serenity. She promptly stopped eating meat.[48]

Students at Mary's school would follow a strict Graham diet (based largely on fruits, whole grains, vegetables, and water), for which they would be charged $2 per quarter. Again she advertised the branches of study standard to common schools ($2 per quarter), but she also expanded the curriculum to include "higher English branches" ($3 per quarter) and French ($4 per quarter). She refined her newspaper announcement further by capitalizing "NEEDLE WORK," perhaps thinking parents would be more inclined to pay for their daughters to learn practical skills. "Particular attention will be paid to the habits and manners of those children entrusted to her care," read this revised advertisement. She ran a similar ad in the *Graham Journal of Health and Longevity*.[49]

The students Mary recruited came from a variety of religious denominations, and the friendships she formed with their families troubled Hiram, who preferred that Mary associate only with Quakers. Yet when he once returned from a trip to find Mary and Elma happily playing checkers with a literary man from town, Hiram did not care that the man was a member of the Society of Friends. He was "struck with horror," as Mary recalled. "I was playing a game with a young man in the presence of our daughter. His jealousy was roused, and his coarse and violent language was most revolting." Mary began to find even the slightest physical contact with her husband a source of agony. "In the first years of my marriage I had spent nearly whole nights often at my sewing, to maintain our family; later I was kept awake from illness; last of all, a continued thwarting of taste and will, and the constant oppression of petty tyrannies, had robbed me of rest. My body seemed at last only a medium and receptacle of pain."

That she was earning considerable money, living near her parents, enjoying her teaching, and making new friends provided Mary some solace. In moments of strength, she even began to imagine leaving her spouse: "I often thought it was possible that [Hiram] might engage in some useful occupation if I left him, but then again his utter weakness forbade me to think so, and admonished me to sustain him. . . . All my hours of study and rest were invaded. . . . I could never know the blessing of being alone."[50] She threw herself into her work.

As Mary taught her students and continued to write for an increasingly wide audience, she began to consider the possibility of public speaking. Though extremely shy as a child, Mary had grown increasingly restive; she found the constraints of Orthodox Quakerism and legal marriage suffocating. Her secret fantasy of offering public lectures on the laws of health became a firm decision when it met with the sanction of Joseph John Gurney, an English Quaker minister who visited with Mary sometime in 1838. After sitting in silence for a time in the company of a few other Friends, Joseph Gurney told Mary that she had a great purpose in her heart, that she should follow it—that she would bring a blessing to the world.[51] His words, though spoken with no knowledge of her intentions, sealed Mary's resolve. Whereas other Quakers had snubbed Mary for her bookishness and her meticulously grammatical Quaker speech, this foreign minister recognized her yearning and sanctioned her ambitious reach. The following week Mary offered a local lecture. She met with immediate and intense censure from the Society of Friends. Soon she offered another lecture.

LECTURES

Like almost all women of her era, Mary had never spoken publicly before adults. Audience-seeking was considered unwomanly in the extreme. Yet women in a variety of causes were nudging this barrier back. Ten years earlier, the Scottish reformer Frances Wright had shocked the nation by lecturing to packed houses in New York, Philadelphia, Boston, Cincinnati, and other cities, advocating political rights for women and a national system of public education. One newspaper had accused Wright of violating "the unalterable laws of nature" with her public speaking, an act that invited the "unhinging" of society. Her name became an epithet; by the 1830s any social radical risked dismissal as a "Fanny Wrightist." In Mary's case, the content of her lectures—anatomy and physiology—provoked as much comment as the fact of her speaking. One contemporary noted that Mary's Quaker garb "rendered her lectures the more acceptable, as the public tolerated a Quaker woman as a public speaker."[52] Still, no woman in America had ever publicly described the workings of the human body.

At twenty-eight years old, Mary had finally found her mission. The abuse of Lynn's Friends pained but did not discourage her. In the late summer of 1838, Mary accepted an invitation to present a series of lectures before the Ladies Physiological Society of Boston. This group, established in 1837 under the leadership of William A. Alcott and David Campbell, represented a branch of the mixed-sex American Physiological Society (APS), of which William Alcott served as first president. The Ladies Society was founded with two hundred charter members in the same year as its parent organization and gained nearly three hundred members during its first year. Such societies, fortified with bylaws, membership lists, and periodicals, nurtured a wide variety of crusades for social reform. A resolution adopted at the second annual meeting of the APS demonstrates why the group appealed to women: "Woman in her character as wife and mother is only second to the Deity in the influence she exerts on the physical, the intellectual, and the moral interests of the human race, and . . . her education should be adapted to qualify her in the highest degree to cherish those interests in the wisest and best manner."[53] By formally asserting the social importance of wives and mothers, the APS was essentially, if not explicitly, recognizing women's political relevance. Those who denounced female lecturers feared the implications.

The rising popularity of self-improvement circles similarly threatened the status quo. During the 1830s, young female mill workers in Lowell, Massachusetts, gathered every two weeks to share original essays and poetry. Concord transcendentalists struggled to articulate the importance of "self-culture." And beginning in the fall of 1839, Margaret Fuller, who became one of the nineteenth century's most famous female philosophers, began to offer guided "conversations" among women. All of these initiatives encouraged women to gain confidence in their intellectual abilities and to seek application of their ideas. Formulating her vision, Fuller wrote to a friend,

If my office were only to suggest topicks *[sic]* which would lead to conversation of a better order than is usual at social meetings and to turn back the current when digressing into personalities or commonplaces . . . , I should think the object not unworthy of an effort. But my own ambition goes much farther. Thus to pass in review the departments of thought and knowledge and endeavor to place them in due relation to one another in our minds. To systematize thought and give a precision in which our sex are so deficient, chiefly, I think because they have so few inducements to test and classify what they receive. To ascertain what pursuits are best suited to us in our time and state of society, and how we may make best use of our means for building up the life of thought upon the life of action.[54]

Between 1839 and 1844, Fuller led weekly meetings every fall and spring. Participants included writers, reformers, and the wives of literary and socially active men. Each member was encouraged to share her thoughts on such subjects as "poetry as expressed in external nature" or "the history of a nation as revealed in the characters of its great men." Margaret Fuller hoped for active participation but did not require it. "No one will be forced," she wrote, "but those who do not talk will not derive the same advantages with those who openly state their impressions and consent to learn by blundering as is the destiny of Man here below." Like the Ladies Physiological Society, Fuller's conversation circles answered a craving among women for education and meaningful social participation.[55]

On May 17, 1838, mobs, infuriated by a mixed-race gathering of the Anti-Slavery Convention of American Women, had burned Philadelphia's Pennsylvania Hall to the ground. In Alton, Illinois, the editor of an abolitionist newspaper had been murdered for his views. On May 26, 1836, Congress had passed a gag rule forbidding all congressional discussion of antislavery petitions.[56] Yet American society demanded review. Amid these disputes, the health reform movement drew thousands who sought a useful role in social reformation.

On the first Wednesday of September 1838, at three in the afternoon, Mary gave her first Boston lecture in Marlboro' Chapel. Describing the perils of female ignorance concerning the human body, this initial talk served as an introduction to her weekly series of lectures. Mild by modern standards, the anatomy and physiology lessons she presented broke the silence on taboo subjects. An advertisement for her first lecture warned readers that "physiological facts of a delicate nature and which many ladies would not bring themselves to hear from a gentleman, but a knowledge of which is of great importance to the well being of society and individuals, will be brought to view. . . . The course . . . will be given to LADIES and to LADIES ONLY." Mary's lecture series was to be no embroidery lesson; it was a singular opportunity for ladies to better the world by enriching their own minds.[57]

Supportive testimonials from respected male physicians accompanied advertisements for Mary's lectures. That "Mrs. Gove" was "amply qualified" to speak on anatomy and physiology only left the question of her character, which a paragraph by the widely known health educator William Andrus Alcott praised in terms of "her benevolence," "zeal," and "devotion to the cause of truth." Tickets for the entire course cost one dollar. For admission to individual lectures, a lady paid twelve and a half cents. Girls under fourteen were charged half price. Where subjects required it, Mary lectured separately to married and to unmarried ladies.[58]

The topics of Mary's twelve lectures ranged from a description of the bones, muscles, and reproductive organs to the value of a healthful diet, and from the evils of tight lacing and masturbation to the importance of exercise, fresh air, and regular bathing. (Fittingly, the basement floor of Marlboro' Chapel housed a Mr. Blodget's bathing establishment, an extensive public complex complete with separate departments for gentlemen and ladies, where anyone could find a shower or plunge bath, warm or cold.)[59] Certain themes received repeated attention, the most prominent of which all related to *breathing and motion*. Whether she was exhorting women to abandon the wearing of corsets, to unveil their babies' carriages, to get up and stretch, or to wash their bodies, Mary seemed driven by an abhorrence of the restrictive. Lungs inadequately inflated, air inadequately pure, bones inadequately free, and skin inadequately clean all served to weaken the flow of nutritive blood and prevented the body from purging dangerous wastes. All of these ills trapped putrid matter in the system. All caused disease. An understanding of the relationship between the circulatory and respiratory systems had given Mary a medical rationale for condemning all that shackled or confined. Ostensibly talking about nature's anatomy alone, Mary Gove was laying the groundwork for what would soon become a far broader defense of woman's right to freedom. At this early period in her career, she could publicly assert that disease caused misery; soon she would feel bold enough to make the reverse claim. From there she would argue for woman's right to personal happiness regardless of such artificial constraints as propriety or law. But in 1839, Hiram still haunted the outer door of her lecture halls, pocketing the admissions fees, then locking them in a box.

William Alcott—who happened to be one of Mary's neighbors and friends—had admitted the difficulty of his own lecturing to ladies. Though Alcott had spent most of his career as a schoolteacher and had even founded a model school based on progressive educational theories, he recognized that some matters simply did not lend themselves to mixed conversation, regardless of their importance. On paper, Alcott had no trouble addressing women. By the time he invited Mary to lecture, he had already published *The Young Wife, The Young Mother,* and *The Young House Keeper,* all of which reached a wide audience. But after seeing the immense success of Mary's lectures, Alcott grew even more resolute in his belief that women had an indispensable role as leaders in health reform. "Male instructors," he wrote, "never can perform the service to which we refer, in a proper manner, at least till christianity *[sic]*—pure and undefiled—becomes more common among us; but as this can never happen till mothers and daughters are instructed in anatomy, physiology and hygiene, the world has been long involved in a dilemma from which nothing but female instruction and female philanthropy could extricate it."[60] Mary's lectures were each drawing from four hundred to five hundred listeners. When she repeated her lecture on tight lacing at no charge to the public, she drew a crowd of two thousand.

Among these women was Anna Breed, who wrote enthusiastically about Mary Gove to her friend, abolitionist Abby Kelley:

> I have attended three of her lectures, which were both edifying and interesting. The first . . . was upon the formation of bones—the 2nd upon their situation, number, and wonderful use—3rd the evils of *tight lacing*—an excellent lecture—she has, according to my estimation, very correct views of the effects of that horrid practice. I think Abby, thou would be much interested in her lectures; she appears better than I ever saw her in any other situation. She is censured, ridiculed, and misrepresented, of course; but as she has a pretty good share of independence, I think she will not be much affected by the sarcasms inflicted upon her. I have never before seen so intelligent

looking a company of Women together in this place as we meat *[sic]* there. She is giving a second course to a large audience in Boston. More of "aunt Gove" when we meet.

It was during this period in Boston that a local physician invited Mary to attend the first human dissections she would ever see; she recalled in particular the autopsy of a child who had died of tuberculosis. Other area physicians generously loaned her the use of anatomical plates.[61]

In December 1838, Mary contracted to repeat her entire series of lectures in Boston, on Wednesday and Friday afternoons. Surprisingly, the attendance at her second series of lectures surpassed that of the first. Although many had come from neighboring towns to hear the fall series, and although Boston's December weather does not encourage unnecessary travel, increasing numbers of the city's "first ladies" overcame their hesitancy and packed Mary's lecture hall.[62]

The following April, the *New York Morning Herald* announced yet another round of Mary's lectures: "This extraordinary woman . . . (for we have hardly decided whether she is more of heaven than of hell) began a new series of lectures . . . before a more numerous and respectable female audience than any that has yet been attracted together to hear her discourses." This unsettling notice of her efforts troubled Mary less than the *Herald*'s sensational and distorted accounts of the lectures themselves. The paper claimed to quote Mary, yet its presentation of her words painted a caricature: "Where a lady finds the doting husband either ignorant of the importance of temperance and moderation, or so far the slave of passion as to chain his reason and judgment captive at the chariot-wheels of the car of Pleasure, and drive on without caring where his fiery steeds may carry him, it is then the duty of the wife to take the reins into her own hands, stop the fiery horses, make them cool down, and by putting a drag chain on the wheel, prevent them from running to destruction."[63]

The renowned Scottish phrenologist George Combe was lecturing to large audiences in Boston at the same time and took interest in Mary's work. His own daughter had been among the women in Mary's audience. Combe endorsed Mary's character and encouraged her success, condemning the *New York Morning Herald* for its treatment of Mary's lectures: "Bennett's 'Morning Herald,' . . . to its own deep disgrace, has published what he pretends to be reports of her lectures, pandering to the grovelling feelings of the men, and alarming the delicacy of the ladies. . . . I have inquired into the character of the lectures, of ladies who heard them, and they declare Bennett's report to be scandalous caricatures, misrepresentations, and inventions."[64]

Others came to Mary's defense as well. The *Graham Journal of Health and Longevity* reprinted an extended endorsement of her lectures that first appeared in the *Lobelian, and Rhode Island Medical Review,* a monthly alternative journal published in Newport: "The base and corrupt portion of the New York editors, whose moral sense is so blunted as to be incapable of seeing the difference between gratuitous obscenity and physiological truth . . . , who visit theaters and applaud and puff in their journals the most revolting dancers . . . assail [Mary Gove] . . . on the plea that these physical truths are wanting in decorum, and as improper for women to know! Oh detestable hypocrisy! or moral sense wanting, or altogether perverted!"[65] The *Lobelian* and the *Graham Journal* both bade Mary "God speed."

The Ladies' Physiological Society of New York had sponsored Mary's first course in that city. Before seeing her off from Boston, the students of Mary's first lecture series expressed their respect and gratitude by presenting her with a valuable silver watch. (Out of consideration for Mary's Quaker avoidance of decoration, the women had revised their original decision to purchase a highly ornamented and less practical gold watch.) The second class of students gave Mary a gift of money for the purchase of anatomical plates.[66] Within his legal rights, Hiram had confiscated every cent of Mary's earnings and the silver watch as well (which he wore), but he did not know of this second gift. Mary felt herself forgiven for ultimately using this secret money to escape life with Hiram rather than to buy anatomical plates.

Not long before Mary began lecturing, Elma had suffered through a case of scarlet fever. Though Mary relied predominantly on water to treat her six-year-old daughter, she also allowed an allopathic doctor to administer small doses of drugs. Elma's condition must have terrified her; it was the last time in her life that Mary tolerated allopathic medicines in her family. It is not clear whether Elma stayed with her grandparents or whether she joined her parents when they traveled to Mary's lecture engagements in Haverhill, Albany, New York, Newark, Providence, Nantucket, Millbury, Worcester, Bangor, Portland, Philadelphia, and Baltimore.[67]

It was during one of these many lectures that Mary suffered a dramatic tubercular attack. Her eldest brother, the one who had admonished her for having an interest in Bell's *Anatomy*, had died of the disease not long before. For four years he had struggled with tuberculosis, pursuing every allopathic remedy recommended by his training—all poisons, as Mary believed. The rough coughing and bleeding lungs characteristic of tuberculosis left its sufferers weak and pale. Contagious, untreatable, and often deadly, consumption often seemed to run in families. What we now understand as a bacterial disease looked in the nineteenth century like an inherited constitutional frailty. A consumptive person's coughing fits came in sudden, attacking waves. When Mary first felt the blood rush through her trachea in the middle of a lecture, she recalled her brother's and sister's deaths and felt sure that she too was going to die. But more than ten years later she wrote that the initial sense of doom was abruptly displaced by tenacity for life. "The thought of leaving my mission unfulfilled, of leaving woman to suffer and die under the black pall of ignorance that enveloped her then, was more than I could bear." She fainted. A group of women carried her out of the crowded auditorium and into the fresh air, where she soon regained consciousness.

Following this episode, Mary took a break from lecturing and treated herself without medicines. Through "constant" bathing, simple diet, outdoor exercise, and much rest, Mary eliminated her cough and regained strength. Soon she resumed lecturing. It would not be the last—or the worst—of her tubercular attacks. She describes a subsequent relapse that resulted in the loss of almost three quarts of blood in four days. A German water-cure and homeopathic physician attended Mary through this most severe episode. His treatments relied primarily on cold water rather than medicine, and she developed respect for his unusual methods.[68] Again, she resumed lecturing.

On February 16, 1839, the *Graham Journal of Health and Longevity* quoted a letter sent from the newly founded Providence Health Society describing Mary's January lectures in that city: "Yesterday and this day the lecture room was crowded full, and it is confidently said that it will comfortably seat 750. The window seats were all occupied, the aisles were filled, and indeed all the room was occupied."[69] It must have been a challenging evening for Mary, who always awoke with coughing after spending time in a crowded or poorly ventilated hall. She had arrived in Providence with letters from prominent Boston physicians encouraging their medical colleagues to lend Mrs. Gove anatomical plates and preparations for use in her public speaking. Dr. J. V. C. Smith, editor of the widely respected *Boston Medical and Surgical Journal,* had written to a Providence colleague: "Pray, oblige [Mary Gove] with the use of books, drawings, or preparations while she remains in the city, should she require them, fully believing she is entitled to respect. . . . Our physicians fully approbate her course."[70]

Of all the cities she toured, Mary found Philadelphia the most progressive. "It is a city of *women*," she wrote to a friend. "I have found *more* intelligent women here than I have ever found in any city." Mary had given her first Philadelphia lecture at the Saloon of Peale's Museum and, despite the stormy weather, had drawn a good audience. In the same letter, Mary admitted that in addition to delivering a series of lectures to women, she had also delivered two talks before mixed audiences:

> I have given two Lectures on the Circulation of the blood and tight Lacing to men and women. I did it by the advice of medical men and others who stand high in my estimation and because I think I have a *right* to speak on proper subjects, in a proper manner, before a mixed audience. They would let me cry fire with no disgust at all but now when an evil worse than a thousand fires is abroad, some will cry "*shame* on a *woman* for speaking before men, setting herself up as a *teacher* when Paul expressly forbids a woman's teaching."[71]

That Hiram traveled with Mary, at least to Philadelphia, seems very clear. In a diary, Mary had written, "Last night I gave my second lecture to a mixed audience. I *redeemed* myself. I rose out of myself, and above myself. My friends were delighted; even my husband, who would not praise, or hardly approve me, for his right hand, lest he should make me vain, *smiled!*"[72] But Philadelphia's liberalism was not echoed in other cities. "In Philadelphia . . . there seemed next to no prejudice against [my speaking to mixed audiences], but my friends in other places with their everlasting dread of innovation were half killed," wrote Mary.[73]

Mary Gove's lectures consisted of far more than general counseling against common habits such as gluttony. Although impassioned by the desire to reform the lifestyles of her listeners, Mary grounded each recommendation in the mechanisms of the body. An attendee at one of her Boston lectures took careful notes on a variety of topics: "the manner in which the brain is protected by two layers of bone with cancelli, or net work of blood vessels between"; "the atlas and dentatus, those curious provisions for nodding and turning the head"; and the "internal villous or mucous coat of the stomach with its fine nervous and vascular papillae from which exudes the gastric juice."[74] A female correspondent published synopses of each of Mary's lectures in the *Graham Journal of Health and Longevity*, with the exception of the tenth lecture (given to unmarried ladies) and the eleventh (given to married ladies). These summaries portray the lecturer as confident in her assertions, detailed in her descriptions of physiology, and relentless in her attacks on quack medications and stimulants.

As for diet, a subject to which she devoted considerable attention, Mary seemed determined not to be understood as a vegetarian fanatic, a target for ridicule like Sylvester Graham. In describing the action of the digestive system, she emphasized moderation in consumption above the avoidance of meat. "I am far from pleading for the use of animal food, but I would have people rational and not like a horse that gets frightened on one side of a bridge and runs off the other." Excessive consumption of vegetables and water could overtax the digestive organs with far more damaging consequences than a small portion of healthy, lean flesh, she argued. Still, animal food incited inflammation and bloating. Relying on authorities from London's Royal College of Surgeons, Mary described both physiologic and anatomical evidence that humans were intended to be vegetarians. Personally, she abstained from meat eating. Her warnings against red and black pepper, horseradish, mustard, vinegar, catsup, pickles, coffee, tea, alcohol, tobacco, and overheated food left a very bland menu indeed.[75]

Mary's lectures derived added strength from their testimonial quality. She could describe nearly losing her life as a result of the tight lacing of her youth. She could speak with deep personal knowledge of the perils in store for a baby born to a weakened mother. She had seen more than one child delivered from her body, only to die within hours. And, given her life with Hiram, one can easily imagine the passion with which she separately spoke to married and unmarried ladies.

Desperately, Mary hoped to spare other women and their children from becoming the indirect victims of their husbands' sexual disorders. Believing that "premature and excessive development of the sexual instinct" constituted disease in itself and that its gratification led to further disease, Mary warned her listeners that no marriage ceremony could "save people from the consequences of venereal excesses." Fundamentally, Mary believed Hiram to be more ill than malevolent—plagued by libidinous imbalance resulting from wrongful upbringing. The terror of her nights with Hiram might be inferred from the metaphor she chose to characterize the stakes involved: "As well may we drop a living coal of fire into a magazine of powder, and beg, and pray, and exhort it not to explode, and expect to be obeyed, as to train our children in a manner directly calculated to produce impurity, and expect them, by the mere force of precept, to counteract the immutable laws of nature and remain pure."[76] The implications of these scarcely masked revelations were not lost on her female audiences. These lectures did not merely teach the proper hygienic means of child rearing; they taught women to see sexual victimization as pervasive, unnatural, unnecessary, and fully woman's business to prevent and avoid.

Female sexual powerlessness might be the state of civil law, Mary argued, but not the state of God's law: physical and mental self-ownership were women's holy birthright. Over the years, Mary's rhetoric would grow even more sharply honed with this message. Yet in the early lectures, she felt the difficulty of articulating so radical a view. Mary *knew* she proposed nothing less than social revolution. Writing to a friend in the middle of the night, Mary struggled to place herself in the long scope of history: "The world misunderstands and abuses me but I shall yet have a *name* and a *place* among the benefactors of our race."[77]

A Professional Escape

ლ   ლ   ლ

IN 1839 MARY GOVE published a short work entitled *Solitary Vice. An Address to Parents and Those Who Have the Care of Children.* A treatise on healthy sexual development, its eighteen pages document a litany of ills resulting from "self-pollution," or masturbation. Notice of this work in the *Boston Medical and Surgical Journal* expressed shock that the evil of masturbation could be as widespread among females as Mrs. Gove asserted—yet "she is a woman," granted the reviewer, and therefore likely to be well informed. Though Mary claimed to have first learned about the prevalence of female masturbation from a medical text, her impassioned exhortations against the crippling vice derived their force from the testimonials of women who had trusted the female lecturer enough to share their dark secrets. These anonymous women elaborated soulful remorse at the depths of their own degradation or that of their family members—a debasement wrought first by ignorance and then by compulsion. "The sufferers are personally less offenders than victims," Mary wrote with sympathy. Her pages demonize the behavior of masturbation without demonizing its practitioners. Sin and disease, suffering and inequity—all could find their antidotes in education. Therefore, she directed her work to those responsible for advising children. By speaking to caretakers, Mary hoped to bring her message to a greater number; she also hoped to protect very young children who might initiate the vice before growing old enough to read independently of its dangers.[1]

The hazards of masturbation loomed ominously in the minds of Jacksonian physicians, clergy, and health reformers. The 1830s yielded a mass of anti-masturbation literature. It was essentially a new genre, preceded by a century of near silence on the topic. Only two texts addressing "onanism" were published in the United States during the eighteenth century: Cotton Mather's 1723 pamphlet entitled the *Pure Nazarite,* and the 1724 reprint of *Onania: Or the Heinous Sin of Self-Pollution, and All Its Frightful Consequences, in Both Sexes Considered,* a book originally published anonymously in London in 1714. Although both of these texts wielded theology to attack self-pollution, nineteenth-century writers attended less to God's written injunctions than to nature's physical punishments. To Mary, the destruction wrought on the human body and mind by habitual masturbation proved beyond all doubt that such a practice violated natural law. Medical arguments displaced their moral counterparts. Readers learned that self-polluters had a great deal to fear in this life as well as the next. Generalized weakness, headache, dyspepsia, epilepsy, insomnia, inability to concentrate, poor vision, diabetes, diseases of the spine and reproductive tract, impotence, premature ejaculation, nocturnal emissions, incontinence, leukorrhea, sterility, consumption, idiocy, insanity, and death all threatened those who indulged in "the solitary vice." As Mary succinctly warned: "Almost every form of disease may be produced by it." Small children reflected the most poignant tragedy, since they adopted the practice unaware of its risks. "Be not guilty of the blood of your children," pleaded Mary.[2]

Like other reformers anxious about a perceived epidemic of masturbation, Mary Gove suspected children of learning the vice from their peers in boarding school or female seminaries. Other writers accused servants or nursemaids. Rather than focus on the details of treatment, Mary devoted her text to the need for prevention. Inevitable doom would result from offended denial or embarrassed avoidance of the problem. Mary believed that knowledge of the vice would repel rather than tempt children. "The silent course has been tried till our world has become one vast pit of corruption," she wrote.[3] Bolstered by the authority of other medical writers, Mary, though publishing anonymously, was growing increasingly brave in tone.

Hers was neither the first nor the loudest voice to incite alarm over the widespread practice of masturbation. In 1832, seven years before Mary Gove published *Solitary Vice,* a new edition of a 1758 text by Samuel A. Tissot, M.D., entitled *A Treatise on the Diseases Produced by Onanism* was published in New York. This publication coincided with (and was perhaps in response to) the publicity surrounding one of Sylvester Graham's lectures, a talk that would be published in 1834 and that would see ten new editions over the following fifteen years as well as translation into several languages. Entitled *A Lecture to Young Men, on Chastity, Also Intended for the Serious Consideration of Parents and Guardians,* the work was the only text that Mary Gove recommended by name in her own tract.[4]

Unlike Tissot, who urgently pointed out that "the loss of one ounce of [semen], enfeebles more than forty ounces of blood," Graham emphasized the debilitating quality of inner arousal, not so much the loss of any particular bodily fluid. Orgasm in particular posed a threat to the system, whether experienced during intercourse or when alone.

> The convulsive paroxysms attending venereal indulgence, are connected with the most intense excitement, and cause the most powerful agitation to the whole system, that it is ever subject to. The brain, stomach, heart, lungs, liver, skin, and the other organs, feel its sweeping over them, with the tremendous violence of a tornado. The powerfully excited and convulsed heart drives the blood, in fearful congestion, to the principal viscera—producing oppression, irritation, debility, rupture, inflammation, and sometimes disorganization—and this violent paroxysm is generally succeeded by great exhaustion, relaxation, lassitude and even prostration.[5]

Graphic and alarming, the lecture reached a wide audience. Its specifically male focus may have inspired Mary not only to write her own book but also to foreground discussion of masturbation's threat to females.[6]

Mary's increasing fame as an unashamed lecturer to ladies established her as the natural conduit of delicate information from the male medical world to women. Tissot had devoted considerable attention to the solitary vice in females and is very likely the source from which Mary claims to have learned about female masturbation. Perhaps she chose to write about the subject because she sincerely believed it to be the single greatest health threat looming over vulnerable youth. Perhaps she noted the attention Graham's work had attracted and desired similar influence. Conceivably she suspected Hiram of the solitary vice and privately attributed his violent outbursts to this diseased habit. And despite her claim that she had no "intimation" of the pernicious habit in females prior to reading of it, one can legitimately wonder whether she was also motivated by personal anxiety over her daughter or herself. Obviously Mary and Hiram did not share a happy sex life. She may have attributed her own stillbirths and frequent sickness to a secret practice she would never admit. There is, however, absolutely no evidence in regard to masturbatory habits in the Gove family.

Solitary Vice was Mary's first and only monograph devoted to a single physical affliction. The work received additional notice in 1845, when Samuel Gregory, M.D. published a widely reviewed and inexpensive pamphlet on the same subject: *Facts and Important Information For Young Women, on the Subject of Masturbation; With Its Causes, Prevention, and Cure.* (Gregory had never actually earned a medical degree, but chose to append the "M.D." to his name anyway.) In this text he quoted *Solitary Vice* at length. The health reform movement, a crusade obsessed with reforming the private habits of others, took great interest in masturbation. As her career developed, Mary Gove would find herself increasingly preoccupied with the nature and social management of passion, pleasure, sex, and reproduction.

Like Graham, Mary Gove suffered mockery and reproof in proportion to her increasing notoriety. The strongest rebuke came, as she knew it would, from the Society of Friends, which condemned her decision to speak on worldly topics before large audiences. Lynn Quakers had spread false rumors about Mary's activities. One lie in particular stung Mary to the core: that she used the skeleton of her own child to illustrate points in her public lectures. Mary's hometown buzzed with invented stories of her licentiousness and crimes. She found her name "blackened." Rather than attempt to refute each rumor, Mary resolved "to *live* down every aspersion, and to take no notice of any."[7] Such a strategy may have spared her much defensive pleading with a variety of critics, but it did not improve her reputation.

In 1839 the Weare Monthly Meeting of the Society of Friends issued a formal complaint against Mary. As they worded it, Mary Gove had "lectured to the dissatisfaction of Friends and others, and to the reproach of our Society." Efforts to disown Mary from the Society of Friends required that the complaint be tried in both the Quarterly and Yearly Meetings. Judging committees refused either to read or to hear Mary's lectures in making their determination. Whether her lectures met with "dissatisfaction" did not, in their view, require knowledge of their actual contents. Mary was expected to submit a certification that she no longer considered herself a Quaker and that she wished to be excommunicated. After fourteen years, Mary once again found herself without a religious home.[8]

As word of Mary's excommunication reached a broader audience of Quakers, several rose to her defense. Testimonials in the Worcester-based periodical the *Reformer,* published by Joseph S. Wall, reflected a more progressive wing of Quakerism.

> Could they [the judging committee] not see that the same principle by which Mary S. Gove is to-day disowned for advocating the great principles of temperance and purity, to-morrow may deprive them of their membership, for spreading the principles of Abolition? But the general plea of the Weare Friends seems to be, that public opinion is against her. . . . If public opinion is to be our standard, then let us unhesitatingly acknowledge that Quakerism consists in wearing a plain dress, speaking the plain language, and sitting in silence twice a week—for this is the opinion of the majority of mankind.[9]

Thus, the paper expressed frustration with the narrow-minded conservatism of the Weare Meeting.

Beginning in the 1820s, a rift had divided the larger Quaker community into two factions: the Orthodox and the "Hicksites." The Orthodox vested tremendous authority in the Society's elders to block troublesome abolitionist Quaker Elias Hicks from speaking at the Yearly Meeting. The "Hicksites" defended his right to speak as the spirit moved him. Hicks preached against a "new evangelicalism" that had overtaken many of Philadelphia's more worldly Friends. He beseeched his fellow Quakers to attend to the inner Christ rather than to the rituals surrounding events in this life. To the elders, Hicks's attacks on Quaker observance of the Sabbath (as opposed to the early Quakers' recognition of every day as holy) sounded blasphemous. The debate over the elders' authority to censor Hicks resulted in a new, relatively liberal branch of Quakerism. Most likely Mary Gove would have fared better in a Hicksite Meeting than in her own Orthodox community. Also at issue in the 1830s was the extent to which Friends should involve themselves with the larger political world— particularly with the antislavery movement. Joseph Wall's paper condemned the Society of Friends as unchristian for discouraging activism on behalf of the nation's sufferers. He called the "non-intercourse recommendation" both "fallacious and unsound." It followed naturally that he should defend the right of a woman to lecture on preventive medicine.[10]

Subsequent issues of the *Reformer* came even more pointedly to endorse Mary Gove's character and work. Aggressive editorials attacked those who criticized Mary's forthright expression: "If they would not hear the names of certain vices mentioned, they should not suffer those vices to exist." A Methodist minister named B. F. Tefft submitted a lengthy letter to the editor of the *Reformer* on behalf of Mary Gove, whom he claimed to know. As a non-Quaker, Tefft expressed no opinion regarding the action of the Weare Meeting, but he felt compelled to share his impression of the slandered educator: "That Mrs. Mary S. Gove possesses talents of a rare order, no person can question. To doubt it, would place in jeopardy one's own reputation for good sense and careful observation. That her moral character is unimpeachable, would be saying but little in her case. She seems to possess a great soul—a conscience quick and powerful—a moral courage absolutely invincible—a philanthropy unbounded." As a teenager, Mary had turned to the Quakers and away from the Methodists. Ironically, this Methodist minister would prove one of the rare, brave allies who would defend her name to the Quaker world.[11]

The publisher of the *Reformer*, Joseph Wall, would later experience his own break from the Society of Friends. Sympathetic both to Mary's reform agenda and to her plight, Wall would soon become Mary's friend as well. Early in 1840, after a renewed attack of tuberculosis left her unable to continue public speaking, Mary moved to Worcester, Massachusetts, to revise her lectures for publication. In April of 1840, Wall launched a new weekly journal to succeed the defunct *Graham Journal and Advocate of Physiological Reform*. It was called the *Health Journal and Advocate of Physiological Reform*, and Mary S. Gove served as a co-editor. Work on her lectures would have to wait.[12]

A WIDER PUBLIC

In addition to writing *Solitary Vice*, Mary Gove also ventured into the prestigious *Boston Medical and Surgical Journal* in 1839, submitting articles as "A. B." She published four articles there between December 1839 and August 1840, during which time she was also lecturing twice a week to a small class. In February she wrote to a friend that the *Journal*'s editor, Jerome van Crowninshield Smith, had sent "A. B." the following note: "Dr. Smith regrets exceedingly that A. B. deems it expedient to conceal his name since the articles written by *him* would be creditable to any professional man in our country" (italics Mary's). She was obviously pleased, but did not know how to respond. "I want to write," she explained to her friend, "and what respect should I get when once known as a woman."[13]

Her first article sharply reviewed a piece entitled "Dr. Durkee's Remarks on Scrofula." "It may be said that therapeutic, rather than prophylactic, means should be used by the physician," she wrote. "But it is surely better to prevent the evils which might be caused by injudicious theses, than to undertake to cure them when they are caused."[14] She then went on, with like irony, to challenge the suggestion that scrofula tends to appear more regularly "in the arms of beauty." She exhibited no patience for the notion that the disease courts a pretty face. Any suggestion that women naturally harbor a tendency toward disease provoked Mary, who fought against a cultural understanding of women as the "weaker sex." Mary had recently observed the autopsy of an infant who had died of scrofula, and the experience seems to have emboldened her pen.

In this article, Mary deliberately pressed for health reform principles ordinarily relegated to alternative medical journals. "I know a practitioner runs the risk, in these days, of being *dubbed* a Grahamite," she wrote, "if he recommend the antiphlogistic regimen in any case, or if he dare dissent from the long received opinion that 'animal food is more nutritive and stimulating than vegetable. . . .' Now I, for one, will not surrender the right of private judgment, through fear that I shall be ranked with this or that class of real or supposed fanatics."[15] Mary demanded evidence for Dr. Durkee's claims that animal food will yield "more and richer blood" than will a vegetarian diet.

Her final article defended Professor Charles P. Bronson, the first president of the Ladies Physiological Institute of Boston and its first lecturer to ladies in April of 1848. Bronson was a teacher of "elocution" with whom Mary had once studied and who, in an earlier issue of the *Journal*, had been condemned as a quack. Demolishing that harsh review with a line-by-line critique, Mary challenged the arrogance of the medical pro-

fession—an arrogance that scorned valuable medical educators merely for
lacking full credentials. Her disgust was personal. "May [Bronson] not
teach what he has *discovered,* to the 'great majority,' even though physicians do the same? 'We found one casting out devils, and we forbade him
because he walked not with us.' Is this liberal? Is this worthy of the profession?"[16] By preserving her anonymity, Mary had found a way to reach
and even to chastise a large audience of physicians.

In between these two "responsive" submissions, Mary published two
columns inviting readers to analyze a series of quotations taken from
François Magendie and John Eberle that together denounced excessive
blood-letting on the basis of empirical observations. To the extended
warnings of these medical experts, Mary appended her own blunt advice:
"Every day's observation convinces me that truth is simple; that the causes
of disease are not as remote and obscure as they are deemed by many. It
is not enough that a physician is able to give beautiful descriptions of
pathological phenomena—that he can talk learnedly of effects, if he
knows nothing of causes. . . . Physicians are a class of men upon whom
rests a fearful responsibility. They should never feel that they are educated."[17] In 1840, what physician would ever accept such cold, direct treatment from a self-taught woman, only thirty years old, undisguised?

For Mary Gove, lecturing to large audiences of women had required
enormous courage. Speaking with equal authority to mixed-sex audiences
required far more. Mary had made the initial brave step of publishing
medical advice for male readers—yet she had published *Solitary Vice*
anonymously and had written under false initials for the *Boston Medical
and Surgical Journal.* Her two lectures in Philadelphia to mixed audiences
had also encouraged further action. When a relatively progressive Quaker
minister proposed a new lyceum in Lynn that would welcome female participation, Mary took an interest. The year was 1841.

The Quaker religion had long allowed women to preach in meeting,
and thus the prospect of female participation in lectures and debates did
not stir undue controversy. Recall that it had been Lynn's Quakers who
had invited Sarah and Angelina Grimké to deliver their antislavery lectures to mixed audiences, a move for which the Friends received harsh
censure from other New England clergymen and which also complicated
the Grimkés' subsequent lecture arrangements elsewhere. As Lynn's new
lyceum took shape, a few women read their own essays aloud, though most

gave their work to the clergyman founder to read for them. Mary noted that if these same pieces had been written and read by male authors, they "would have been termed 'lectures.'"[18]

When the minister solicited a composition from Mary, no one in town knew of her troubles with Hiram. Mary used this opportunity to deliver a stinging attack on the social injustices borne by women. While speaking from the pulpit on the "Sphere and Condition of Woman," Mary noticed the collection of highly educated men filling the steps on either side of her: a poet and historian, a teacher, doctors, lawyers, and merchants. The room was packed. To hear a woman speak publicly offered rare entertainment for the town, which had supported the lyceum series with great enthusiasm from the start.

The text of this lecture has not survived, though Mary claimed to have sold it several years later to a man who delivered it as his original work. As she spoke that night, Mary felt divinely inspired—full of calm and magically unified with her listeners. She later recalled, "I numbered [woman's] curses, almost for the first time, in the hearing of men and women in our 'free country.' . . . I spoke of marriage as annihilation of woman, as often the grave of her heart and the destruction of her health and usefulness." But she did so with grace and poetry rather than with rancor as she desperately sought to reach the men who "if their hearts had not been touched as with a live coal from Heaven's own altar, if the ideas had not been clothed in the beauty, and power, and poetry of an inner world, would have hurled me in wrath from my high place. . . . But they were rapt." At the close of the evening, many listeners congratulated the plain-dressed speaker. Mary, who had been expelled for disrespect before, had struggled to find an acceptable voice for her evolving political beliefs. That night, she succeeded.[19]

It is difficult to imagine Hiram's attendance at that particular gathering. Were he there, his humiliation must have been acute. Likely he had either sought to prevent the lecture or had known little of its content regarding marriage. For her part, Mary felt convinced that she had truly communed with the audience, if only for the short duration of the lecture. The evening glowed brightly in her memory. She would soon lose much, if not most, of that hard-won sympathy.

RETURNING HOME

In 1841 the *Library of Health and Teacher of the Human Constitution*
published a brief notice that an association of approximately forty women
in Bangor, Maine, had begun meeting regularly for the purpose of physiological inquiry; that they had been inspired to such action by the work
of Mrs. Gove; and that they had already begun to schedule guest lecturers. Knowledge of such influence must have been powerful stimulation to
Mary, who had reached the end of her rope with Hiram. In February of
1842, she unburdened herself in a letter to her esteemed friend, John Neal.
How Mary came to know the famous writer is not clear, but the reasons
for her affection and trust loom large. Born in 1793, Neal had, by the mid-
1840s, published eight novels; written widely for American and British literary periodicals; edited newspapers; publicly encouraged young writers
like Poe and Whittier; made a fortune by investing in Maine's granite
quarries; and, most tellingly, defended women's rights with vehemence.

In confidence, Mary wrote, "I will here say to thee that I think my husband's phrenological developements are such, and he is the subject of so
much disease, that *scarcely* any blame, if any, attaches to him. I am as
satisfied of this fact as I am of my existence and tho this knowledge will
not enable me to support existence with him, it takes all anger and vin-
dictiveness from my feelings and I can at all times say, Father forgive him
for he knows not what he does." Her denial of anger may have been enabled by distance—for by the time she wrote these words to Neal, Mary
had finally left Hiram. The years of lecturing, of publication, of lucrative
independence, and of listening to her own exhortations nourished Mary's
self-confidence and fortified her resolve. Weighing her existing misery
against the prospect of misery should she risk all, she decided to do the
unthinkable: she took Elma, left Hiram, and returned to her parents. It
was August 1841. Elma was nine years old; Mary was thirty-one.[20]

William and Rebecca Neal had known absolutely nothing of Mary's unhappiness with Hiram. She had suffered in silence for many years. In her
autobiography, Mary described her final confrontation with Hiram:

> I spoke to this taskmaster of a separation; I was told by "my husband,"
> who lived in idleness on my labor, I might almost say on my bloody
> sweat, that the law left me no redress; that if I left him, public opin-

ion would blast my name, and that my child, in whom alone I lived, should be taken from me. The law gave her to him, he said, and he should take her. And more than this, he told me that the brand of infamy should fall heavy and hot upon me. He *could* blast me, and he *would*, if I left him. These were his words.

One can imagine William's outrage upon learning of his daughter's plight. What exactly he learned is unclear, but he and Rebecca learned it first from Hiram, in July of 1841. Mary describes her parents as "horror struck" when she divulged that "the same state of things had existed from *the day of my marriage.*" That she returned to their home the following month suggests that Mary had parental encouragement to shun all propriety and abandon her husband.[21]

Here, Hiram's ineptitude as a breadwinner served Mary well: Hiram owed William Neal money—money he did not have. To protect his daughter and granddaughter, William threatened to claim his debt (and have Hiram face the legal consequences) unless Hiram left Mary and Elma alone. William made it clear that Hiram was not to pursue custody. He was not to darken their door. In fact, he was to leave town. In this confrontation, Mary remembered her father telling Hiram that "it would be a symptom of manhood" for him to return the silver watch on his wrist to Mary, since it had been a gift to her from her students. Though he did leave town, Hiram refused to part with the watch. Later, when Mary suggested to William that Hiram "does as well as he knows," she met with the "fiercest look that I ever saw shoot from his perforating eyes." She would vividly recall that single look years after her father had died.[22]

When Mary wrote to John Neal in February 1842, she had been living with her parents for seven months in Lynn, Massachusetts. Through December and January she had suffered with her most severe bouts of tuberculosis. Fever and cough kept her bedridden. She had lost a great deal of blood. Despite it all, Mary felt fundamentally rescued. Living safely at home, protected by her parents, Mary steadily gained emotional strength. From this distance, she even paid Hiram's tuition at the Washington University School of Medicine in Baltimore, where he had enrolled.[23]

Mary's primary concern during these months was how to obtain a legal divorce. She told John Neal that she wished she were a lawyer. To avoid hurting her reputation, Mary sought advice clandestinely. She knew that publicity regarding her marital desertion would tarnish her name and diminish her influence. Hiram was already threatening to take Elma and to "blast" Mary's name if she refused any longer to submit to his will. Mary needed answers. To Neal she summarized her plight in one question: "If I absolutely refuse to leave my father's house can my husband take my child[?]" Laws differed from state to state. Mary had recently received an invitation to join the staff at a New Jersey seminary, but was concerned only to know the custody laws of that state in considering the offer. Mary explained to Neal that her parents were willing to move anywhere "rather than I should suffer as I have heretofore." In this lengthy, confessional letter, Mary described her predicament:

> I want the privilege of educating my daughter tho I by no means wish to shut her out from the kindest intercourse with her father. I am very desirous that a separation should be effected so that the kindest feelings may exist between my husband and myself, tho I fear he will not be able to keep any kind feeling if he finds I am resolved to be separated. I am willing to maintain him if my exertions can do it. . . . A Divorce will be my *last resort,* but I must do some thing for life, for his horrible malady is wearing me into the grave. When I am with him nervous fits, terrible convulsions are immediately bro't on, and his letters shake me in every nerve and fibre. I have not been able to sit up but very little for the last two months. My medical adviser tells me that no medicine but that of the soul will do me any good. . . . I am satisfied that the dreadful hectic fever and cough *etc* with which I have been afflicted for two months past might be relieved immediately could I be assured of two things—that my chil[d] would be spared me, and that the vultures of o[ur] corrupt press would not prey upon my vitals.[24]

Mary was preparing to publish her collected lectures in book form—simply titled *Lectures to Ladies on Anatomy and Physiology.* She was also working on a novel, writing poetry, and grinding out a series of articles for the *Genesee Farmer* "on production, the currency, monopolies' antagonism of interests in Civilization with a criticism on the present state of Europe and America." It was not a time for bad publicity. Being one of the era's most prominent and successful literary figures, John Neal would understand. His responses to Mary's letters must have provided her solace. She wrote to him with concern for her own professional reputation and for Elma's future. She sought support for her desertion of Hiram. Mary knew that her physical problems derived from psychological anguish. If she wrote to female friends with equal candor, the correspondence has been lost.[25]

During these months of sickness, Mary filled her time with writing. William and Rebecca Neal must have marveled at the literary and professional success of their once shy, bookish daughter. Meanwhile, Hiram was spreading false rumors of Mary's infidelity, and many local publications that had previously accepted Mary's stories and poems no longer made room for her prose. That scandal followed her name probably disturbed William Neal less than it would have disturbed most fathers; familiar with slander himself, he may even have felt a bit proud.

LECTURES TO LADIES

As Mary regained strength and began to plan her future, she did find a number of people who supported her actions. Some, she felt, lent her greater sympathy because she had seemed to be dying of consumption. A few non-Quaker friends even sent her money. During and after her illness, however, she found her closest ally in Elma. Mary sustained herself with fantasies of their future together. She imagined raising her daughter to embrace a life of freedom. Marriage to Hiram had enabled an epiphany: "I saw that the law gave him . . . power over me, and then again I was sensible that my own weakness gave the law its force."[26]

Lectures to Ladies on Anatomy and Physiology reached the public early in 1842 and met with praise, even from the regular medical press. The *Boston Medical and Surgical Journal* found fault primarily with Mary's tendency to quote "too much from those who are altogether her inferiors in knowledge" and to overworship Sylvester Graham, whose physiologic theory the reviewer called "a sinking ship." Overall, however, the review recommended Mary's work, asserting that "all liberal-minded medical men have given countenance to her efforts." Even Bennett's *New York Herald*—the paper that had so abused Mary for her public lecturing—admitted that the book "contains some very sound and valuable advice that many may benefit from."[27]

The frontispiece of *Lectures to Ladies* presented readers with the image of a skeleton, lowered on one knee, praying. Its hands, clasped together, reach upward. Its head tilts back as if gazing toward heaven. Its teeth, by their very complete exposure, seem clenched in a passionate plea to God. Apart from a thin cushion that pads the figure's knee, the entire drawing floats in white space, without context. A woman could pick up Mary's book and gaze at this opening drawing without fully departing the comfort of her proper "sphere." Though a scientific study, the engraving is also a religious picture—innocence and devotion incarnate. To study the bones of this drawing is to contemplate one's relationship to God; the figure's pose allows no scientific detachment.

Mary had always considered the study of anatomy and physiology to be a form of worship. To follow God's will required an understanding of God's intentions, a knowledge of his laws. Mary had been raised in a religious culture. Despite her father's cynicism, she devoutly believed in the perfectibility of humanity. Health reform offered a bridge between the fiery religion of her childhood community and the scientific rationalism that would, by century's end, depict its skeletons upright and inanimate. In 1842 Mary's *Lectures to Ladies on Anatomy and Physiology* enabled women to pursue a traditionally male field of study without "unsexing" themselves. To preserve the health and morality of one's own family— and by extension one's own society—a woman, Mary argued, needed to understand her own body. The text opened invitingly: "God is paid when man receives; T'enjoy is to obey."

Likely few of Mary's readers had ever encountered a text so powerful in its depiction of women's strengths and rights. In 300 pages, with illustrations, *Lectures to Ladies* presents fourteen chapters whose organization and content derived from Mary's oral lecture series. The book begins with a general argument for the study of anatomy and physiology, followed by chapters on bones, muscles, circulation, respiration, digestion, dietetics, nerves, spinal disease, and, lastly, the importance of education. Mary relied heavily on personal stories as well as on the use of metaphor to illustrate her points. She posed rhetorical questions to her readers, encouraging thoughtful participation rather than passive absorption. A conversational tone suffuses even her technical explanations, while vivid word scenes enliven Mary's didactic commentary: "Even professed connoisseurs, who lounge and dawdle in the galleries of art, and labor to express their weak rapture at the Jove-like stature and sublime strength of Hercules, or at the majestic figure of Venus, beneath whose ample zone there resides the energy which prevents grace from degenerating into weakness—even they will belie, in dress and contour, all the power and beauty they profess to admire."[28] In Mary Gove, readers found a teacher bold enough to mock hypocrisy and smart enough to win respect.

Although it did not treat the subjects of reproductive anatomy or the physiology of sex, *Lectures to Ladies* still introduced women to tantalizing secrets—access to interior and personal spaces previously the domain of men alone. It also assumed an intellectual competence in women rarely granted by most literature aimed at the "weaker sex." From their youth, girls were taught to preen their looks and sweeten their dispositions, not to study their innards. For example, 1842 saw yet another new edition of Hannah and Mary Murray's already classic children's book, *The Young Lady's Toilet*, which metaphorically presented female character strengths as cosmetics, emphasizing the importance of appearance for girls: "A Wash to Smooth the Wrinkles: Contentment"; "Genuine Rouge: Modesty"; and "The Most Approved Head Ornament: Discretion," etc. By contrast, Mary wrote of arteries and marrow.

"If girls are taught to reason," wrote Mary (echoing many other social reformers of the day), "they will not spend their days reading fictions, and their nights in morbid dreams of love—a love that bears about as much resemblance to the true and healthful sentiment of love, as the blasting simoom does to the refreshing breeze." The thrust of Mary's work for women was to foster self-examination. If women could be made to understand their bodies, their passions, and the consequences of their behaviors, then they would—Mary fervently believed—make choices in the direction of strength and happiness. "Let woman once know her own organization, and she will tremble at the thought of sacrificing herself, for she will know that she is doing it."[29] Repetition plays an important role in these lectures. Again and again, Mary argues that women's miseries stem from ignorance.

Of the many legal, economic, social, and physical constraints placed on women in antebellum America, Mary chose to emphasize the one she believed had killed her sister and had induced the consumption that recurrently threatened her own life: the corset. She tells the story of one former pupil, a girl devoted to "tight lacing," who was stricken with fever and congested lungs. "A few days, and she was a corpse," wrote Mary, "*as much murdered as if she had drawn the cords about her neck.*" Rage bubbles through her lengthy discussion of the subject. Mary was taking on a formidable opponent: the height of fashion, the "death grasp." She begins by explaining the fragile anatomy of the lung, the physiology of circulation and respiration, and the chemical constituents of air. Throughout, she underlines the vital role of oxygen and the complexities of its exchange in the body. After examining a diagram of the heart and contemplating the relationship between the thoracic duct and the pleura, readers encountered Mary's blunt objective: "My object is to make you understand the mischief that arises from the ruinous practice of compressing the chest."[30] Seeking to change her readers' behavior, Mary offered physiology as a scriptural guide to personal conduct.

Many other medical writers had described the dangers posed by tight lacing, and Mary did not hesitate to draw on their authority. She included in her book an illustration from the popular textbook *The Class Book of Anatomy* by Dr. J. V. C. Smith (whom we have already encountered as editor of the *Boston Medical and Surgical Journal*). The drawing depicted the torsos of two female skeletons, one compressed by years of lacing, the other naturally broad. Framing the illustration is a vignette that captures Mary's disgust with the image: "Not long since, I took up a newspaper . . . which contained a story. I read . . . , 'Rising, she displayed a delicately slender waist, rather smaller than ordinary.' Let the dissecting knife display the ulcers in the lungs, within that waist, and it would not seem desirable, to the most vain and sickly sentimentalist."[31]

Mary did not let readers forget that she had been witness to dissections and was respected by many doctors as an educator in the field. Oblique references to her own friendships with physicians bolstered Mary's credibility. "So general is the distortion of the female form, and death from this cause," she wrote, "that when I asked a physician in Philadelphia, if he had a female skeleton, distorted by tight lacing, 'No,' said he, 'we have no need to save them; we can get one when it is wanted, at a week's notice.'" His response, as told here, reminds readers that Mary's request for a skeleton did not strike the physician as odd or unreasonable. She grafts this detail onto the potent and disturbing image of male physicians taking for granted their access to deformed female cadavers. Would women, fortified with knowledge of the risks, continue to compress themselves in corsets? Mary's answer appealed to all possible motives for reform: "Let all those who have the least love for science, for philanthropy, or Christianity, answer, *No: resolutely, and firmly,* No."[32]

The reviewer who praised *Lectures to Ladies* in the *Boston Medical and Surgical Journal* noted that Mary expressed herself with greater force and interest when speaking "untrammeled" before an audience than when writing on the page. If so, Mary must have expressed herself formidably from the podium. Her writing at times practically dares her reader to resist: "What I have learned I would leave to the world; and I am confident that it will be well received by the virtuous and intelligent." Mary argued that "it is [woman's] right, by God's intendment, to be hardy and robust." She sought a potent amalgam of health, freedom, and happiness—an imaginative feminism not centered on suffrage.[33]

Mary's lack of animosity toward men also widened her audience. No woman who recommended *Lectures to Ladies* could be justly accused of endorsing revolution or of despising the opposite sex. "I am not one of those who charge man with injustice to woman," Mary established. "Man is no more unjust to woman than he is to himself." Instead, Mary blamed "society." She encouraged women's anger without inciting division. "I do not wish to leave my subject to enter into argument about the equality of the sexes," wrote Mary. "I know full well, as woman is educated and enslaved by circumstances, that she is not equal to man. Whether she would be in a better state of things, I stop not to inquire." In subsequent books, Mary grew bolder. She later asserted that "the conditions of health being equally secured to both sexes, there will be found greater equality in the progress of boys and girls in scholarship." She advocated coeducation and even wrote that "the feminine intellect is quicker than the masculine, and girls often grasp by a sudden intuition what boys acquire slowly by study."[34] However, in *Lectures to Ladies,* Mary emphasized the *distinct* contribution women could make to society and specifically avoided the inflammatory question of gender equity: "That there will always be a dissimilarity between the sexes, whether their education be the same or different, I think no one will deny," she asserted. "But dissimilarity is no proof of inferiority. Man has more of intellect, woman more of affection. But I have yet to learn that wisdom is *superior* to love."[35]

Like the body, Mary argued, society required full health of all its members. Nature intended balance—between organ systems, between inborn

passions, and between men and women. The reiterated medical thesis of
Lectures to Ladies served as metaphor for Mary's political aims: "There is
a sympathy between all the organs of the body; however great, complex,
or minute, 'all are but parts of one stupendous whole.' If one wheel in a
clock is injured, all will go wrong, because all the parts are dependent on
each other." Women needed to recognize their own significance. "For the
sake of the race," wrote Mary, "I ask that all be done for woman that can
be done. . . . [I] know that I am not a shadow of what I might have been
had I been rightly educated—educated with wise reference to soul and
body."[36]

Mary longed for control of her own book's copyright. She described this
craving to John Neal in August 1841: "I want to publish my book, and I
want it secured to me." She had even consulted Robert Rantoul, a lawyer
who accepted "two dollars to tell me that my manuscript was not mine
or rather that a woman's manuscript was not hers." From this meeting,
Mary understood that if a married woman solicited a trusted male friend
to take out the copyright, her husband would still have to "transfer his
property right in the manuscript to the man who took out the copy right
or the man could not hold it." In this letter (which Mary requested he
burn after reading it), she described her humbling predicament to Neal
and begged his advice. "Years before my marriage," she wrote, "my husband failed in business. Since my . . . marriage, by my pen, I have paid the
larger portion of these debts contracted when I was a child. A part remains
due. I am willing to pay them, and have written to my husband that I will
do it, if I receive enough for my book past paying expenses, that is if he
will relinquish *his right* (?) to my manuscript, to some one in trust for me,
who shall take out the copy right. I have received no answer from him."
It is hard at times to determine which Mary found more despicable—her
husband's physical claim to her body and child or, as she put it, "*his right*
in my *brains.*"[37]

HENRY GARDINER WRIGHT

Within one year of publishing her lectures, Mary would find a man to
help take her mind off marital woes. Henry Gardiner Wright was twenty-
eight years old and beautiful. Recently arrived from England, he had been
serving as the headmaster of an experimental boarding school called Al-

cott House, located near London at Ham Common. The school had been named after the American educational reformer and transcendentalist Amos Bronson Alcott, the father of Louisa May Alcott. In Cheshire, Connecticut, Alcott had founded the Cheshire Pestalozzian School, a coeducational primary school that rejected traditional rote learning in favor of interactive techniques advanced by the Swiss educator Johann Pestalozzi. Students learned mathematics by manipulating objects; they learned to read by associating words with pictures. They studied the Bible by discussing its messages, rather than by reciting its verses. All students participated in gymnastic exercises. A vegetarian and devoted Grahamite, Alcott believed that "physiology is none other than the study of *Spirit Incarnate.*" His educational experiments had been memorialized in two controversial books: *Record of a School*, written by his assistant, Elizabeth Peabody; and *Conversations with Children on the Gospels,* conducted and edited by Alcott himself.[38]

Henry Gardiner Wright, a devotee of Alcott's methods, was the son of a watchmaker. He had served as a clerk in a wholesale importing house before becoming involved with James P. Greaves and Charles Lane—Englishmen full of admiration for Alcott's work. Greaves, a former businessman, founded Alcott House in 1838, thirteen years after studying on the continent with Johann Pestalozzi himself. He became a mystical thinker, writing opaquely that "spirit alone can whole," and attracting as friends a collection of somewhat lost intellectual reformers, including Henry Wright. Unfortunately, Greaves died in March of 1842, two months before Amos Bronson Alcott set sail for England to tour his namesake school and to meet the staff that taught five languages, writing, drawing, music, singing, physiology, anatomy, gymnastics, geography, dancing, mathematics, history, natural history, chemistry, domestic economy, gardening, and more. Though too late to know Greaves, Alcott found sympathetic friends in Henry Wright and Charles Lane. At the end of September, these men, along with Lane's young son William, traveled to the United States to join Bronson Alcott in founding an experimental "consociate family farm."[39]

Henry Gardiner Wright had deep blue eyes, full lips, and fine clothes. Mary met him at a picnic sometime in the autumn of 1842. She gazed at Henry's curly golden hair, which fell seductively over his open Byronic collar. He took an equal interest in his observer. That they were both vegetarians suggested a likely compatibility and opened up conversation. At the time, Henry was struggling with the adjustment to America. He had left a wife and new baby in England, with plans to send for them once he, Lane, and the Alcotts had succeeded in establishing their new utopia. But a suitable site for "Fruitlands" had not yet been found; and in the meantime Henry, Charles, William, and the six Alcotts were all living together in Dove Cottage, the Alcott's cramped Concord home. Though he probably did not yet know it at the time of the picnic, Henry was also ill with lung cancer.[40]

Over the months that followed, Henry grew closer to Mary and more distant from his colleagues back in Concord. The Englishmen had spent their first week in the United States at the home of Alcott's good friend Ralph Waldo Emerson, but had voluntarily returned to the less luxurious accommodations at Dove Cottage. Emerson had never shown support for the experimental utopian communities that were sprouting throughout New England and the Western states during the 1840s. His lack of enthusiasm likely influenced their departure. Though in a position to support the venture financially, Emerson refused to participate. The enthusiastic Alcotts, on the other hand, had no money to speak of. Conditions at Dove Cottage strained relationships in many directions. Charles Lane had a naturally controlling manner and a profound mistrust of the conjugal family structure—a mistrust that would eventually destroy his friendship with the Alcotts. He and Bronson spent most of their time lecturing throughout the Boston area, seeking recruits for Fruitlands. Henry also gave lectures independently, though with less success than his peers. The men promoted a vision of agrarian self-sufficiency, communal harmony, and hygienic living. Vegetarians who would wear canvas shoes in place of leather, and home-spun linen instead of slave-grown cotton, residents of Fruitlands would live a pure life. They would eat only "aspiring" vegetables, like asparagus or corn—ones that grew upward. They would shun the downward root-crops. But still in Concord, the founders soon irritated one another.[41]

Henry began to complain of the cold potatoes and the absence of milk with dinner. Bronson attacked Henry's "disorderly habits," his "love of food," and his "unsteadiness of purpose."[42] During the period when he was getting to know Mary, Henry was lonely and frustrated. He had come to America to join a family farm that still existed only in promotional conversation. In reality, he was living in a small, unheated bedroom in a house full of other people's children. He began to visit Mary regularly. In January he moved to Lynn and became a boarder in William Neal's own house. That he and Mary both had legal spouses did little to inhibit their affair. Mary simply hung curtains in the parlor of her parents' home to grant their scandal-courting relationship the privacy they desired.

In her autobiography, Mary makes no apologies for the love she shared with Henry Gardiner Wright. At the time, however, she did want to avoid further damage to her reputation. *Lectures to Ladies* had won her new respect. Interest in health reform created an instant bond between Mary and Henry. Before coming to the United States, Henry had coedited with Charles Lane a reform journal called the *Healthian*. Mary's previous experience in Worcester editing Joseph S. Wall's *Health Journal and Advocate of Physiological Reform* gave the two more common background and naturally suggested the possibility of a joint project. By January of 1843, Henry and Mary had launched a new journal: *The Health Journal and Independent Magazine*. Charles Lane, absorbed with plans for Fruitlands, agreed that the new journal should subsume the *Healthian*.[43]

The *Health Journal and Independent Magazine* was edited by Mary, Henry, and David Hatch Barlow, a Harvard Divinity School graduate who also lived in Lynn. The two surviving issues of the *Health Journal*—possibly the only two ever to exist—belie their editors' forced optimism. Full of enthusiasm for a different version of experimental utopia, the second issue of the *Health Journal* delivered a recruitment call to those interested in founding a new joint-stock community in the West. (Henry, apparently, felt little pull to return to his family in England.) Soliciting shares at twenty-five dollars each, Mary, Henry, and David proposed a community "where communal and individual property are both secured—where attractive occupation shall be provided" and where men and women would receive equal payment for their labor. But few if any readers responded, and Henry's cancer was getting worse. The *Health Journal* soon faded away.[44]

It was clear that Henry needed surgery. He had avoided the fact as long as possible. Over the months he lived with Mary's family in Lynn, Henry futilely pursued alternative means of treatment based on regular exercise, fresh air, a vegetarian diet, and many baths. He was practicing the "water cure," having learned its complicated methods from Vincent Priessnitz himself.

Mary had only vaguely heard of Vincent Priessnitz, the Silesian peasant-turned-healer who treated his patients with cold water. Henry, a devoted follower, was eager to teach her all about the man and his miraculous techniques. He loaned Mary books that explained the origins and methods of "hydrotherapy." The formal water cure originated in 1826, when Priessnitz suffered a rib-crushing wagon accident. Doctors offered him no hope of full recovery. Left with this dire prognosis, Priessnitz soaked a towel in cold water and improvised a dripping bandage, which he wrapped around his torso after fully inflating his lungs to reposition the broken ribs. This treatment, along with extensive drinking of water and ten days of rest, produced swift and dramatic healing. It even seemed to work on injured farm animals. Capitalizing on his discovery, Priessnitz soon founded the Grafenberg Water Cure, and in 1829 he began to receive foreign invalids for treatment. They came from Prussia, Hungary, Poland, Russia, Sweden, Belgium, Switzerland, and even America. By 1840 nearly seventeen hundred patients per year were seeking treatment there. Among others, these guests included royalty, generals, high and low civil servants, physicians, artists, and divines.

Soon the popularity of water cure spread to England, where in 1842 Dr. James Wilson opened Grafenberg House at Malvern. By the time of his death in 1850, Priessnitz—who never articulated a systematic theory of pathology—had acquired international fame as the father of modern hydropathy. People marveled at his seeming ability to diagnose disease merely by studying the quality of a patient's skin. Henry Wright, who had received treatment at the original Grafenberg, was an important proselytizer in America. His informal New England student, Mary Gove, would devote the rest of her life to promoting the water cure.[45]

Henry demonstrated as well as explained the practice of drinking twenty to thirty glasses of cold water every day. Priessnitz had enforced strict measures at Grafenberg, where patients ate no spiced, heated, or over-refined food and received no medication at all. Daily cold baths and frequent exercise, combined with wet bandages and a variety of sitz and rubbing baths filled patients' days. As another Grafenberg patient remembered,

Priessnitz's dress was of the plainest kind; his coat a gray frock, loosely and badly cut, pantaloons of the same material, vest double-breasted, and buttoned up to the throat; his complexion was fair and slightly pitted, (I afterwards heard him say, that he had the small pox before he had a knowledge of the water-cure, or he would not have been marked,) hair light, and shortly cut, the forehead expansive and well formed, expressing high perceptive and intellectual power—moral sentiments well developed—eye restless, brilliant, and strikingly penetrating—nose prominent, mouth large and square—lips firmly and handsomely set together—the figure erect and manly—all together, his appearance was impressive. I felt that I was in the presence of no ordinary man.

Dr. Wilson, a man so taken with Priessnitz's methods that he founded his own hydropathic establishment, recalled drinking more than thirty glasses of water before breakfast while a patient at Grafenberg. In eight months, he had taken nearly one thousand baths and had spent 480 hours wrapped in a wet sheet.[46]

Henry taught Mary about Priessnitz's most original contribution to cold water's long history of therapeutic uses: the wet sheet pack. It treated non-localized disease by either heating or cooling the patient as each case required, and it involved wrapping a person mummy-style from the neck down, first in a wet sheet and additionally in several dry blankets. Other specific treatments ranged from hip baths to eye baths, from head baths to foot baths, from rubbing wet sheets to whole body plunges. A favorite treatment was the repeated sitz bath, which required a patient to soak her or his hips and lower pelvis in water (usually cold) for approximately fifteen minutes (though some prescriptions—intended to be more tonic than decongesting—called for much longer baths). All patients received individualized treatment plans based on their symptoms, strength, and allegiance to the water cure.

Henry Wright's final decision to call a surgeon reflected dire circumstances. He had applied Priessnitz's methods to no avail. The twenty-minute operation took place, without anesthesia, in the parlor of William Neal's house. But it did not do any good.[47] Slowly dying, Henry decided to return to England. His ship would depart from New York on the first of July 1843. Mary traveled with him to the pier, dressing his incision daily and planning for his eventual return, when the two would either form or join a harmonious community of like-minded reformers. But Henry did not return. He died in England, only thirty-two years old.[48]

Fruitlands fared little better. On May 25, 1843, Charles Lane had purchased a ninety-acre farm with the financial assistance of Bronson Alcott's brother-in-law, the Unitarian minister, temperance man, and abolitionist Samuel May. Located in Harvard, Massachusetts, fourteen miles from Concord, the farm was deceptively bucolic. Its soil proved to be depleted and rocky. Lacking experience, the new farmers planted crops late in the season and met with unusually fierce summer storms. In autumn the hopeful inhabitants of Fruitlands harvested little more than damaged barley. For a brief time the community had enjoyed the philosophical discussions and healthful lifestyle originally envisioned. Visitors to the farm found members dressed in linen tunics over bloomers, working in the fields or reflecting on difficult questions such as "What is the highest aim?" and "What is man?" But it was an exceptionally cold winter as well. By January the communal experiment had utterly failed, and the Alcotts' marriage had come close to final disaster as well. Charles Lane and his son joined a nearby Shaker community, writing to a friend back in Ham Common that "Mr. Alcott's constancy to his wife and family and his inconstancy to the Spirit have blurred his life forever."[49] Mary had also suffered tremendous disappointment. But she would soon face even worse.

KIDNAPPED

On December 1, 1844, William Neal died of consumption. He was seventy-six years old. Though he had shown signs of deterioration for at least two years, Mary had maintained faith in his resilience and had grown comfortable under his protection from Hiram. Too comfortable. Less than four months after William Neal died, Mary left Elma with her mother and embarked alone on a trip to Ohio. Traveling by coach and steamboat, Mary toured a range of experimental communities in the West. She was exploring possible new living arrangements among social reformers, seriously considering the plans she and Henry Wright had envisioned together. It was during Mary's well-publicized absence that Hiram reclaimed his right to Elma. Rebecca Neal had no legal right to refuse his demand for his thirteen-year-old daughter. Hiram took Elma away on March 20, 1845, amid a scene of tears and protests.[50]

That fathers automatically possessed custody rights to their children left Mary with few options. Retrieving Elma would prove to be no easy task. Mary returned home as quickly as possible, only to spend the following weeks in an agony of panic and rage. She had no idea where Hiram had taken Elma. She had no right to challenge his action in court. Soon, however, a letter arrived from a stranger, describing a brief conversation with Elma on a New England railroad. Elma's tears had drawn the woman to her when Hiram had stepped away, and Elma had begged the woman to write Rebecca Neal in Lynn and let her know that her granddaughter was being taken to stay, temporarily, with Hiram's brother. Mary pursued her daughter immediately.[51]

What followed were many consultations with lawyers and a drawn-out custody battle that would drain Mary of most of her income. The first lawyer that Mary found was a sympathetic man who attempted to reassure her with the fact that Elma would soon reach the age of legal independence and could not be held thereafter. When she was not pursuing additional lawyers and contriving schemes of rescue, Mary filled the following months with fiction writing. Her friends encouraged her to return to Lynn so that Hiram might grow complacent and relax his watch over Elma, opening up new opportunities. When she followed this advice, it was only to learn that her mother could no longer afford to keep the family house. "I can not describe the feeling of homelessness, of utter loss, that entered like an iron into my spirit when our dear home passed into the hands of strangers," wrote Mary. She and her mother moved in with friends. Their days revolved around the mail, as they waited for word of Elma. During these months, Mary suffered prolonged trouble with her eyesight, making it impossible for her to read or sew. Her hair began to fall out. She hardly slept. Looking back on that time, Mary felt as though she had aged thirty years.

Eventually a letter did come, instructing Mary to return to the Quaker village where Hiram was keeping Elma. When she arrived at the hotel, a gentleman soon appeared who introduced himself as the business partner of the very first lawyer she had consulted. He encouraged her to stay with his wife while he perfected plans for Elma's recovery. During the time that

Mary stayed in this lawyer's family, she met with many "mercenary" offers to relay messages between mother and daughter or to bring information about Elma. That people cared so little for the tragedy of her situation as to derive profit from it left her sickened; yet she did learn that Hiram had been treating Elma to all sorts of gifts. Elma was living with a young widow who had only one child of her own—"a gentle, sweet woman, who doubtless believed that she was saving a soul from perdition in keeping my child from me," wrote Mary.

Mary made one bold attempt to see Elma herself, but of course found the doors locked. Word of her aim flew through the town more rapidly than Mary could. It required enormous inner preparation and strength to walk through streets peopled by a sect that had disowned her. Though she did not fear for her personal safety, she knew from many Quaker meetings how painful a silent, steely gaze could be. "The people of the village, almost as one, regarded me as a woman of ill fame, or a poor wretch of a novel-writer, without character or reputation, and fit only to be an outcast from all mercy, here and hereafter, as I was from their faith and fold." Only by distracting herself with writing did Mary endure her obsessive worry.[52]

Eventually, however, the business partner presented a solution. He ultimately decided that an overt move would prove more unexpected than any of their covert operations. Together with two strong men, he devised a relatively simple scheme and liberated Elma. One of the men waited in a carriage stationed half a mile from Elma's new home. A steep and impassable embankment separated the house from the road. The lawyer and the second assistant approached the house from the back and conveniently found Elma picking strawberries, guarded only by the widow's young son. They quickly thrust into Elma's hand a letter from Mary. While the boy ran to the front of the house to call an alarm, the rescuers guided a willing Elma up the hill and into the carriage. The boy could not even indicate the direction in which the men had taken Elma.

In a small town, everyone recognizes everyone. The wife of the assistant captor was expecting Hiram to come angrily to her house—which he did, immediately. The woman stalled and fretted and used as much time as possible before misleading Hiram. At ten o'clock that night, Elma was returned to Mary near a hidden cottage flanked by large elms. They traveled through the night. It was June 16; Mary and Elma had been separated for three months. That very year, Margaret Fuller had written about the kidnapping of children by their fathers:

> [There are] innumerable instances in which profligate and idle men live upon the earnings of industrious wives; or if the wives leave them, and take . . . the children, to perform the double duty of mother and father, follow from place to place, and threaten to rob them of the children, if deprived of the rights of a husband. . . . Such instances count up by scores within my own memory. . . . I have known these men steal their children, whom they knew they had no means to maintain, take them into dissolute company, expose them to bodily danger, to frighten the poor woman, to whom, it seems, the fact that she alone had borne the pangs of their birth, and nourished their infancy, does not give an equal right to them. I do believe that this mode of kidnapping—and it is frequent enough in all classes of society—will be by the next age viewed as it is by Heaven now.[53]

Mary and Elma spent the following two weeks in hiding, staying with the family of a kind lawyer who, when neighbors inquired, described his unexpected guests as cousins. Fearing discovery and also needing to earn money, Mary resolved to move on to a larger town, where she might go undetected by Hiram even if she were to teach classes.

For a time, Mary and Elma moved from one boarding house to another, often meeting with ill will. Meanwhile, Hiram, rather than pursue his daughter, pressed charges of abduction against one of the men who had kidnapped her. Under the laws of coverture, he could not bring suit against his own wife. Legally, marriage transformed a woman. No longer allowed to negotiate her own business transactions, a wife lost control of her property and earnings as well as her right to make contracts, to sue, or to be sued. Still, Mary naturally felt compelled to pay the defendant's legal fees. A lower court awarded Hiram heavy damages, and the appeal process dragged on for two years. Though a higher court ultimately exonerated the defendant, Mary had still accrued substantial legal expenses. She desperately needed to earn some money.[54]

CHOOSING THE WATER CURE

In June of 1845, Mary learned that Dr. Robert Wesselhœft had just opened a new water-cure establishment in Brattleboro, Vermont. Though she had been advocating many of hydropathy's principles in her lectures and writings, Mary had thus far received no formal training in water cure. Desperate to escape from debilitating gossip, to find safe haven, and to secure a means of earning steady income, Mary decided to go to southern Vermont and seek training as a water-cure physician. Many of America's leading intellects had begun to respect and publicly endorse the practices of hydrotherapy. Margaret Fuller had just published *Woman in the Nineteenth Century*, a text that would become a landmark in the history of feminist thought, where she wrote:

> The praises of cold water seem to me an excellent sign in the age. They denote a tendency to the true life. We are now to have, as a remedy for ills, not orvietan, or opium, or any quack medicine, but plenty of air and water, with due attention to warmth and freedom in dress, and simplicity of diet. . . . Every day we observe signs that the natural feelings on these subjects are about to be reinstated, and the body to claim care as the abode and organ of the soul; not as the tool of servile labor, or the object of voluptuous indulgence.[55]

Brattleboro, Vermont, was a town of 2,300 people when Mary arrived in 1845. Located on the western bank of the Connecticut River, twelve miles from the Massachusetts border, Brattleboro seemed a fine site for a water-cure establishment. The town maintained a paper mill, a tannery, a machine shop, a woolen mill, and factories producing cabinets, silk, and shoe-pegs. It supported banks, taverns, churches, three native newspapers, and the Vermont Asylum for the Insane, founded in the 1830s. Every evening people watched the sun's last rays linger on the summit of Chesterfield Mountain, a peak of 1,600 feet that sat opposite Brattleboro on the river's eastern shore. Forests of beech, maple, and pine surrounded the town, amidst meadows, brooks, hills, gorges, and waterfalls. All but the weakest residents of Wesselhœft's Water Cure grew familiar with the "four-mile circle," a favored walking route that overlooked the village. And all who could manage the effort hiked in the local mountains.

The Brattleboro Water-Cure Establishment opened its doors to patients on May 29, 1845. Though it quickly grew to accommodate nearly two hundred patients, the bucolic retreat initially welcomed only eighteen people for treatment. Located just off Main Street near the center of town, the water-cure establishment included separate buildings for men and women, each supplied with hot and cold running water and equipped for a variety of baths. The plunge baths—twenty-five feet long by fifteen feet wide and four feet deep—were continually renewed with a constant flow of fresh water. Half a mile away, in a wooded area, patients found an outdoor spa. Showers (called "douches") plunged from as high as twenty feet. There, the establishment also maintained an eye bath, an ear bath, twelve running sitz baths, two "rising douches," and access to a "river douche," warmer in temperature than the springs that supplied the outdoor baths and located just below the "wave-bath," which was fed by a small millpond. This diversity of baths invited Americans to explore a highly unusual practice. Only ten years earlier, a subscriber had written to the *Boston Moral Reformer:* "I have been in the habit during the past winter of taking a warm bath every three weeks. Is this too often to follow the year round?"[56]

In summer, Brattleboro's springs ran at 49 degrees; in winter, 44. The combination of baths and exercise, along with a plain (though not vegetarian) diet, would "strengthen the system and rouse it to such a degree of activity, as will enable it to throw off disease by those various natural modes, which have been provided for the relief of the body."[57] As Mary would learn, water cure required considerable skill to administer. In exchange for this practical education, Mary offered physiology lectures to the guests of Dr. Wesselhœft's establishment.

Robert Wesselhœft advanced a rigorous treatment program designed to provoke "a vast acceleration in the change of substance which is always taking place in the system." Hydrotherapy literally washed the body of morbid matter, assisting nature in its continual quest for renewal. When "waste matter . . . is constantly thrown out of the system, by the pores of the skin and other channels, the substance of disease passes away, and the body, freed from its oppression, is built up," explained the establishment's first report. Such rehabilitative purges induced "crises," which, though physically dramatic, confirmed a patient's progress toward cure: "These crises consist sometimes in the appearance of large boils, discharging great quantities of matter, sometimes in eruptions and humors, either in the common forms of scrofula, erysipelas, &c. or in others peculiar to the water cure, sometimes in critical vomiting or diarrhoea, and sometimes in the recurrence and consummation of a previous disease, which had been suppressed but not cured by the administration of drugs." Water-cure theory held that chronic disease reflected an internal congestion of trapped, toxic matter; cure demanded its liberation. As the *American Journal of Hydropathy* explained it, "The first effect of the Water Cure processes is to relieve the more apparent and external symptoms of the disease, such as morbid heat, irritability, pain, symptomatic fever, disquietude, etc. . . . At length, a grand rally of all the vital powers takes place. The organic powers, experiencing a pleasurable degree of newly recovered freedom, try to throw off the tyranny of disease, and achieve their independence by a single battle." Many hydrotherapists, however, were quick to reassure prospective patients that they believed these most extreme crises to be quite unnecessary and wholly avoidable.[58]

Most of those who traveled to residential facilities suffered from chronic diseases like asthma, dyspepsia, gout, spinal distortion, and dysmenorrhea; they tended to stay one to three months. Typically they were asked to bring (or rent) several sheets, blankets, comforters, towels, and linen bandages for personal use. Retreat from the pressures of regular work and urban living was said to assist recovery, enhancing the appeal of rural establishments. As Mary later reflected, "The great trouble with Americans is, they are in too great a hurry. They are in a hurry to eat and drink, and to get rich. They get ill as fast as they can, and they want a short cut to health. Chronic disease that has been . . . induced by wrong-doing through half a lifetime, cannot be cured in a day by any process now known to the world." Yet not all water-cure patients required extended absences from home. Acute disease—which was thought to reveal the throes of a natural, curative crisis—required prompt intervention "to govern and regulate" the crisis by mitigating its "too violent symptoms." Tonic therapies to strengthen the patient would follow. Whether for months or days, this treatment demanded close attention to diet and behavior. Wesselhoeft's staff discouraged any "constraining etiquette" among residents, and intentionally scheduled patients' days so as to make impossible "great display of dress."[59]

Catharine Beecher recalled the treatment she received at the Brattleboro Water-Cure in the summer of 1847:

At four in the morning packed in a wet sheet; kept in it from two to
three hours; then up, and in a reeking perspiration immersed in the
coldest plunge-bath. Then a walk as far as strength would allow, and
drink five or six tumblers of the coldest water. At eleven A.M. stand
under a douche of the coldest water falling *eighteen feet, for ten minutes*. Then walk, and drink three or four tumblers of water. At three
P.M. sit half an hour in a *sitz* bath (i.e., sitting bath) of the coldest
water. Then walk and drink again. At nine P.M. sit half an hour with
the feet in the coldest water, then rub them till warm. Then cover the
weak limb and a third of the body in wet bandages, and *retire to rest*.
This same wet bandage to be worn all day, and kept constantly wet.[60]

Treatment protocols varied considerably from case to case, responding
to each patient's symptoms, stamina, and age. From Wesselhœft, Mary
learned the art of individual prescription. "The efficacy of water cure depends upon the amount of vital energy or re-active force of the patient,"
she wrote, "The same treatment that would cure one might fail entirely
with another." By "re-active force" Mary meant the ability to regain
warmth after bathing in cold water. She described the plunge bath as "a
great luxury" for those with easy access to abundant water. Its method was
straightforward: "Fill the long tub about six inches deep; first wash the
face and head, and then quickly immerse the whole body, rubbing vigorously in the water for a few seconds. If the water is cold, half a minute is
enough. Follow with a good rubbing with soft and hard towels." Her clinical training in Vermont gave Mary profound respect for the healing
power of pure, cold water: given adequate time and unfaltering devotion,
hydropathic treatment would fortify the skin, purify the blood, eliminate
accumulations of toxic medications, and cure nearly all disease.[61]

After three months in Brattleboro, Mary traveled with Elma to the New
Lebanon Springs Water Cure, about twenty-five miles southeast of Albany, New York. The elaborate aqueducts and various baths of the establishment had cost more than three thousand dollars to construct. It had
been built by David Campbell, a former publisher of the *Graham Jour-*

nal of Health and Longevity, which had enthusiastically promoted Mary's original lecture series. Mary served as resident physician at New Lebanon Springs for three months, where she managed patients with apparent success. On December 1, 1845, Dr. Joel Shew, who was a part owner and advisory physician of the New Lebanon establishment as well as the editor of the *Water-Cure Journal,* published notice of Mary's appointment and endorsed her skill. By the end of that month, however, Mary's health began to suffer under the physical demands of her work, which included vigorous friction-rubs of patients, lifting of dripping wet sheets, and assisting people of all sizes in and out of baths, beds, and blanket-wraps.[62] It would be easier, she concluded, to teach classes in anatomy, physiology, and water cure. Just before the holidays, with the hope of attracting a pool of paying students, Mary and Elma moved to New York City, where they would remain for the next six and a half years.

Though she had acquired new skills and made important professional connections, Mary felt the pressure of her situation. Not only did she have herself and a teenage daughter to support, but she also had a lawyer's bills to meet and a reputation to revive. The hydropathic community eased her transition to New York. She and Elma found immediate temporary lodging at 47 Bond Street in the home of Dr. Shew and his wife, Marie Louise Shew. Had she been able to afford the six-dollar-per-week rent, Mary would have stayed longer than ten days. The Shews had converted their home into a water-cure house and accommodated a stimulating and diverse collection of people—some rather bizarre—who would become Mary's friends.

Joel Shew had earned his medical degree in 1843 after working in a Philadelphia daguerreotype shop. He was twenty-seven years old. At some point, he and his wife began to take interest in Priessnitz's use of water, and by 1844 they found themselves devout converts to hydrotherapy. Though only one year out of medical school, Joel Shew founded the *Water-Cure Journal* in New York City and edited a *Hand Book of Hydropathy.* Meanwhile, Marie Louise Shew published *Water-Cure for Ladies: A Popular Work on the Health, Diet, and Regimen of Females and Children, and the Prevention and Cure of Disease; with a Full Account of the Processes of Water-Cure* (1844). They also opened their house to patients.[63] When Mary met the Shews in December of 1845, Joel was obsessively involved with the production of his *Journal,* and Marie was happily overworked with the care of her full household, her father's nearby household, and three children, including a new baby boy.

Mary found Marie warm and genuine—not at all the showy flirt that Marie's reputation had suggested. She liked her hostess and bristled at Joel Shew's dismissal of Marie from the parlor when he desired use of the room. Why Marie became childlike in the presence of her husband, Mary could not understand. She considered Joel Shew's worst quality his "being everywhere present" like "the frogs of Egypt" and found his hawk-like supervision of the kitchen unbearable. She saw that other boarders abhorred him. The man was chronically finding his way into debt and irritating those around him with his mutterings about "the *Journal.*" Though she did not take to Dr. Shew, Mary found friendship with Marie and with the interesting people in the house.

Several residents stood out for Mary. One man wore long hair; one grew a moustache "when half the people about him had never seen another"; and two wore their collars "à la Byron, with a black ribbon instead of a close neck stock." These few were the artists, musicians, poets, and philosophers of the house, young men who struck Mary as "unconsciously determined that the world should not conquer them." All seemed devoted to Marie, and each had somehow modified his behavior—abandoned cigars, adopted cold bathing—to win her approval. With the exception of Marie, none of the house's women made any impression on Mary.[64]

Elma, who was fifteen years old, found the landscape, portrait, and miniature artists fascinating; she determined to become an artist herself and asked her mother for lessons. Mary had arrived in New York City with thirteen dollars during the middle of the holidays. To establish a class, she would have to wait until after New Year's when people would be relaxed enough to read her advertisements. She calculated the need for three weeks' rent, ten dollars in advance for a classroom, ten dollars for promotional circulars, ten dollars for presentable clothing for herself and Elma, and a bit of money for food. It came to about fifty dollars—and all for the highly uncertain prospect of attracting a class. Still, pencils and drawing paper cost less than a dollar. Perhaps remembering the lack of parental support she had received as a child wishing to write, Mary bought the art supplies for Elma.

Anticipating her need for money, Mary had submitted three stories to the popular women's magazine, *Godey's Lady's Book.* They had been accepted for publication but would not appear for nearly a year, at which point Mary would be paid. Desperate for cash, Mary wrote to the editor, Sarah Josepha Hale, asking for advance payment. The fifteen dollars that arrived in the mail enabled Mary to pay her debt to Joel Shew and to acquire new accommodations on the fourth floor of a boardinghouse on Broadway in a small room not normally available for rent. The arrangement cost a dollar and a half per week and included no meals. Mary spent her second week in New York making plain dresses for herself and Elma of pale brown mousseline de laine. She and Elma survived on inexpensive Indian mush and molasses. They also consulted A. B. Durand, who referred them to an elderly, asthmatic, yet still-talented art instructor, who charged only five dollars for a quarter's lessons. With building confidence, Mary submitted an article and poem to the editor of the *Democratic Review* and was astonished to receive prompt acceptance and a check for twenty-one dollars. Ecstatic, she ordered her circulars and began drafting her lesson plans.[65]

THREE

Passion Unleashed

☙   ☙   ☙

THOUGH THEY HAD moved out of the Bond Street house, Mary and Elma maintained ties to Marie and her circle. One boarder at the Shews', a favorite of Marie's, was especially attracted to Mary. Marx Edgeworth Lazarus was a young Jewish medical student with long hair, alluring dark eyes, and a mysterious vocabulary. At the time Mary encountered him, he was deeply absorbed in the philosophy of Charles Fourier. "Characters are distributed in categories," he declared to Mary on their first meeting. He brushed his hair from his eyes. "I flatter myself we may have affinity." Mary found his affectation endearing and listened with amusement as he launched into a convoluted dissertation on "passional harmony"—a subject Mary herself had studied and one that she had published on. There was no question that the two shared an affinity.

The night before Mary moved to her new boardinghouse, Marx left a potted rose bush in her room. He had a reputation for both wealth and abstraction. Soon after Mary and Elma moved, he invited them to the theater, along with his younger sister. It was not long before Marx began looking for a large house where he, Mary, Elma, and an association of compatible friends might live together in harmony. Mary, he planned, would head the household; he would pay for it.

While he developed these plans, Mary began to offer classes. Women and girls eagerly came to learn as they had eight years earlier when she gave her first lectures. Mary earned money but found her income consumed by the "bottomless pit of litigation" that persisted in New England. Though she did not like to owe anyone, the choice to accept Marx's generous living arrangement must have been an easy one. With only thirty dollars in her pocket, Mary moved, with Elma, into one of the largest bedrooms in a spacious house at 261 Tenth Street. Their house-mates included poets, musicians, a novelist and his sister (both orthodox Calvinists), and a woman who translated George Sand—probably eight to ten people in all, plus a servant. Water-cure devotees and vegetarians, the group fashioned a small gymnasium before they even bought furniture. "Not one of us had health," recalled Mary. "All were waifs and strays from a sick world, seeking to go higher. . . . Not one of us, with the exception of [Marx], had a dollar, except what he earned from day to day." Some wrote regular reviews of concerts and theater productions. Discussions of art, politics, and philosophy revealed stark differences in opinion among the housemates, but all got along well. "General toleration was the strong bond that bound us together, and personal liking forgave heresies," wrote Mary.[1] Still, by mainstream standards, 261 Tenth Street was occupied by a cabal of radicals.

The house, Mary quickly perceived, had all the makings of a success-ful water-cure establishment. The main parlor could accommodate a class of forty women, and the empty bedrooms could be furnished for inpa-tients. "Immediately I began to throw out threads in every direction," she later recalled. "I formed classes, and gave four lectures a week; I wrote for two reviews and one magazine at three dollars a page. I wrote the edito-rials for two weekly papers for five dollars a week. I took patients, and pupils from my classes. . . . My room was a hall of entry for all inmates, for questions, consultations, and the processes of water-cure; and I wrote articles, with interruptions almost at every line." Many of these articles appeared in Shew's *Water-Cure Journal*.[2]

Approximately twenty women paying five dollars each attended her first home-class, a series of twenty two-hour lectures, complete with il-lustrations, that covered the structure and function of the human body. It was May of 1846. They met in the empty parlor, sitting on mismatched chairs. Mary, wearing a plain gray gingham dress, lectured to elaborately ornamented women arrayed in rich fabrics. One evening, a box was left for Mary. It contained an elegant bonnet, adorned with white ribbon and artificial violets. Soon students began to deliver other gifts. "One after an-other brought me something beautiful, till at last my asceticism was fully conquered," Mary recalled, "and [I] became 'vain and worldly' in the eyes of those who thought me evil, but only simply and prettily dressed to myself. . . ." Her commitment to Quaker plainness waned. Mary began to allow herself beauty.[3]

The aid and friendship of Marx Edgeworth Lazarus had seemed a divine providence. So involved with his philosophical musings that he seemed as impersonal "as the rain or the dew," Marx filled the house with talk of Fourier—a man of increasing fame among New York's intelligentsia. The combination of Marx's support and Fourier's philosophy would profoundly influence the rest of Mary's life.[4]

What was so compelling about Fourier? The ideas of François Marie Charles Fourier, who had died in 1837, were first introduced to the United States in 1840, when Albert Brisbane published *Social Destiny of Man; or, Association and Reorganization of Industry*, a distillation of Fourier's complex blueprint for utopian socialism. Between 1827, when he was eighteen, and 1834, when he returned to New York, Brisbane had traveled and studied in Europe and Turkey. Disappointed in the conservatism of Hegel, with whom he had studied, Brisbane found his way to Paris and to the side of sixty-year-old Charles Fourier, a "thin, short, tight-lipped, . . . bitingly sarcastic, solemn" man, "never known to laugh," whose family had lost its small wealth in the French Revolution. For two years, Brisbane absorbed firsthand the theories of a man obsessed with remaking society. He returned to the United States an ardent missionary of Fourierism.

In the spring of 1842, Horace Greeley's *New York Tribune* began to publish regular columns by Brisbane, the first of which was titled: "Association; Or, Principles of a True Organization of Society." For more than a year, Brisbane enjoyed access to the *Tribune*'s large audience under a special arrangement whereby his columns would be entirely his own—not under Greeley's editorship and not officially endorsed by the paper's stockholders. It was no secret or surprise, however, that Horace Greeley was personally sympathetic to Fourierism. Relentless propaganda, meetings, festivals, and lectures soon made household words of "associationism," "phalanxes," and "passional affinities." By October of 1843, Brisbane had rallied enough popular support to launch a new journal, the *Phalanx*, which ran until the end of May 1845. Throughout the decade, inspired by the promise of "association," thousands of Americans eagerly participated in experimental living arrangements.[5]

Ultimately—pared to its core—Fourierism promised happiness. After analyzing the complexity of human nature, Fourier developed a model for

society that sought to render labor attractive to workers, to eradicate boredom, to allow full expression of passion, and to ensure personal fulfillment. Civilization, he believed, encouraged vice, poverty, misery, evil, and
boredom by repressing natural instinct at every turn. As Mary herself expressed it in a letter to the *Phalanx* in February of 1844: "Civilization very
much resembles an obstructed stream, which if it cannot flow on regularly to its home, overflows its banks, and checks and dams and all manner of appliances are continually needed to keep the mischievous waters
somewhere." It was a philosophy she had expressed with even greater force
in *Lectures to Ladies:* "The natural degree of activity should be given to all
our passions or propensities. *Excessive* or deficient action produces evil. . . .
God has not implanted evil passions within us, but we have destroyed the
healthy balance that should exist in us; we have . . . wrought for our race
. . . *total depravity.*" In short, God had endowed each human being with
only *good* instincts; these healthy instincts grow "mischievous" only when
unnaturally constrained. "As soon as we wish to repress a single passion
we are engaged in an act of insurrection against God," wrote Fourier. "By
that very act, we accuse Him of stupidity in having created it."[6]

Fourier—who had no use for books and only scorn for established sciences—devoted his life to the promulgation of an extremely complex plan
for society. He envisioned a world of organized associations so precisely
crafted that only harmony could result. Like hydrotherapy, Fourierism
claimed to work *with* divine law, rather than against it. Mary was one of
thousands who in the mid-1840s found herself drawn to this system pur-
portedly derived from an understanding of human nature. Fourier argued
that God had granted every person twelve passions, each of which fell into
one of three categorical groups: the luxurious, the group, and the serial.
Luxurious passions included the five senses, each of which has both internal and external manifestations. For example, a person might be born
with a great love of music (internal manifestation), but, depending on
wealth (an external manifestation), might or might not be able purchase
concert tickets or master an instrument. Fourier despised poverty and argued that its elimination would enable internal senses to flourish. The second category, group or "affective" passions, also varied from person to person in intensity and in proportion to one another across time. They
included the desire for (1) respect, (2) friendship, (3) love, and (4) parenthood. The last category, serial or "distributive" passions, included the

passion (1) to make arrangements (the composite passion), (2) for intrigue (the cabalist or discordant passion), and (3) for variety (the changeling or "papillon" passion). Fourier argued that by suppressing the serial passions, civilization prevented the healthy expression of the luxurious and group passions. Reason and passion existed in each person in the ratio of 1:12. All passions were considered positive and inherently harmonious. Fourier proposed to remake society in a way that would psychologically nourish rather than starve humanity. Mary endorsed this social philosopher who recognized the intellectual, emotional, and physical complexity of women as well as of men.

Fourier imagined a society formed of independent "phalanxes" or "phalansteries"—self-sufficient agricultural communities of sixteen to eighteen hundred people who would live in a common building. Each phalanx would occupy three square miles of orchards, fields, and gardens. Architecturally, a phalanstery would form a square, surrounding a central outdoor plaza. One side, the central building, would be flanked by two balancing wings—all residential. Barns, workshops, and warehouses would occupy the fourth side of the structure. Families could live in private apartments within the common building, each apartment also designed for balance, with a central portion and two wings. Community dining rooms, libraries, schools, nurseries, and theaters would prevent isolation, as would the phalanstery's highly regimented way of life. They would also eliminate the wasteful redundancy of effort inherent to isolate households.

As in the military, the phalanstery's population would be subdivided into units, each "series" consisting of at least five "groups," which in turn would consist of at least seven people each. These series would provide the community with every imaginable occupation. Individuals would naturally be free to move from one group and series to another, since the passion for variety abhors monotony. Meanwhile, the passion for intrigue (the discordant passion) would foster alertness, interest, and energy among the population. Competitiveness between groups (e.g., between the cabbage growers and the rose gardeners) would heighten sensory and emotional life without causing social destruction, for one's morning agricultural competitors might well be one's evening orchestra mates. Friendship, not rivalry, would bloom in an environment built solely of attraction. Each member would only pursue work suited to her or his personal pleasure and would change activities as frequently as desired. Fourier anticipated that periods of work would likely last about an hour before people would seek change. To ensure the completion of all necessary work, each phalanstery's population would include the 810 personality "types" Fourier believed to exist. This community-style system of labor appealed to many abolitionists for promising an economically viable alternative to slavery; it also drew adherents from the emerging working class, who resented their own exploitation by capitalists.[7]

Fourier believed that human passions remained constant across historical time and that only the social repression of passion varied from culture to culture and across the eras. "Since customs and morality are conventions which vary," he wrote, "there is only one way to arrive at moral stability: rallying custom around the desires of the passions, for these are invariable. In what century, in what place, have they bent before our systems? . . . What is the use of beating against this rock?"[8] In a phalanx, children would have the freedom to pursue the messy work they naturally enjoyed (like cleaning stables or spreading manure on crops); young adults would wallow undisturbed in their obsessive love relationships; and the older generation would pursue the intellectual, agricultural, and family lives more appealing to their age group. Works of extraordinary genius and creativity would naturally pour forth from so happy and inspired a population. Traditional marriage would fade out of existence, replaced by a liberated sexuality, immune to the deadening powers of inequity, tyranny, and boredom. Fourier believed that "Civilised love, in marriage, is, at the end of a few months, or perhaps the second day, often nothing more than pure brutality, chance coupling, induced by the domestic tie, devoid of any illusion of the mind or of the heart." Because he considered the slightest repression antithetical to harmony, Fourier advocated equal rights for all people. A society's progress, he argued, could be measured in the social position of its women.[9]

Albert Brisbane's columns in the *New York Tribune* promised many things to a readership increasingly desperate for satisfying work, rich personal relationships, and escape from monotony. But significantly, few American Fourierists had actually read their prophet's own work. Because Brisbane carefully glossed over the more controversial aspects of the texts he promoted, most had no idea of Fourier's extreme position regarding sexual freedom in the phalanx, which tolerated polygamy as well as cross-generational sex (with the exception of children). They also knew nothing of Fourier's most bizarre notions, which included the belief that the earth was progressing through thirty-two stages, of which civilization had reached only the fifth. The "Great Harmony" would be reached in the eighth stage, when "men will grow tails, with eyes on the tip. Dead bodies will be turned into interstellar perfume. Six new moons will appear. The sea will change into lemonade, and all fierce and noxious animals and insects will be transformed into sweet and gentle anti-lions, anti-rats, and anti-bugs."[10]

Instead, Brisbane's readers encountered a rational, if radical, social reformer whose theories seemed to deserve greater influence. Mary's housemate Marx Edgeworth Lazarus became a prolific advocate of Fourierism. "The harmonic epochs," he wrote, "we can immediately enter by organizing industrial partnerships embracing all classes . . . ; distributing functions in minute subdivisions according to capacity and attractions; operating in small groups of spontaneous formation, and interlocking those groups by short sessions, which shall alternate the occupations and social combinations of the individual, and connect his interest with many others whilst attaining for him the most integral development." Or, more succinctly: "We must not nail one man for life in his office, another in his field, another to his joiner's bench, another to his desk; the man to the thing, as we do now. A fine dramatic piece which lasts for four hours, wearies the spectators; if it lasted six hours they would be wretched."[11]

Fourierism pervaded the Saturday-night soirées held at 261 Tenth Street. Albert Brisbane, who was only a year older than Mary, became a regular at these popular gatherings of young intellectuals and artists. In her autobiography, Mary recalled Brisbane as oppressive in his earnest associationism. "He did not converse—he talked. His utterance was a monologue always, and his endurance only measured by the attention he received." Mary described him as "tall, pale, [and] graceful" with a searing intensity of expression. "If you would listen ten, twenty, thirty hours, it was all the same to him; he would talk so long." Fortunately, Mary liked what he had to say. This was the man who had written that "nature made [woman] the equal of man, and equally capable of shining with him in industry and in the cultivation of the arts and sciences—not to be his inferior, to cook and sew for him, and live dependently at his board." His sentiments bore repeating. Besides, there was no question that Brisbane's formidable friends were able to hold their own in his presence. Edgar Allan Poe, Herman Melville, Horace Greeley, Frances Osgood, and a regular collection of thirty to forty visitors devoted Saturday nights to relaxed conversation, good music, and dancing. Mary had finally found invigorating friends, intellectual stimulation, and a paying career. She was surrounded by artistic genius and liberal thought. Never before had she felt such energy.[12]

LIVING THE CURE

Mary worked in the face of rumors spread by Hiram that she was keeping a brothel in New York City. This was annoying. But a more serious blight on her happiness was the behavior of one of the home's original members, novelist Charles Wilkins Webber. A struggling alcoholic with a history of mental illness, Webber had fallen passionately in love with Elma, who believed herself equally in love with him. It was two years since they had moved into the house; Elma was now seventeen. "I had two things to accomplish," determined Mary, "to uncoil a serpent from my child, and save the loved one from . . . the venom." Mary, who could not bear to see Elma repeat the mistake of a bad marriage, sent her teenage daughter to stay with friends. This separation worked a cure on Elma, who soon came to see the "evil that was upon all his beauty, through drunkenness and an insane revenge." But it had a deranging effect on Webber, who threatened Mary "with the vengeance of a maniac fiend." In 1853 he would publish a novel called *Yieger's Cabinet. Spiritual Vampirism: The History of Etherial Softdown, and her Friends of the "New Light,"* which depicted Mary as a consumer of human souls. The book opens with Shakespeare's question, "Be thou a spirit of health, or a goblin damned?" Mary claimed never to have read the book, having been warned of its contents.[13]

With the exceptions of this episode and Hiram's relentless slander, 1846 and 1847 were very good years for Mary. At long last, a second trial had exonerated the man accused of abducting Elma from Hiram and had thus relieved Mary of financial and psychological burdens. Still, she felt the legal bonds of her marriage to Hiram, which technically gave her husband ownership of her body, her child, and her income. The laws had not changed. Nonetheless, Mary felt a sense of autonomy displacing the anguish that had suffused a marriage whose worst details she could never bring herself to write. Mary's outrage no longer suffocated; it began, instead, to fuel her new career.

Though she had never attended medical school, Mary was leading a physician's life. The first patients to board at 261 Tenth Street were women who had attended her lectures; soon, however, patients came from as far away as Ohio, Rhode Island, Kentucky, Connecticut, and northern New York. Mary also made many house calls to children suffering from scarlet fever and measles. In 1846 her *Lectures to Ladies on Anatomy and Physiology* had earned a second printing; its new title, *Lectures to Women on Anatomy and Physiology*, reflected an obvious editorial revision, perhaps in response to a generally friendly reviewer's remarks in the *Boston Quarterly Review*: "The only fault we have to find with this book is with the title, that it reads Lectures to *Ladies*, instead of Lectures to *Women*. Woman is a better and a higher term than Lady. Ladies are sometimes very weak and disagreeable. Women are always deserving of honor and respect from every manly heart." Walt Whitman also recommended Mary's book, writing in the *Brooklyn Daily Eagle*: "As respects physiological truths, . . . the more and wider these truths are known, the better." Mary had achieved an extraordinary feat: she had earned a wide reputation as a trustworthy medical expert. Her success bolstered the social position of both women and water cure. That her patients had an exceptional rate of survival only strengthened her position. "People learned to feel assurance of being saved, if they could conquer prejudice so far as to call my aid," Mary wrote. She was reading every new work on physiology or hygiene as fast as it appeared before the public; the booming genre had scarcely existed twenty years prior.[14]

The treatments Mary offered her patients relied almost exclusively on hydropathic principles—pure cold water, cleanliness, and a diet of fruit and grain. But she tempered the cure's rigidity with sensitivity to her patients' desires. "I have allowed my patients, at times, to amuse themselves with homeopathic medicines, upon their own responsibility, whilst they obeyed all my directions," she admitted. "I allowed this, because they were earnest to try the effect of infinitesimal doses, and I had no fear or faith for Homeopathy. The genuine article is to me *nothing,* and, at the same time, a great negative good, because it takes the place of the positive evil of allopathy. I believe, however, if there is any potency in the infinitesimal poisons of homeopathy, it is an evil potency." Mary navigated among

competing medical systems with skill. Even while condemning allopathy as "one of the greatest evils that now rests on the civilized world,"
Mary reserved praise for individual practitioners. "Monarchy and despotism are . . . gigantic in their badness, but kings and despots may be good
men," she explained.[15]

As an advocate of the water cure, however, Mary believed simply that
disease resulted from one fundamental cause: lack of nervous energy in
the system. Nervous energy preserved health by constantly renewing the
body—casting off all "morbid matter" and continually supplying life-
giving nutriment and fresh air. Mary argued that this theory of disease
causation reconciled two allopathic schools of thought: humoral pathology (which attributed disease to changes in the blood) and nervous pathology (which blamed the exhaustion of "nervous influence"). Lack of nervous energy would result in contaminated blood. Likewise, hydropathic
theory validated the homeopathic claim that *psora*, or irritated skin, induced disease, but it did not consider it a first cause. The fundamental
difference between the water cure and its competitors lay in hydropathy's
absolute rejection of medication. The nervous pathologists, Mary wrote,
"have had a correct theory of disease. Their error has been in introducing
medicines into the system, which they thought increased the nervous or
contractile power. The medicines being poison, and recognised as such
by the vital organism, have aroused all the energy left in the body to cast
them out. . . . Increase of action has been mistaken for increase of
power."[16] Because Mary wrote clearly, rationally, and prolifically, her
efforts greatly enhanced the popularity of water cure. To a lay audience,
her many familiar references to the works of Hippocrates, Galen, Celsus,
Boerhaave, Magendie, Hall, Hoffman, and other medical giants implied
a deep knowledge of medical literature and invited confidence in Mary's
advice. Her first-hand descriptions of dissections, anatomical museums,
and difficult cases further strengthened Mary's credibility as a well-
educated, if unlicensed, physician.

Like other advocates of water cure, Mary appealed to the intelligence
of her readers. Rather than adopt an inaccessible medical jargon, hydrotherapists sought to recruit practitioners and educate their patients.
They spoke plainly. "The water-cure is the scientific application of the
principles of nature in the cure of disease," wrote Mary. "The applications
of water . . . are cleansing, exciting, tonic, or sedative." The stronger a pa-

tient, the more able to withstand an exciting treatment. Thus, no standard protocol applied to all cases of the same disorder. In her popular 1850 handbook *Experience in Water-Cure,* Mary recalled the case of a robust ten-year-old boy who suffered with croup. Because the boy was "of a full habit," Mary had applied a "proportionally active" treatment:

> Placing him in a tub, I first poured over his throat and chest two pails full of cold water, and then rubbed the parts until the skin was quite red. He was then packed in the wet sheet, and well covered with blankets. With the glow and perspiration came the relief to his breathing, and freedom from the choking distress. As soon as the perspiration was fully established, he was taken out of the sheet, and drenched with cold water, followed by rubbing with coarse towels, after which he was put into bed, quite free from the croupy symptoms.[17]

Sometimes vigorous response to acute disorders resulted in prompt cures. More often, however, the water cure required time, patience, and a diligent reform of lifestyle. Common diseases such as dyspepsia, consumption, and gout challenged regular medicine with their chronicity; hydropathy promised a definitive cure.

Mary explained to her patients that recovery often demanded months and even years. Success depended on each patient's determination, endurance, and faith in the process. Water cure thus gave people substantial responsibility for their own outcomes. If a person followed the cure's dictates precisely, recovery would almost inevitably follow; at the same time, any lapse in hygiene, diet, or treatment regimen could drastically undermine progress. With this burden of responsibility, however, came empowerment: "If a patient thoroughly understands his or her disease, and has the requisite energy to accomplish a cure, it may be done almost anywhere, and with very meagre advantages. I have known delicate and feeble women, who have done wonders for themselves, at home, with no physician but their own clear understanding, and no help but their own indomitable energy." To free herself from dependence on expensive physicians, all a person needed was knowledge, "skill, patience, perseverance, pure living, cold water, proper exercise, pure air, and good food, in proper quantities." By the beginning of 1847, twenty-one water-cure houses were operating in nine states. The numbers continued to grow. While affluent patients sought the personalized care available at these residential retreats, most water-cure patients relied on the *Water-Cure Journal* and an expanding library of hydropathic texts to guide self-doctoring.[18]

Though Mary wrote for the general readership of hydropathic literature, she always spoke most passionately to women. Unlike the famous Frances Wright, who publicly beseeched men to remove the chains of female oppression, Mary believed that woman's advancement was primarily woman's burden. "Men cannot concede to us our position, but they can help us to secure it, when the purpose to attain it has come fully into our hearts," she wrote.[19] In advocating the cause of women physicians, Mary emphasized the need for practitioners with whom female patients would feel comfortable—particularly in the case of gynecological problems. Uncounted women, too embarrassed to consult male physicians, were suffering and dying of treatable disorders. In 1836 Eliza W. Farrar had published a popular and wide-ranging manners book called *The Young Lady's Friend*, explicitly written for girls between fifteen and twenty. In this text, the author encouraged her readers to approach their male physicians with less anxiety:

> In all your intercourse with a physician, remember that his whole course of study and practice leads him to consider the human body as a curiously complicated machine, all the parts of which are familiar to him, and equally honorable to his view. . . . The real indelicacy is in that embarrassment and difficulty which some feel in mentioning such things where it is necessary and proper to do it; thus calling a person's attention to the subject under a more degrading view of it, than that taken by the physician.[20]

Nothing mobilized Mary to action with more force than the silent suffering of women. She *would* see women trained as physicians. "[Woman] sees and comprehends with a rapidity that makes the conclusions of reason seem intuitions," she believed. "There is a propriety, a delicacy, a *decency*, in a woman being the medical adviser of her own sex—which most people can see."[21]

Elizabeth Blackwell, the first woman to graduate from an American medical school, earned her degree from Geneva Medical College in 1849. Neither her success nor the existence of the Boston Female Medical School markedly advanced women's professional training, however; with rare exception, admissions committees continued to deny women access to medical school. Advocacy for female physicians extended beyond the bounds of the water-cure movement and flourished within it. "We cannot receive a diploma from an Alma Mater, that has borne us through a course of study like an infant in arms," Mary wrote. "No long established institutions, no ancient and honorable societies offer us support and facilities on our untried way. Single-handed, we must grapple with iron prejudice and a time-honored custom, grown hoary in a dotage of error. We have work to do to strengthen our hands."[22]

GODEY'S

Mary Gove did not limit her feminist agitation to medical subjects. Between 1844 and 1848, she published several short stories in *Godey's Lady's Book*, the premier ladies' magazine of its era, edited by Sarah Josepha Hale. Written under the pseudonym "Miss Mary Orme," these short pieces supplemented Mary's earnings, satisfied her penchant for creative writing, and offered a public identity different from the one she simultaneously cultivated as a water-cure physician and health lecturer. She had always loved to write. By producing the sort of sentimental domestic fiction characteristic of *Godey's,* Mary found a way to reach "ladies" as well as "women."

Sarah Hale, who preferred to coddle male anxieties and promote women's rights in only the most demure and nonthreatening fashion, would not have welcomed Mary Gove "in the rough."[23] Margaret Fuller, the most famous woman's rights advocate of her time, would not deign to publish in a periodical like *Godey's*—and surely *Godey's* would not have wanted her to. Hale advised women to leave politics to the men. That was not to say, however, that women should exert no influence. On the contrary, "influence" was woman's weapon par excellence; woman represented the moral beacon of family and society. Woman's "influence" would shape future generations of male leaders and revive a deteriorating world. This view was shared by the Female Moral Reform Society, which since its founding in 1834 had strongly identified religion and morality as the rightful domains of female power. The organization specifically challenged the culture's double standard toward the sexual conduct of men and women. But while members of the Female Moral Reform Society published, financed, and typeset their own periodical and even braved dangerous neighborhoods to rescue "fallen women," *Godey's* encouraged domestic work. It celebrated motherhood, not political action. Such publications saturated America with the rhetoric of "separate spheres" and "woman's place." They reached thousands.[24]

Four of Mary's moralizing stories turn on a protagonist's decision to marry; the fifth portrays a young woman sick with unrequited love. Marriage takes many forms in these pieces—from the miserable to the sublime, from the alienated to the truly companionate. Interestingly, none depicts abuse. And in several, the most sympathetic character is the husband. It seems that Mary used her stories to imagine alternative scenarios to the one she endured with Hiram. They represent the sugarcoated beginning of her intense struggle against the legal institution of marriage.

"Marrying a Genius," published in September 1844, surprises the reader by presenting Horace, who is struggling with his general aversion to the idea of marrying a genius. After opening the story by declaiming, "I will not say I hate talented women, but I will say I fear them," Horace soon wonders, "Whence comes the prejudice against talented women?" He is visiting with his brilliant and beloved Aunt Mary, a spinster. (The name *Mary* appears with notable frequency in Mary Gove's creative writing.) Aunt Mary suggests two reasons for the culture's widespread disapproval of ingenious women: first, that women who pursue their own interests may neglect their household responsibilities; and second, that women of genius often marry "men of much will and little talent" who find their wives' strengths a constant and embarrassing rebuke to their own flaws. Granting that a woman's primary responsibility is to her family and not to her novels, Aunt Mary describes her love for a man Horace had never heard of, a man traveling in China. As the story unfolds, Horace does not take Mary's advice to seek a woman of talent, but instead marries a woman of average intellect who provides him every material comfort. She cannot, however, stimulate him with her company. Over time, Horace grows desperately unhappy and isolated in his marriage. Meanwhile, Aunt Mary's beau returns and the two establish an ideal marriage. Horace cries to her, "Oh, aunt, I wish to Heaven you had married first, then I should have known that a woman who has a soul could make her husband happy."

Fortunately for the narrative, Horace's wife soon dies, and Horace has a second chance to heed his aunt's advice. Though friends urge him to remarry quickly, Horace opts to wait for the woman who will prove a true wife to him. This woman soon appears in the form of Jane Crawford, a schoolteacher who has published magnificent stories under a pseudonym, stories that Horace has long loved. They marry. Quickly, their lives together develop into a romantic, if limited, collaboration: "They studied, read, wrote and worked together—for many were the cares and labours that the loving husband learned to share and lighten. At Aunt Mary's last visit, she found them in the library. Horace had written out a scientific paper. Jane was copying, polishing and beautifying his work." The story closes with Horace declaring, "Thank Heaven, I do not hate or fear women of genius."

No conclusion could be farther from the reality of Mary Gove's life with Hiram, who would not read a word of Mary's writing unless she presented it to him as the work of someone else and who, as a strict Quaker, rejected fiction outright. For Mary, the story form prettily packaged aggressively reformist politics. Readers of *Godey's* finished the piece with much to think about. What is the difference between making a husband comfortable and making him happy? Why do men fear talented women? Can joint effort yield fulfillment for both man and woman? It is significant that in this story, Aunt Mary finds the couple working in the library—a male domain within the female domain; woman has entered the larger world without leaving her house. Intellectual collaboration (if not wholly equitable, with the wife editing her husband's original work) proves exquisitely romantic. As Jane works on a manuscript, Horace, unthreatened, "twined his finger in one of her rich dark curls."[25]

In her second story, "The Artist," published six months later, Mary Gove attacks those who marry for reasons other than true love, which she understands to mean passionate fellowship. Sophia mistakenly forsakes the poor artist Gilbert Ainslie for the elite Edward Montague. Her married fate is grim: Edward commits suicide after the two have produced an idiot child. Sophia ultimately dies alone and unloved, at which point the noble Gilbert reemerges to provide for Sophia's abandoned child until the child, too, dies at only twelve years old. Gilbert is rewarded for his devotion by meeting Mary: "Mary—it was his favorite name. I hardly ever saw any one who did not love this name." Gilbert had encountered the fictional Mary awash in wildflowers by the banks of the Hudson River, where he was wandering with his sketchbook. The two live happily ever after, owing to the fact that "the deep marriage love of her parents was incarnated in her."[26]

This story, like its predecessor, offers a sympathetic male protagonist who is forced to endure—or who, like Gilbert, is nearly won by—shallow beauty devoid of deeper passion. Thus, Mary Gove seems to advocate women's independence for the sake of their men. This is precisely the strategy that many have detected in the larger agenda of *Godey's Lady's Book*. Tucked elsewhere into "The Artist" is a sentence rebuking much that *Godey's* ostensibly promoted. Sophia Wilton's mother lives by *Godey-esque* standards—or rather, by the superficial *Godey's* ideal: "As it was very fashionable just now to be very moral and sentimental, Mrs. Wilton preached morality constantly to Sophia, and overflowed with love and kisses for a shaggy little fright of a Portuguese lap dog, who wore a blue ribbon round his neck, and was gouty from consuming as many luxuries as would have sustained two or three poor children, had their cost been expended for bread." Mary Gove has condensed her scorn for Sophia's society-conscious mother into a lap dog's bow. That such a sentence appeared in a magazine devoted to fashion and the promotion of female morality reveals the ambiguity of Hale's mission and perhaps the ambivalence of her readers as well, who would not identify themselves with Sophia's mother, but who might well be wearing blue ribbons themselves.[27]

The word most closely considered by Mary, however, is not *morality*, but rather *love*. Harriet Beecher Stowe had defined love as "self-sacrifice," declaring that "its very essence is the preferring of the comfort, the ease, the wishes of another to one's own."[28] That Mary's idea of love differed is not immediately apparent from the *Godey's* prose. Her stories have a canned, predictable shape. Yet their characters reveal Mary's belief in liberated love. In the mid-1840s this belief was already starting to take radical form.

In "The Evil and the Good," published in July 1845, Mary contrasts two friends. Florence is "pale and delicate and slight . . . shrinking, timid"; Sarah, "proud . . . radiant . . . beautiful . . . bright . . . joyous." Their friendship thrives on meek Florence's reverence for her selfish friend. It is easy to predict an outcome of misery for Sarah and bliss for Florence. Before anticipated events unfold, however, the reader listens to the two friends discuss love. Sarah projects scorn for marriage; while Florence, though lacking in Sarah's experience with the opposite sex, has deep faith in the possibility of happy marriage and perfect love. Sarah finds her innocent friend amusing, calling her "a precious little transcendentalist." Soon Florence falls in love with Herman Liston, a good-looking man who deserts Florence for Sarah practically the minute he meets this charismatic friend. Florence, though suffering deeply, forgives Sarah for stealing Herman away to marriage.

Eight years later Florence develops a friendship with a printer, who later becomes her husband. Unlike Sarah and Herman, who met at a party and ambitiously "conquered" one another as prizes, Florence and Charles had met many times "before they thought of aught but friendship. Their friendship slowly ripened into love." The contrast is significant. Not only does it protect Florence from dangerous impulse, but it also gives her time to articulate her experience of true love: "This sentiment that I can so calmly analyze, and find that it contains esteem, confidence, reverence, and an indefinable tenderness that can never be analyzed—which is made up of the mysterious attractions of our being, in a mysterious combination." This passage represents an early attempt by Mary Gove to define *love*. Its clumsy striving suggests the many elements missing in her relationship with Hiram, the most important of which was the least well articulated: mysterious attractions. Mary was seeking to understand how passional affinities or attractions shape one's life and health.

But to finish the story: considerable time passes before the happily married Florence visits the declining Sarah, who is now the mother of three boys. Though wealthy materially, Sarah declares herself broken and wretched. "My heart has no home," she mourns. Florence perceives that Sarah's selfishness has prevented love from growing in marriage; her cold nature has given no warmth to her fame-seeking husband. Florence advises her friend to express more love toward her husband, to be less proud. This, of course, proves the solution.

Once again, *Godey's* has offered a story that seems to preach a woman's selfless devotion to her husband. "Have you been gentle and kind?" asks Florence. "Have you let him know that you have a woman's heart?" But it is really the relationship between the two women that matters most. Florence has loved Sarah faithfully and has ultimately saved them both from misery by knowing how to feel and express love. The men are rather peripheral to this lesson about the power of true love. In fact, it is the early, innocent musings of Florence that serve as Mary's central moral: "All this outward beauty . . . speaks to my heart that there must be spirit beauty, for whence is all loveliness but from the ever-living, all-pervading spirit of beauty that lives in God, in angels and in man?" Awakening to one's internal magnificence could sustain a person through the darkest hell, through the most grim enslavement. Mary had faith in love *as a force*. Love did not float ethereally through her protagonists' lives; it almost took physical form.[29]

False love, however, festered like disease. In January of 1846, Mary published her next *Godey's* story, "Mary Pierson." Opening with a general admonition against idleness, the story describes a love-struck young woman, Mary Pierson, who has become physically ill as a result of her unrequited longing. Her mother, desperately concerned, consults a doctor, who simply prescribes regular activity for what appears a terrible disorder. In a new twist, Mary Gove has allowed this male doctor to narrate her story. (Only four months later, Mary Gove would anonymously publish "Passages from the Life of a Medical Eclectic" in the *American Review*. Probably she was already working on that lengthy personal narrative at the time she wrote "Mary Pierson," thus fully immersing herself in the physician's voice.) Before allowing the doctor to launch the tale, however, Mary Gove bluntly preaches a full column of text against the lolling life: "Oh woman, in thy idleness thou has sought out many inventions, besides making pin-cushions, working worsted, and getting up fairs for everything conceivable! But industry is better than idleness, however frivolous . . . for it is the idle who brood over that sickly sentimentalism misnamed love. . . . Cast about you for some occupation. . . . Better [to] spoil the beauty of those hands and win quiet for your soul, than live on a prey to misery." It is almost as though Mary did not have the patience to rely on the story form as a vehicle for her message. Better to blurt out the thesis at once and then relax in the knowledge that the argument would not be shadowed by the fiction. The story stops as suddenly as it starts, with the doctor abruptly declaring, "But I will abridge my tale by saying that I saw Mary faithfully follow all my directions." Once her point has been reiterated in parable, Mary Gove ushers her narrator quickly off the stage. Perhaps as a writer she was feeling exasperated by the limitations of the *Godey's* format— and also by her imagined reader: "My dear lady reader, have you taken my story and lolled on to the sofa or couch to read for the sake of having something to do?"

The chiding tone adopted in her opening remarks is echoed by her narrator, who instructs the suffering girl, "I will tell you what you do not know. You do not love him. . . . You love an idea." This is a fascinating story, for one can see each of the characters presented as Mary Gove. Not only is she the physician—carefully prescribing a full regimen of study, housework, exercise, writing, and reading for the moping girl, but she is also Mary Pierson, ill with passion for unrealistic love. It is not Mary Pierson's relationship to her love object that most strongly underlines her similarity to Mary Gove, however. It is her relationship to her mother, Mrs. Pierson, who dominates the midsection of the story, her own life saga summarized and blamed for the dissipation of her daughter. For Mrs. Pierson "was not at peace." She had long ago married Mr. Pierson for practical reasons (including his property) only to discover soon thereafter that they shared nothing in common. The distance that grew between them, even as they produced children and an "exquisite" home, left Mrs. Pierson irritable and hollow. Because she "never confided in her children," her daughter learned never to confide in her. Meanwhile, Mary Pierson "shunned her beautiful virago mother most sedulously . . . because there was nothing in common between them." One is reminded of Mary Gove's relationship to her own mother. Yet in this story, Mary Gove identifies with Mrs. Pierson as well as with her daughter: "Oh, had the springs of Mrs. Pierson's heart been unlocked, had she loved as she was capable of loving, the sweet Mary would have had a resting-place on her bosom unlike any other out of Heaven!" The sympathy for Mrs. Pierson intermixes with a bitter blaming. Had the mother herself found a true love—and shown her daughter how to express and feel that love—then Mary would not need a doctor, would not shrivel in her room, pining after a romantic fantasy.

The doctor has enormous affection for Mary Pierson, advocating what might today be termed "tough love": "Be sure it is a thousand times better to fight than yield. The very activity of the soul necessary in resistance, is health restoring." For Mary Gove, writing constituted a vital, resisting, health-restoring activity of the soul. Mary used her pages, which were autobiographical in the extreme, to advise and understand herself, to delineate a meaningful narrative of her life that she would rewrite again and again.[30]

One month after "Mary Pierson" appeared in *Godey's,* "Mary Orme" published, this time in the *United States Magazine and Democratic Review,* a poem entitled "Providence." The brief, optimistic poem includes a verse nearly identical to one penned by the fictional Florence in "The Evil and the Good":

> Struggles give strength to every soul,
> And light is shed athwart thy gloom,
> Dark, tho' the waves that round thee roll,
> Land ho! To sink is not thy doom![31]

Mary must have been pleased with this verse, revising only one word: "waves" replaced the earlier "shades." Things were going well in 1846. Mary had finished a new novel, *Agnes Morris, or The Heroine of Domestic Life.* The *American Review* had accepted her series of personal articles, "Passages from the Life of a Medical Eclectic." And the *Water-Cure Journal and Herald of Reforms* continued to publish her columns regularly.

During these years of creative writing, Mary enjoyed steady work and lively friendship. She was surrounded by intellectuals and reformers who did not shun her status as single mother. On the contrary, it gave her more dimension. Her friendship with Edgar Allan Poe intensified in 1846. Poe did her an enormous service by favorably reviewing her talents in his series, "The Literati of New York," published in *Godey's Lady's Book,* where, by way of personal description, he wrote:

> She is, I think, a Mesmerist, a Swedenborgian, a phrenologist, a homoeopathist, and a disciple of Priessnitz—what more I am not prepared to say.
>
> She is rather below the medium height, somewhat thin, with dark hair and keen, intelligent black eyes. She converses well and with enthusiasm. In many respects a very interesting woman.[32]

CHRISTMAS, 1847

Mary had come to know many prominent writers in New York as friend and as physician. Though initially shy among strangers, she quickly overcame her reserve and joined conversations. Among her illustrious friends was the prolific author Frances Osgood, who sometimes wrote under the pen names "Florence," "Ellen," and "Kate Carol." Osgood had much in common with Mary Gove. However, her greatest significance to Mary lay in her matchmaking ability: Frances would introduce Mary to Thomas Low Nichols.

Only one year younger than Mary, Frances Osgood had also grown up in New England. With family encouragement, she had begun publishing her stories at fourteen. In 1835, she married Samuel Stillman Osgood, a Boston artist. Their first child, Ellen, was born the following year, four years after Mary had delivered Elma. When they moved to New York City's Astor House in 1839, they had a new baby, May Vincent, in tow. For the next ten years, Frances would publish widely in most of America's leading periodicals. When she first met Mary Gove is not clear, but the two made natural companions, as their daughters likely did. Frances gave birth to a third daughter, Fanny Fay, in the spring of 1846. After this youngest baby died in October 1847, Frances suffered increasingly from tuberculosis, an affliction that had dogged her for years but that even at its worst had not stopped her from writing. In addition to hydrotherapy, Mary Gove could offer Frances empathy in her grieving, in her illness, in her literary ambition, and in her bad marriage. Samuel Osgood would set out alone for California in February 1849, the year before Frances died, two years before the deaths of Ellen and May Vincent.[33]

Before this string of tragedies, Mary and Frances had a great deal to share. Ironically, both Mary Gove and Frances Osgood have survived time's erasure less by their own achievements than as a result of their respective relationships with Edgar Allan Poe. Mary chronicled a visit to Poe's Fordham cottage that has served Poe historians well as the best detailed description of Poe's poverty and desperation during his wife's fatal illness.[34] Frances, on the other hand, spent so much time with the celebrated writer that their relationship drew suspicious remarks. After meeting for the first time early in 1845, the two were often seen together in literary salons; they exchanged letters regularly. To read Mary's account of her friends' involvement is to suspect what contemporaries might have described as the worst: "That he loved [his wife Virginia], and sorrowed for her, as few can love and sorrow, I *know*. That he loved other beautiful and loveful spirits also, will be his honor, and not his condemnation, when our race becomes *human*. Till then, his memory can wait."[35] On February 2, 1847, Virginia Poe, cousin and wife to Edgar Allan Poe, was buried. By then, Frances had distanced herself from Poe, in response to nasty gossip begun by Elizabeth Ellet, a woman who sought Poe for herself. Here, too, Mary must have proven a valuable friend—one who had personal experience with public censure for her conduct in marriage.

Rather than projecting the image of a downtrodden, struggling writer, Frances Osgood struck others as a graceful and vivacious woman, fully aware of her own charms and talents. She played the piano beautifully, writing and publishing her own music. Full of creative energy that matched Mary's own, Frances awed her friend with a social sophistication that Mary had never had the opportunity to cultivate.[36] After suffering in bed on and off for months after the death of her youngest child, Frances decided to shake off the gloom. She proposed a Christmas party—a big one.

Social gatherings at Mary's house regularly included about thirty people. This time Frances aimed to invite seventy, and she counted on others to help pay the bills. She seemed to be one of those people for whom confidence generates success. Her vision included all of New York's most prominent editors, artists, poets, and writers. Each would not only attend her party but also contribute something toward it—be it prose, poetry, music, or something practical, like tables. She expected that Poe would read "The Raven." She asked Mary to write a spoof letter from some literary lion, expressing regret at being unable to attend the affair. In her effort to warm Mary to the whole extravagant idea (after all, the party would be held at Mary's house), Frances teased, "I have unearthed that protean prodigy of yours and propose to invite him."[37] Without releasing his name, Frances described the man whose anonymous writing Mary had long admired in the New York journals. He was very tall, she said, with black eyes, auburn hair, and military whiskers. Mary liked the idea of tall and of auburn, but the black eyes and military whiskers did not appeal to her at all. Still, her curiosity was piqued.

The party went just as planned, with Frances acting as hostess and

Mary gratefully hanging back, like a child. At first the rooms lacked adequate light, creating a "funeral seeming" to Mary. Frances retreated to the kitchen and returned with a dozen raw potatoes. With the help of "a poet and a philosopher, whose names have won a world-wide celebrity," Frances carved a hole into each potato and let them do service as candle holders around the rooms. In Mary's description of the evening, Frances herself shines like a lamp. "[She] knew how to welcome every one, according to character and need. She was dignified to those who deserved it, pleasant and patronizing to the humble and diffident, frozen to the frigid, formal, and fastidious, and a perfect manners-book, if any had a demand for frost-work that would not melt." Poe did recite "The Raven." Charades were a success. And finally, Frances led two tall gentlemen across the room toward Mary, one of whom wore military whiskers. "'Madam,' said he, 'will you pardon a busy man for being kept out of Paradise much longer than he wished or intended to be?'"

Mary was repulsed.

Thomas Low Nichols had dressed flawlessly that night. Though slender and attractively built, he carried himself with an immediately irritating "crystalline precision." His polished speech did not help matters. "A fop," thought Mary. Thomas, who was five years younger than Mary, did not improve his first impression quickly. His flattery had a saccharine quality that Mary distrusted. She chatted with him for a while, perceiving too much interest on his part. Uncomfortable, she introduced him to a pretty woman and excused herself to another part of the room. But he seemed to reappear by her side throughout the evening. Thomas both annoyed and disappointed her: "Could it be so? Could the earnest, democratic, and philosophic spirit I had admired and fraternized with in his writings, be really walking about under a white waistcoat and white kid gloves, a coat of faultless Parisian fit, with a figure as graceful as a gymnast, and yet with a manner so formally genteel, that one felt that he never committed a breach of etiquette in his life?" Mary dismissively lumped Thomas Nichols into the cultured sphere embodied by Frances Osgood. When he sang an accompaniment to Frances's piano music, Mary saw herself utterly outclassed. In her autobiography, she admits, "I had decided that I could not please Mr. Vincent [Nichols], and that therefore he should not please me." But her conclusion that she could not please Thomas Nichols met a forceful opposition. Before the evening was over, he and a few other gentlemen had publicly declared their intention to call again on New Year's Eve. When, saying good night, Thomas Nichols lightly touched Mary's arm, the physical attraction that electrified her body could not be denied.

On New Year's Eve, Mary welcomed to her already crowded home Nichols, Poe, and Albert Brisbane. It was customary for women to dress up and stay at home on New Year's, serving food and wine to gentlemen visitors. Poe and Brisbane made a mild impression that evening. Nichols, on the other hand, tirelessly strained to win Mary's approval. "Wherever I went, he came. Whatever I said, he understood and improved. Whatever I liked, he appreciated with an analysis which gave me more to like, and at the same time proved his sincerity." All this attention both aggravated and enticed Mary. Technically she was still married to Hiram. Though her newfound community had forgiven her separation, she did not take their approval for granted should she consider pursuing another man. Her water-cure practice had earned her a wide respect, one she would not casually risk. Mary did all she could, within the bounds of courtesy, to discourage Thomas's flirtation.

During this New Year's visit, however, Thomas revealed to Mary that he knew she had written the many articles published anonymously in his journal over the previous few years. She had thought her identity was a secret from him. When he praised her writing, Thomas discovered her vulnerability to his charms. In his exuberance that evening, he improvised waltzes, sang songs, and initiated games of twenty questions. At two in the morning, he was among the last of the guests to leave.[38]

LETTERS

Mary's growing craving for Thomas is evidenced by her autobiography, which at this juncture practically abandons the narrative form altogether and documents her new marriage year with transcribed love letters alone.[39] Several days elapsed after the New Year's party before Mary received a polite note from Thomas, apologizing for having stayed so late into the night. "He [Mr. Nichols] would have felt bound to make this apology in person," read the message, "but from the fear that a call for that purpose would have proved an irresistible temptation to repeat the offense for which he hopes to be excused and forgiven." Mary interpreted the be-lated note as a generous way of saying he'd gotten her message—she wasn't interested in him. This thought made her internally admit that she was, indeed, very interested in him. Thirty-eight years old and lonely for love, Mary resolved to submit a draft of her new novel, *Agnes Morris,* to his journal for publication as a serial. Maybe this move would prompt him to visit again.

His editorial rejection note initiated the romance that would dominate the following six months. "I find fault with nothing that is," he had written. "I will find fault, because there is not what there should be." He recommended that she make the work three times as long. "You shall throw your whole soul, mind, and strength into a book . . . and the world shall know you for one of God's blessed angels." Thomas did not praise Mary's beauty or grace or femininity—qualities in which she lacked confidence; he praised those traits she had sought to cultivate: her mind, her spirit, and her strength. He also proposed to visit her again. "I was affected by this note," recalled Mary, "precisely as by [his] personal presence. I was interested, flattered, and offended." Her reply encouraged his visit: "If you were a lady and I a gentleman, I believe I would propose to you, just for the sake of the polite, and kind, and really handsome *no* I should get. . . . Don't you wish I would tell you . . . how I relished your note, and whether it came up to my brain as full of delicious intoxication as you could wish? . . . I shall see you very kindly when you call."

Thomas's subsequent visit was awkward. Mary received him alone in the parlor and watched with pleasure as he struggled to entertain her without the backdrop of music and games. When he left, Mary noted, Thomas looked "mortified and chagrined" at his unsuccessful efforts to win her attraction. "I was well enough pleased at this," wrote Mary, "for I thought he had been too familiar in his notes and his manners; and I like retributive justice in the small particulars of life, as well as in its large affairs." Her cool behavior provoked Thomas to even greater lengths. The following day Mary received a long, revealing letter:

> I used to think that the reason I could not converse was because the people I met were so stupid. . . . Now, I see my mistake, for with you I am no better off. I can tell you nothing you don't know already. . . . Do you know that I would like to have you in the room, and never speak to you at all? . . . [W]hen you talk to me, I always think your voice has

come through some medium, which has stopped a portion of it, as some kinds of glass let the light through, but stop the heat. . . .

I am a fool to write to you, for I don't love, I don't even like, you. I have not the least degree of warm, or kind, or tender feeling in regard to you. Not the least. There is no mother, nor sister, nor friend about it. I have no regard for you; I feel no kind of affection; nothing but a vague strong influence upon my brain, which, in opposition to the habits of my whole life, compels me to see you—for no purpose; to write to you—for no reason; to think of you forever—for no object or conclusion. Now, do you understand? I shall never compliment you—I shall never flatter—I shall tell you the plain truth. . . .

You and I were born to precisely the same destiny, and we shall both do our work. It is not to rule mankind; or be loved by mankind; nor even much known of them; we are schoolmasters—teachers—nothing more. You will teach the women, I the men. We shall both instruct them. They will profit by our work, without knowing it; and without applause or fame, with the simple consciousness of having known our duty and done it, we shall enter upon a sphere of being where that consciousness will be to both an eternal satisfaction. To this I pledge my hand, without a glove; and so far am yours.

It was a rugged love letter. It was perfect. Thomas had not proposed a kiss under moonlight; he had proposed an intellectual partnership in action. He imagined sharing a single "sphere of being" with Mary, a sphere in which their work and destiny would be one. He asked her to sacrifice nothing at all. He was the incarnation of her imagined "Horace," the protagonist who appreciated the value of "marrying a genius," who "studied, read, and wrote" with his new bride in Mary's story in *Godey's* four years earlier.

Mary's reply to this letter adopted the same affectionately sparring tone Thomas had chosen to express his love:

I received your letter when on the steps, going to see a poor sick lady, and now, at 10 o'clock, P.M., I am writing at her desk. I shall answer it sentence by sentence, because it is worthy of it. I am not sure that it does not deserve to be glassed and framed.

First, you say you are not satisfied with yourself; *vous avez raison*, I doubt not. . . .

As to your losing your power to talk, don't you think it may vex you more than your friends? . . .

As to this influence on your brain, I will explain it a little. The first step of all philosophizing is to wonder. You have taken it with me. You are becoming a philosopher, Heaven help you. I believe they generally repudiate the affections. . . .

Thank you for your promise to never compliment or flatter me; I am afraid there is about as much truth in it as in the foregoing assertions about your want of liking for me.

You are greatly mistaken respecting my destiny. I am loved strongly, deeply, by very many. Don't think there are many such barbarians in the world as you profess to be. I don't say that I love strongly or deeply in return, but I know and thank God for the knowledge, that I am deeply loved by many men and many women. Take care, or you will like me before you know it.

I hope you will write me again. You know my life is without condiments or candy, wine or malt liquors; so the spice of your letters is very acrid and delightful to me. Thank you for all.

Mary made her availability clear without overdoing her longing. The letters filled her with love-struck energy. Thomas promised her an appreciation that motivated hours of creative writing. She began to revise her novel.

The letters Mary and Thomas subsequently exchanged gradually replaced sarcasm with sincerity, snipes with sighs. Thomas began to visit Mary every other day. She read her rough drafts aloud to him, and he provided substantive reactions. The intellectual collaboration fueled deeper passions. Before long they abandoned any pretense of a game. "It seems to me that we are to just fill the vacant places in each other's lives," wrote Thomas. But the vacant place in Mary's life was not legally empty. Mary had a husband. "Now as to my visiting you," wrote Thomas, "it is for you to judge and decide. Surely no one with you has any right to find fault, and, so far as I see, no one else need know more than is necessary. I wish you to act wisely, considering *all things*. Be neither too brave for the world, nor too cautious for ourselves." They were in a difficult situation. Mary replied, "I have already had hard things said to me for my acquaintance with you—for this I care not, *only* so far as it may affect my happiness with you, and my business. If I were simply a writer, and had a stipend that would support me, the world might edify itself after its own fashion. But my business, my darling profession of water-cure, must not go into other hands."[40]

Thomas responded with support for all aspects of Mary's career. His respect for Mary's independence and self-sufficiency were truly exceptional in 1848—even for a suitor. He wrote,

> I am very glad that you do not belong to that amiable class of philanthropists who do nothing for their fellow-creatures until they are in the last extremity. They take drunkards out of the gutter; they seek for magdalens in the Five Points; they are very kind to malefactors, and anxiously attend the last hours of the condemned felon.
>
> All this philanthropy is full of excitement; it shows well; it reads well in the newspapers; but it does a very homeopathic amount of real benefit to society. We had much better spend our efforts in prevention than in cure. . . .
>
> You are directing your efforts in the best manner. Follow your profession; it is noble, useful, honorable, and will command the world's respect. The active work, the society, the observation it gives you, are just what you require. It has dignity and independence. It will surround you with grateful and admiring friends. It is the solid foundation of an enduring usefulness.
>
> But do not suppose that this is your greatest work. The least of your writings may accomplish more than all your professional efforts. Your books may not make a fortune, but they will lay up for you treasures in heaven where you will know, and so enjoy, the good you will have accomplished. *You must write.* There is a directness and energy in all you write, a heartiness, and a soul-fullness, that must produce its effect.

Mary's father had discouraged her from learning to write. Hiram had despised and censored her prose. But in Thomas Low Nichols, Mary found more than acceptance. She found insistence: "*You must write.*" Thomas respected Mary for every risk she had taken. It seemed God had delivered to her the very antithesis of Hiram: a sexy, intellectual man who showed his love through genuine empowerment. Who could find such a man in 1847? Awed by her good fortune, Mary felt compelled to write Thomas, "I do not want you to have the most superficial feeling even (a deep feeling I know you will never have) that I wish ever to lay the weight of a hair on you in arbitrary influence. You must do what your heart tells you, if it tell you to go from me. . . . If our love make us one, then we shall have one life only, and one life-impulse. But neither must live falsely or arbitrarily from the other's life."

Marriage to Hiram had taught Mary to suspect and fear permanent vows. At the same time, she was able to write to Thomas, "I love you with an infinite love. . . . I am stilled in this love that wraps, and *is*, my being. I pause reverently before this almightiness of affection." And Thomas was able to reply, "I am filled. I realize fully the answer to the deep craving of my soul . . . the intimate companionship of a kindred spirit, some one to love, and reverence, and adore, all at once. This has been the want of my life; and it is at last so fully, so completely satisfied, that were I to ask any thing of God, it would be only that I might keep what I have found."

Concluded Mary, "This is the greatest happiness of our love, that it is mutual and equal."

"Minna Harmon, or The Ideal and the Practical" was published in *Godey's* in December 1848. None of her pseudonymous stories so closely parallels her life. Creatively, Mary had been obsessing on the narrative of her love life, remembering the first young poet who so enraged Hiram, the short-lived passion for Henry Gardiner Wright, and her unexpected union with Thomas. "Minna Harmon" represents an early, condensed autobiography of these romances, with lengthy dialogue between Minna (Mary) and "Charles Herbert" (Thomas). But the story begins with an unhappy child, mature beyond her years, who seeks fulfillment and knowledge. Sadly, "the dependence, and misery, and monotony of home, the persuasions of friends, the earnest entreaties of a man who thought himself in love, all combined, induced Minna to give her promise to become a wife." The similarity of this account to that of her full-length autobiography could not be more striking. Even the husband's name "Harmon" bears resemblance both to "Hiram" and to "harm."

Soon after her engagement, Minna meets a new young man. "They met to love, wildly, madly." Here is the poet she ultimately forgoes to keep her vow to the first man. During her engagement, Minna prays for death. Mary answers her protagonist's prayer by writing the death of Mr. Harmon. In her new freedom, Minna finds ambition taking hold of her soul: "Not the mean ambition that asks only a name, but the ambition to be useful; to create more of happiness wherever her influence extended. . . . The consciousness that she was useful, came with vivifying power." It is in this phase of independent success that Minna meets Charles. "Without genius, he had talent, judgment, a cultivated mind, and upright heart." They become "lovers." The story, written so soon after the actual events, offers rare insight into Mary's view of her early relationship with Thomas. "There was too much chaos in her soul," she writes of Minna. "The wisdom and kindness of her loved one evoked order from this chaos."

The rest of the story consists of romantic dialogue, which reads much like the love letters presented in Mary's autobiography but with the difference of making Minna the less confident participant, more inclined to seek reassurances. Meanwhile Charles speaks paternally. In short, Minna is more "womanly," Charles more "manly" than their living models. Fitting *Godey's* stereotype, Minna says, "I wish I could always do what you wish, for I am sure you are incapable of wishing me to do wrong." To which Charles replies, "This from *you*, Minna, the proud and independent . . . thinker? Remember that I love a *woman*, not a shadow, or an echo of myself." If such an exchange really did take place between Mary and Thomas, then we see the strengthening appeal he must have had for her. If Mary would never have made so self-evaporating a statement (which is the more likely), then we glimpse the feminist aims of her fiction. As the story closes, Minna has achieved fame in the literary world.[41]

FOUR

The Needful Maturation
of Thomas Low Nichols

❧   ❧   ❧

NOTHING IN SURVIVING documents—either published or personal—indicates that Mary felt any less passion for Thomas Low Nichols
in fact than in fiction. Not a single disillusioned remark endures. No disappointment. No criticism. Mary would live and work closely with
Thomas for the thirty-six remaining years of her life. Whatever conflicts
they shared found no chronicler.

Thomas Low Nichols was born in Orford, New Hampshire, a town
nearly as remote and as tiny today as it was in 1815, the year of his birth.
Little is known of his childhood or lineage, save that his family roots extended back to the early colonists of Massachusetts and that his maternal
grandfather was an active Whig in the American Revolution. Family lore
held that this grandfather had not only fought in the battle of Bunker Hill
but had even helped throw the tea into Boston Harbor. "Full of patriotism," wrote Nichols, "my grandfather invested his savings in Continental
paper-money, and, by its depreciation to utter worthlessness, lost all he possessed." Thomas's father had been born on the coast of Massachusetts, and
his mother in Boston. Their names and occupations are unknown. Thomas
wrote almost nothing to or about his family that has survived. In a letter
written when he was twenty-four, Thomas described his sister:

> [H]ad I another sister to choose, of all the world, it should be you.
> That's frank. I know not what alteration two years and a half may have
> made in my own sister, but when I saw her last, I thought her beauti-
> ful; but, better than that, she was ever amiable, kind and affectionate,

the soul of gayety and good nature, yet full of feeling and spirit. Oh! I have seen her dark eyes flash so beautifully. There was something sublime in her momentary passion. I loved her as a brother loves sister, and the world has no such love beside. Indeed she was the light and joy of my existence.

In this letter, Thomas also referred to a brother named Ned, of whom no details are known.[1]

As a young boy, Thomas attended a country academy. One of his classmates, the son of a Boston merchant, described to Thomas the city he would finally explore himself on a visit to his uncles in 1824. It was the first city he ever saw. Within an hour of his arrival in Boston, nine-year-old Thomas climbed alone to the cupola of the statehouse, while his father waited below. From this high vantage, Thomas could gain a sense of the sprawl created by 60,000 inhabitants. He watched the commercial activity at the wharves. He examined the rooftops. He squinted over the sea to the horizon. Thomas had probably never seen so much at once in his life. From the statehouse, the two wandered throughout the city, visiting Fanueil Hall, the ships at dock, and the battleground of Bunker Hill. The air smelled of bituminous coal and saltwater. The next morning Thomas rose early enough to discover that before dawn, delivery boys had filled the city's front stoops with sweet loaves of fresh bread, new milk, and the day's newspapers. Town watchmen had cried the hours through the night. "Twelve o'clock, and a cloudy night; all's well!"[2] Before long, Thomas Low Nichols developed a passion for descriptive journalism, and as soon as he was old enough, he became an avid traveler. Though his later descriptions of rural New Hampshire would depict an idyllic wonderland and glorify the nobility of the New Hampshire farmer, Thomas seems always to have sought a larger society. The polished mannerist Mary met in New York City had never really wanted to farm the land; he preferred ink to soil.

In the fall of 1834, possibly to please his mother, Thomas enrolled at Dartmouth Medical School, where he intended to study the standard course of anatomy, physiology, obstetrics, and *materia medica*. However, New Hampshire required no degree or license to practice medicine, which meant that students had small incentive to persevere through the two-year curriculum. Hanover was a cold, secluded place for anyone, but probably especially isolating for an ambitious young man who wanted to see the world. Like the majority of his classmates, Thomas abandoned the study of medicine around Christmas-time, after only one term. His true love, he discovered, was writing. He also took an interest in preventive health when one of his professors, a vegetarian, invited a provocative lecturer named Sylvester Graham to deliver twelve lectures at a church in Hanover. Graham, whose talks would later be published as *The Science of Human Life*, converted Thomas to the cause of health reform. While the medical-school faculty obsessed over disease, Grahamites sought to preserve health. Like trains on parallel tracks, Thomas and Mary would spend the next fourteen years living two versions of the same experience.[5]

At the age of nineteen, with a very limited medical background, Thomas adopted a strict vegetarian diet. He renounced not only meat but all stimulating condiments as well (with the exception of salt). Inspired by Graham, Thomas spent the next year and a half traveling through New England and giving his own series of public lectures on phrenology and physiology. On these trips he stayed at luxurious hotels, graciously refusing the extravagant meals "with which the tables groaned." Instead, he dined on mashed potatoes, sweetened with a bit of milk. These were good months for Thomas. He felt healthier and stronger, equipped with greater clarity of mind, and, of course, the appreciation of his audiences. "I was indescribably light and cheerful. I enjoyed all my powers and faculties up to their point of development, and felt, every day of my life, that mere existence was a luxury." Over time, however, he began to backslide. Living in a boardinghouse of congenial fellows who dined almost exclusively on flesh, Thomas allowed himself a thin slice of lean roast beef. Though he found the consumption of this meat "repugnant," he managed to eat a bit more the following day. Soon he had returned to a diet of flesh, washed down with coffee and tea and even the occasional spirits. Thomas later credited his stint of vegetarianism with warding off debility during this initial period of self-abuse. After five years, however, he found himself devoid of stamina. The thought of abandoning coffee appealed to his intellect but horrified his sensory dependence. He postponed the action. It was not until 1847, under the influence of Mary Gove, that he returned to his "purer life."[4]

Around 1835 Thomas was living in the manufacturing town of Lowell, Massachusetts, twenty-five miles north of Boston. Famous for its mills, which were staffed by legions of young farm girls who traveled miles from home to live in dormitories and earn their own money, Lowell fascinated Thomas. With a population of 10,000, two-thirds of whom were these very young female operatives, Lowell had special charms. Thomas described the scene at town churches on Sundays: "There would be a thousand girls from fifteen to twenty-five—rarely one older—all dressed with neatness and even a degree of elegance, and, scattered about, a hundred men perhaps, who seemed quite lost and unprotected."[5] Other than the obvious appeal of such company, we do not know what drew Thomas to Lowell. By the following year, he was spending time in Boston.

Thomas had launched himself into the world of publishing, writing anonymously for the most part. His later reminiscences of these first post-Dartmouth years take the form of travel narratives and give a better sense of Thomas's surroundings than of the young man himself. However, in 1835 he did produce a revealing little newspaper called the *Standard*. Thomas never explicitly referred to this aggressively anti-Catholic newspaper in any of his later writings. It makes sense that he would not: an ugly bigotry pervades the columns of this paper, supposedly "Devoted to American Principles, Literature and General Intelligence." The paper did not advocate forced suppression of Catholic schools or monasteries by either law or violence, but it did seek that end through persuasion. That Thomas Nichols ultimately became a Roman Catholic in 1855, spent years lecturing at Catholic institutions, and published a series of addresses defending Catholicism from the slanders of Protestantism would astonish any reader of this early production.[6]

How Thomas, who was only twenty, managed to publish the *Standard* every Tuesday beginning in September of 1835 and continuing at least through May of 1836 is not clear, but it speaks to his initiative. Each issue offered four large pages of tiny type, without illustrations. With such headings as "Insidious Designs of Papists," the text offers declarations like "Be it known to all the world that *nunneries* are nothing more nor less than *baptised brothels*." In the second number of his paper, published on October 6, 1835, Thomas elaborated his prejudice: "We charge [Roman Catholic priests] with being the subjects of a foreign power, with bitter and unrelenting hostility to our government and institutions, with being Jesuits, and in this word comprehended all that is detestable!" This passage is followed by vilification of the convent at Charlestown, which stood accused by one John Bartlett of quietly welcoming nighttime male visitors. The paper maintained a judgmental fascination with the imagined sexuality of nuns and priests. At one point, Thomas described the Catholic Church's "hellish contrivance" to "cover the licentiousness of its priests. . . . It holds as a doctrine of faith, that demons are able to assume the human shape, disguised as priests or monks, and in this form indulge sensual desires, which they can impart to cloistered nuns; producing conception." Of course, Thomas could not know in 1835 how much a victim of similar rhetoric he would later become.[7]

Sprinkled throughout the *Standard*'s anti-Catholic diatribes appear original and reprinted discussions of health reform and marriage. These passages express sentiments more consistent with the mature Thomas Nichols—advocating cold baths, for example, or encouraging women, before entering into marriage, to think long and hard about the cruel obligation to "obey" one's husband. By January 1836, the paper (which claimed to have about one thousand subscribers from Boston, Roxbury, Worcester, and Lynn) also included poetry, biography, foreign and domestic news, notes on science, and entertaining miscellany. The result created bizarre juxtapositions of text. For example, preceding a lengthy column on "The Influence of Popery" is a paragraph explaining how to wash calicoes to prevent fading. The same number also includes articles in favor of Graham bread and jeremiads against tight lacing. By the spring of 1836, the *Standard* had substantially diversified its offerings, presenting reviews of theater and books, advice on love and manners, crime accounts, editorials on subjects other than religion, and even a few advertisements.[8]

Ten years later, in a liberal address on *Immigration and the Right of Naturalization*, Nichols obliquely referred to his first independent newspaper: "A native of New England and a descendant of the puritans, I early imbibed, and to some extent promulgated, opinions, of which reflection and experience have made me ashamed, but which have not been entertained since I arrived at the age of manhood, or, let me add, to the 'years of discretion.'"[9] He wrote these confessional words more than a decade before his own conversion to Catholicism.

BUFFALO

From Boston, Thomas found his way to New York City and then to Buffalo, New York, arriving by canal-packet in the fall of 1837. Three horses pulled the brightly painted craft across the state at an even five miles per hour—a slow pace, intended to protect the canal's embankments from the wearing slosh of stronger wakes. The trip from Albany to Buffalo took three days. Passengers breakfasted on cornbread, veal cutlets, fried potatoes, ham and eggs, applesauce, and hot coffee before making their way to the open-air decks. The crew arrayed luggage within strict boundaries along the boat's midline, yielding narrow walkways along either side. There, travelers socialized and watched the banks glide by, interrupted only by the steersman's frequent shouts of "Bridge!" requiring all to crouch and at times even lie flat against the floorboards until the boat had cleared some crossroad's dark underbelly. Passengers had many opportunities to relieve claustrophobia by jogging alongside the packet on the tow-path. To maintain a level course, the canal wound picturesquely through farmland and villages. Thomas was in no hurry. He had come to see Niagara Falls—the Great Cataract—and had no intention of settling in the flourishing lakefront city.

For reasons unclear even to him, however, Thomas took a job writing for the *Buffalo Commercial Advertiser* and decided to stay put. He took a room at the newly built United States Hotel, a grand, four-story structure that faced the city in one direction and the lake, the canal, the harbor, and Canada in the other. Few jobs familiarize a person with new surroundings as efficiently as does journalism. Thomas quickly learned the wheres and whos of Buffalo. The *Advertiser* paid him five dollars per week, and he earned another three dollars a day contributing to James Gordon Bennett's *New York Herald,* sending columns back East to the "Patriot News." Why Thomas had abandoned Boston and the *Standard,* New York and the *Herald,* is unknown. It is easy to imagine that he wanted to see more of the world, particularly the burgeoning West. Situated at the union of Lake Erie and the Niagara River, Buffalo had grown quickly since the opening of the Erie Canal. Encroaching railroads promised future miracles of speed and profit, but in 1837 canals still governed a town's prosperity.

Buffalo, accessible by canal-boat from the East and steamboat from the West, offered passage for thousands of westbound settlers and for ton after ton of eastbound crops. Nearly twenty thousand people called Buffalo home when Thomas arrived. The decade had seen tremendous speculation in real estate, with a boom in construction that transformed a quiet lakeshore town into a true metropolis. The majority of Buffalo's expan-

sion resulted from the initiatives of one daring individual: Benjamin Rathbun, the self-proclaimed "Master Builder and Architect" of Buffalo. His
projects included luxurious hotels, retail stores, stately residences, a stage-
coach line, and ownership of banks and territory. For a time, Rathbun
even maintained personal control over the American Falls at Niagara, envisioned as a future tourist mecca. However, Rathbun's strategy as a developer involved enormous risk: though a rich man on paper, Rathbun had
to scrape for every investment cent. Steadily borrowing from one man to
repay another, Rathbun accumulated a long list of creditors as well as a
huge stable of grateful employees. A smart man, Rathbun kept his economic struggles veiled; for many years, he found loans easy to obtain and
public confidence high. As the 1830s progressed, however, Rathbun's ambition to build finally drove his debt beyond his ability to scramble up legitimate credit. When his kingdom crumbled and Rathbun found himself
imprisoned for forging on promissory notes the names of some of Buffalo's
most prominent men, he was not alone in his bankruptcy. Wildcat speculation had thrown America into the Panic of 1837—an economic convul-
sion that left the nation to struggle through a six-year depression.[10]

Thomas, awed by the splendor of Rathbun's public works, considered
the developer wrongly accused. Aware that approximately a third of
Buffalo's citizens depended on Rathbun for their livings, Thomas grabbed
his pen and recklessly began to defend the accused. As he was exploring
details of the case and continuing to write for the *Advertiser* and the *Herald*, an unexpected offer emerged to cofound a new weekly newspaper—
the *Buffalonian*. Thomas readily accepted. The paper, more a tabloid than
anything else, issued its first number on Christmas Day 1837. Dedicated
to "liberal and independent principles," the paper offered sensational
scandal, despite the first column's promise that "nothing of a libellous or
scurrilous character will be admitted."[11]

As editor of the *Buffalonian*, Thomas guarded his anonymity carefully.
Rather than sitting down to write at the printing office, for example,
Thomas composed his pieces in the morning, back at the United States
Hotel (itself a Rathbun production). Asserting that anonymity enabled
him to produce a paper more honest and entertaining than its competi-
tors, Thomas spewed joking egotism through every issue. A typical pas-
sage, entitled "The Wonder Increases," appeared in the third number:
"No paper that has appeared in this city ever attracted so much attention

as the *Buffalonian*. . . .' Its spirit—its wit—its originality and its independence have surprised and delighted the whole community, while those
who have been pierced by the unseen shaft, have writhed in agony, and
wondered the more, that, like the judgments of Heaven, its castigations
have been both just and mysterious." The flippant paper began as a
weekly, but by the following March it was issued triweekly and eventually daily. Sold only by couriers and not by subscription, the *Buffalonian*
rapidly gained popularity. It brutally jibed its competitors: "We tell the
Journal, that it is tame, flat and insipid. We tell the *Commercial*, that it
has not one spark of independence, that it is the mere . . . organ of a
clique." Occasionally the editor included a brief request that no sleuthing
reader unmask his identity. "The mere idea of being known, and therefore held responsible, would destroy all our vivacity," pleaded Thomas. For
a time, Thomas was using the pseudonym "George Arlington"; it was as
Arlington that he chose to be listed in the City Directory for 1838. The
protection of pseudonym ran its course quickly, however, given Thomas's
penchant for editorial attack.[12]

In the very first issue appeared a brief letter from "One Who Bleeds,"
questioning the solvency of Benjamin Rathbun. The Rathbun scandal
would soon land Thomas in the Erie County jail, convicted of libel. It was
a topic he could not resist. He became Rathbun's champion. For Thomas,
Rathbun was a victim—cheated, robbed, and wrongly convicted by a powerful and corrupt "clique." An honest and overly trusting developer, Rathbun had, through vision and daring, basically created the best of Buffalo.
Thomas's version of events offered one hero and many villains:

[Rathbun] employed his brother in the financial department, owning
two or three banks, and raising large loans. . . . His paper, to the amount
of several hundred thousands of pounds, was readily discounted, as,
besides his own credit, it bore the endorsements of Buffalo capitalists
who had been benefited by his operations. These notes were so often
renewed that a clever young clerk, who was an adept in imitating signatures, to save himself trouble began to endorse the notes which were
required to renew others. By some means it became known. Rathbun
went to the endorsers, told them what had been done, placed in their
hands an assignment of his property to the amount of some millions

of dollars, to secure them against loss, and went to work to take up the forged paper.

He was treacherously arrested, on the complaint of the men who had promised him their aid. The temptation of the immense estate he had assigned to them was too strong for them to resist. He was committed to jail. After two years, and on the third trial, held in a distant county, . . . he was convicted . . . and sentenced to five years' penal servitude.[13]

Why Thomas initiated a crusade of defense for Benjamin Rathbun is not entirely clear, although it is evident that he greatly admired the reserved man who created so beautiful a boardinghouse as the United States Hotel. Surely the controversy boosted sales of the *Buffalonian*. Thomas's public praise of Rathbun found its balance in his relentless accusations against many of the town's elite, including a former mayor, Hiram Pratt. The *Buffalonian*'s analysis of the Rathbun scandal drew a great deal of attention and effectively raised doubts regarding the developer's guilt. Thomas saw Pratt, not Rathbun, as the shame of Buffalo and relentlessly pounded Pratt's character.[14]

In March of 1838, a group of ruffians attempted to kidnap Thomas. They probably intended to tar and feather him, but in this they failed. Others succeeded in destroying the offices of the *Buffalonian*, however. Those convicted for the vandalism included Henry P. Darrow, a leader of the First Presbyterian Church, as well as other prominent citizens. In addition to smearing the names of Buffalo's leading citizens in connection with the Rathbun case, Thomas had also outraged a subset of the City Guard by publishing a letter that accused the men of drunkenly harassing citizens, illegally carrying and firing loaded muskets, and making a nuisance of themselves. The editor's comment on this letter granted that a few individuals did commit such offenses, though "Capt. Stanley, we understand, is the only officer that commits, or authorizes such outrages as our correspondent complains of—and he will shortly be cut off by his own company." No wonder that by the following month Thomas was writing that he had been "most wantonly outraged by Capt. Stanley, and members of his company." Fortunately a passer-by interfered and offered protection. In response to the assault, Thomas wrote a plea to the Common

Council, demanding the men's discharge from the City Watch, but "was induced by my then employers to defer presenting it." A certain John Tanahill had even promised to assassinate Thomas if he should ever meet the young editor while on duty. Obviously, Thomas was courting disaster, which finally came, not in the form of assassination, but of prosecution. After calling Pratt a despicable perjurer and printing the claim that Pratt's attorney was "a tool of his employers" who as attorney for Rathbun's nephew had compromised "the honor of his client by inducing him unnecessarily to turn State's evidence, against his relation and benefactor," Thomas, no longer anonymous, was indicted for libel.[15]

Details of his trial filled the pages of the *Buffalonian* during June 1839. He faced a crowded courtroom. Proceedings began on a Friday evening, and the guilty verdict was delivered after midnight on Sunday morning. The judge set a ridiculously low bail—an invitation, Thomas presumed, for him to leave town, which he would not do. For two days after his conviction, Thomas wandered Buffalo freely. His sentence: four months in the jail of Erie County and a fine of one hundred fifty dollars, which was ultimately paid from the proceeds of a theatrical company's benefit performance made in his behalf. Even after his conviction and imprisonment, Thomas continued to write for the *Buffalonian*, complaining bitterly in his journal that the jailer was required to screen his prose for libelous passages. Ironically (and perhaps deliberately), Thomas spent his four-month sentence in cell number twenty—the very same cell that had held Benjamin Rathbun before his transfer to the state prison at Auburn.[16]

Though he included the story of Rathbun's downfall in an 1864 memoir, *Forty Years of American Life,* Thomas made no reference to his personal involvement with the case or to his incarceration. He even claimed to have taken his first steamboat excursion on the Great Lakes during the summer of 1839—an impossibility, since he spent that summer in the Erie County jail. He actually took that trip in October, very soon after his release. Thomas loved steamboats. His *Journal in Jail* laments the deprivation of a particular July cruise on the steamer Chesapeake, which would have taken him to Sault St. Marie and the remote upper regions of Lake Huron.[17]

An unusual text, *Journal in Jail* invites special attention for being the closest thing to a diary that remains from Thomas Nichols's life. Entries exist for most days of his sentence, the first on June 18, 1839, and the last on October 15, 1839, including transcriptions of letters he received in jail. The first few entries wail with self-righteous indignation. "There is no act of my existence—no deliberate act—that I regret. . . . [A] sense of right has ever been with me," he declares, outraged at rumors that he had been "the calumniator of female virtue!" Then, "What must a mother, a sister, feel? Grieve not, beloved ones. . . . Four months . . . and then I will be with you." In his entry for July 21, 1839, Thomas includes a letter from his sister that assures him of the family's faith in his innocence, their anguish at imagining him wrongly imprisoned, and their wish to come visit him, though neither she nor his parents could make the trip. "It seems to me that a prison would not be dreary with you," she writes. "Happy is it for us both, that we do not depend entirely upon outward circumstances for pleasure. . . . You have your books for your companions. . . . And even should they take away your books, you could think."[18]

Thomas claimed—unconvincingly—to have kept the journal for personal amusement alone, without any intent to publish, and said that he changed his mind only after being encouraged by friends and needful of money. It is impossible to know how he actually revised his journal for publication. From its pages and those of the *Buffalonian* emerges a rabble-rouser who craved attention, who never hesitated to speak his thoughts, and who fancied himself a true patriot—as well as wit. It is easy at times to share Mary's initial repulsion.

In his newspaper, under the cloak of anonymity, Thomas had written his intention to attend "4 balls, 6 parties, and 3 prayer meetings. A great many things want to be noticed." But his journal entry for July 2, 1839, claims "I attend no parties." Likewise, he insists that he avoids gossiping calls and that he despises a male flirt. Yet his columns for the *Buffalonian* could not be more flirtatious or gossiping. And what can explain the fact that a married woman came to visit him during his first week in jail, kissing his lips through the grating of his cell door? Why did women send him flowers, and strawberries and cream? Why had three or four women revealed that he had occupied their dreams? More callow preening than sincerity suffuses his apparent mystification: "I have acquired the reputation, the Lord knows how, for no one was ever more innocent of it, of using every art of seductive flattery, and of being something very near an accomplished rake: when every one, who is acquainted with me, knows that I am the plainest hearted mortal living, and little less than a palpable personification of . . . moral reform." He then wisely adds, "I hope this may never fall into the hands of any of my readers of the *Buffalonian*, who 'like it, all but its egotism.' Good Heavens! if that were taken away, I wonder what there would be left! The advertisements?" Thus, even as a young, loud-mouthed, arrogant, sarcastic editor, Thomas Low Nichols seems to have kept a bemused eye on himself. The journal passage regarding his reputation as a ladies' man followed the transcription of love letters from more than one woman, written to him while he languished in jail. Though calling himself "but tolerably good looking," Thomas always evidenced tremendous self-esteem.[19] Married women liked him; single women liked him. He liked himself.

Thomas left Buffalo soon after his release from jail. It seems that he accepted a cash bribe and the promise of relinquishment of all suits against the *Buffalonian* if he left town and stopped publishing his paper. In his *Journal in Jail*, Thomas defended this action by explaining that members of "the clique" had concocted false evidence against his friends that would have proven extremely hurtful had they proceeded with their insinuations. It was more honorable, he concluded, to take the fall himself. In truth, it was probably something of a relief as well.

Though Thomas wrote nothing further about his Buffalo disputes, one of his adversaries did. In 1839 an anonymously written twenty-eight-page pamphlet appeared, entitled "Vindication of the So Called 'Clique.'" And it was just that. "When a human fiend of desolation, revelling in his scathing and blighting power, and sardonically smiling at the dreadful ruin he has made, has at length ceased from his demoniack attacks upon the great, the wise, the good, and the virtuous of our fair city," cried the author, "it seems necessary that some one . . . should attempt to undo the mischief that he has done, and vindicate the fame and actions of those who have for almost two years been the subjects of incessant slander and abuse." The pamphlet describes Thomas Nichols as "an unknown adventurer, who first came to Buffalo under an assumed name, and in the character of a strolling lecturer and ventriloquist! . . . Since his residence in Buffalo, he has never received an invitation to dine, unless at some publick house; and has never been invited to a single fashionable party, given by the *beau monde*. . . . Even those—the pitiful few who pretended to be his friends . . . have left him now."[20]

Thomas had made fierce enemies in Buffalo, and despite consistent bravado, he had suffered personal repression. His cell had measured eight feet long by five feet wide. Its only light struggled through the grating of an iron door. The place was filthy. Though Thomas did not write another explicit word about this confinement after publishing *Journal in Jail,* he would ultimately devote many hundreds of pages to a more mature defense of personal liberty. While in jail, he brewed a concentrated passion for freedom. During that same summer, his future wife was articulating the same desperate passion in the context of her hateful marriage.

EASTWARD BOUND

From Buffalo, Thomas headed to Rochester, New York, where he accepted a job at a political journal whose name he did not record. He claimed to have no personal ambition for public office, asserting absolutely no desire "to make laws or execute them."[21] However, 1840 was the election year in which Harrison defeated Van Buren; in all likelihood, Thomas campaigned for Harrison, since he harbored contempt for Van Buren's earlier defense of neutrality regarding the Canadian independence uprisings. Thomas found the official neutrality position to be profoundly hypocritical. While Northern frontiersmen flocked to the aid of the rebels, Van Buren sought to appease the South, a constituency that not only relied on Britain for much of its cotton trade but that also dreaded the thought of Canadian land being added to the Republic, augmenting Northern political influence.

The Canada War had occupied Thomas's attention from the moment he settled in Buffalo. He rallied to the support of Canada's "patriot" insurgents who occupied Navy Island, preparing for a war of independence. Thomas had delivered a rousing address at Niagara Falls on the evening of December 29, 1838—the one-year anniversary of a British attack on Canadian rebels. On December 29, 1837, only a few months after Thomas had arrived in Buffalo, the British set fire to a rebel supply boat, the *Caroline,* which was docked at night in the Niagara River. British troops then cut the burning ship loose to crash down the rapids and over the falls, taking the lives of sleeping crewmen. Thomas later recalled dining on Navy Island with the Patriot governor (Mackenzie) and the commanding general (Van Rensselaer) during the Canadian Rebellion, or "Patriot War," as he preferred to call it. The group ate pork and beans from tin plates to the background sounds of bullets and shell bursts.

When he arrived in Rochester—dragging the baggage of his reputation as an egotist and thrower-of-stones—Thomas initiated a creative experiment in self-promotion. Capitalizing on his recent fame as the imprisoned editor from Buffalo, he solicited advance subscriptions for a series entitled "My Notions on Matters and Things." If more than one installment of this series ever existed, it has not been preserved. A reading of the first part strongly suggests that Rochester's citizens would not have financed part two. *My Notions on Matters and Things* strings together thirty-six pages of disconnected, rambling reflections on all manner of mundane subjects, from the value of firemen to the charm of the local cemetery. Thomas considered his brief volume "philosophical." It included short quotations from Scripture among lengthier observations about human nature. "A belief or confidence in success, in whatever manner produced, is the finest incentive to exertion," Thomas wrote.[22] Throughout his life, Thomas would draw energy from this elusive incentive more reliably than most other mortals.

"It is apparent that the charge of egotism will remain good against me," Thomas acknowledged. "There is a secret about this. Criticism must have something to carp at—so I give it that." Rochester's eagerly subscribing populace showed greater interest in Thomas's *Notions* than he had anticipated—and for reasons that did not settle his soul. It dawned on Thomas that subscribers expected his book to entertain them with caustic personal attacks. Rather than satisfy this craving, Thomas chose the more cautious route: he recognized it and boldly declined the dare. "Am I a Don Quixote, tilting at wind-mills, and roaming about this bright and beauteous world, for the sake of getting up quarrels and scrapes?" he asked. "Am I a monster . . . ? Would it not be the extreme of folly for me to make enemies unnecessarily?" Buffalo may not have silenced Thomas's song, but it revised his lyrics.[23]

My Notions on Matters and Things makes clear that Thomas considered himself a liberal, that he loved to dance, that he sought a future of economic equality for all, that he loved to be on the water in the moonlight, and that, personally, he had some trouble forming close friendships with women that did not suffer from romantic complications. In this last context, he advocated marriage from affection as the only way to avoid the contamination of friendship by courtship. As in Buffalo, he found the ladies of Rochester lovely. Still, the city soon bored him, and by the end of 1841, he was back in New York. There he resumed newspaper work, accepting the position of editor for the New York *Aurora*, a brand new twopenny daily. In February of 1842, he left the *Aurora* and immediately began to produce another daily, the New York *Arena*. He also initiated the *Nichols Weekly Arena*. Over the next five years, he published three novels and also wrote for the *Young Hickory Banner*, a political journal devoted to the election of James Polk in the 1844 presidential race.[24]

Ellen Ramsay; or, The Adventures of a Greenhorn, in Town and Country appeared in 1843, one year after Mary had published *Lectures to Ladies on Anatomy and Physiology*. Thomas had written the brief and racy novel to earn money. He claimed it was a true story, based on true characters and settings. Its adventurous protagonist, Edward Freeman, leaves the bucolic New England town of his childhood and travels by steamboat to New York City, where he takes lodging at the elegant Astor House hotel. Quickly, however, the naïve Freeman—who hopes to make his living as a writer—discovers that publishing houses will not risk capital on unknown, untried authors when they can simply reprint proven European works without compensating anyone. The periodicals likewise rely on a stable of known writers and are always flooded with submissions from those who would be gratified with publication alone. Only the newspapers pay for original writing, but they pay little and are already well staffed. Soon Edward Freeman finds himself enmeshed in the city's underworld, swindled by men and women alike. Mortified by the insincerity and vice he encounters, Edward ultimately returns to his hometown and marries Ellen Ramsay, whose honesty and devotion he has finally come to appreciate.

Though fictional, *Ellen Ramsay* documents many of Thomas's early struggles. The novel articulates feelings about personal relationships that would find fuller expression in Thomas's later work. Written when he was only twenty-eight, *Ellen Ramsay* tells the story of a young man who has gained enough life experience to reflect on the differences between the brothel, idle courtship, and true love. During this time in New York City, Thomas socialized with a number of prostitutes and may for a time have rented a room inside a brothel. Details are sketchy and evidence questionable, but it seems clear that as a single young man, Thomas moved in "morally questionable" social circles. Though *Ellen Ramsay* ends with a traditional country wedding and does not come close to advocating anything like the radical free love of the phalanstery, the book does address issues that came to dominate Thomas's later life as a social reformer: "Men and women dress, and act, and play their parts to deceive and trap each other. What must a woman feel when she finds the gentleness of her lover assumed to cover the natural bearishness of a brutal, selfish, unfeeling beast, who cares only for his own sensual pleasures, and compels her to submit at all times to his desires, whether in the humor or not?"[25]

In the autumn of 1845, an old friend from Rochester wrote to Thomas in New York City, begging him to return to western New York. The man was dying of tuberculosis. He asked Thomas to travel with him, under his doctor's orders, to a warmer climate. He did not want his wife and children to watch him die; he preferred that they remember him with whatever health he could muster on his departure to Florida or the West Indies. Thomas, who must not have had overly pressing commitments in New York, agreed at once, and the two set out immediately on a slow, elaborate journey that took them through Philadelphia, Baltimore, and Washington, D.C., over the Allegheny mountains to Pittsburgh, Cincinnati, Louisville, Memphis, and New Orleans. Presumably, Thomas's companion died during this journey, or the two parted ways at some final destination for the friend. Mysteriously, the narrative Thomas has left of this trip begins with his companion by his side, but it evolves into the story of a lone traveler, who winds throughout the South as a journalist, with not another mention of his dying friend.[26]

NEW YORK CITY AND MARRIAGE

Thus, Thomas Low Nichols happened to be leaving New York City just a few months before Mary Gove and her daughter arrived. By the time they met two years later, Thomas had established himself once again as a journalist, and Mary had developed a successful hydropathic practice. Though both were lonely, neither was desperate or dependent. Elma was studying art. Hiram, despite his continual distant slander, had become to Mary more an ugly symbol of male dominance than an immediate threat. Mary had lived half of her life. The second half would prove to be far happier.

"I do not wish that I had known you before," Thomas wrote to Mary in an early love letter. "It is just right. I was never before so likely to profit by your—sympathy. I paused for the word, but that comes very near it. . . . Yours ever is hard to say and mean. I am yours *now.*"[27]

Both Mary and Thomas had come a long way from their provincial New Hampshire childhoods. From their common origins to their common destination, the two had traveled similar paths. Each had experienced personal repression, and each had rebounded. They shared the strengths of sassiness and self-confidence; both found fault with authority structures before finding it in themselves. Each had staked hope in the promises of Sylvester Graham and Charles Fourier. The two met because they liked the same people, wrote for the same journals, held the same opinions, and shared the same roots. Only five years apart in age, Mary Gove and Thomas Nichols seemed more than compatible. They seemed destined.

The reality of Hiram both postponed and ensured this union. Because Mary admitted to having left her husband, the State of Massachusetts had granted a "Legal Separation for Voluntary Abandonment," but this designation did not allow either Mary or Hiram to remarry. As the victim of abandonment, only Hiram had the clear right to sue for divorce; and Mary doubted this would ever happen, for Quakers did not sanction divorce. The chains of this marriage did not stop her affair with Thomas, but they did enforce limits. Mary resolved that she would wait a full year before moving in with Thomas and abandoning all respect for appearances or law. Perhaps she was hoping for some unexpected change in circumstances with Hiram; perhaps she was simply using caution in the new relationship. Mary would not impulsively sacrifice reputation or risk career in the gamble of this new love, no matter how ideal it seemed. "No man on the broad earth could more fully sympathize with me [than Thomas] in the holy fear I felt of bonds," she wrote.[28]

A few months passed. And then, a miracle. Mary learned that Hiram had fallen in love with another woman and that he wanted a divorce. Suddenly, unexpectedly, Mary was free. Thomas Low Nichols, thirty-three years old, opened his arms to her and Elma. In her autobiography, Mary described her firm words to Thomas: "In a marriage with you, I resign no right of my soul. I enter into no compact to be faithful to you. I only promise to be faithful to the deepest love of my heart. If that love is yours, it will bear fruit for you. . . . If my love leads me from you, I must go. . . . I must keep my name—the name I have made for myself, through labor and suffering. . . . I must have my room, into which none can come, but because I wish it." Thomas objected to nothing. In the same year that Mary published her autobiography, Thomas wrote: "The model husband gives to his wife her rights as a human being; her privileges as a woman; the respect and deference due to a lady; the devotion of a lover to his mistress; and the protecting care of the father of a family."[29]

They decided on a Swedenborgian ceremony. The choice made sense. Emanuel Swedenborg, an eighteenth-century Swedish mystic whose diverse writings were experiencing a popular American renaissance in the 1840s, had articulated a theory of "conjugial love" that both Mary and Thomas valued. Ministers of Swedenborg's "New Church" taught that a deeper love existed than the pretense typically expressed by traditional marriage—an eternal, spiritual union of souls so profound that it transcended death. This love was extremely rare. Those who could not find it on earth would perhaps find it in heaven, where permanent True Love between men and women would flourish. Thomas described Swedenborg's conjugial love as a "pure monogamy" that "supposes the existence of two imperfect beings, each the half of the other, the male and female portion in body and soul, which require to be united to make up the perfect human being. Each of these parts is created for the other, and can fit no other half. . . . [S]uch marriages are made in heaven. . . . The two souls unite to make a single angel in the spiritual world."[30]

Swedenborg's writings also supported Mary's decision to leave Hiram. "The love of domination to be exercised by one party over the other completely banishes conjugial love," he had written.

> When one party wills or loves what the other does, both enjoy liberty . . . : but where domination is assumed, neither enjoys liberty: one party is confessedly a slave; and so is the ruling party too, because led as a slave by the lust of domination. . . . Domination subjugates; and the mind that is subjugated has afterwards no will at all, or else a contrary will; . . . if a contrary will, instead of love, there is hatred. The interiors of those who live in such a marriage, are in such mutual collision and combat, as ever exists between two opposites. . . . The collision and combat of their interiors display themselves openly after death.[31]

Because so many unfortunate people married under the mistaken impression that they had found conjugial love, Swedenborg argued for the freedom to divorce and remarry—a tenet obviously important to Mary and Thomas.

While Elizabeth Cady Stanton, Lucretia Mott, and Mary M'Clintock formulated the Declaration of Sentiments in Seneca Falls, New York, Mary was planning her wedding. While they composed the terse and powerful document that would spark a formalized movement for women's rights in the United States, Mary was choosing a dress.

The history of mankind is a history of repeated injuries and usurpations on the part of man toward woman, having in direct object the establishment of an absolute tyranny over her. . . .

Flowers, rather than cake and wine, would be given to the guests.

He has compelled her to submit to laws, in the formation of which she had no voice. . . .

He has made her, if married, in the eye of the law, civilly dead.

He has taken from her all right in property, even to the wages she earns. . . .

In the covenant of marriage, she is compelled to promise her obedience to her husband, he becoming, to all intents and purposes, her master—the law giving him power to deprive her of her liberty, and to administer chastisement.

Elma would be the bridesmaid.

He has so framed the laws of divorce, as to what shall be the proper causes of divorce; in case of separation, to whom the guardianship of the children shall be given; as to be wholly regardless of the happiness of women—the law, in all cases, going upon the false supposition of the supremacy of man, and giving all power into his hands. . . .

Mary would wear a headdress of cape Jessamine, with white roses and geranium leaves.

He has monopolized nearly all the profitable employments, and from
those she is permitted to follow, she receives but a scanty remunera-
tion. . . .

He has created a false public sentiment, by giving to the world a
different code of morals for men and women, by which moral delin-
quencies which exclude women from society, are not only tolerated but
deemed of little account in man.

The minister would recite the Lord's Prayer while everyone kneeled.

He has usurped the prerogative of Jehovah himself, claiming it as his
right to assign for her a sphere of action, when that belongs to her conscience and her God. He has endeavored, in every way that he could to
destroy her confidence in her own powers, to lessen her self-respect,
and to make her willing to lead a dependant and abject life.

Mary and Thomas would each hold her ring together with the minister
before placing it on Mary's hand. The historic Woman's Rights Convention of Seneca Falls—the first of its kind in the United States—preceded
the Nicholses' wedding by only nine days. Had Mary been less in love at
the moment, she might have shown more interest.[32]

[1] Advertisement for Mary Gove's Graham Boarding School. During her grim first marriage, Mary Gove supported her family financially with a school that taught reading, writing, arithmetic—and physiology. *Lynn Record* (28 March 1838), Lynn Museum.

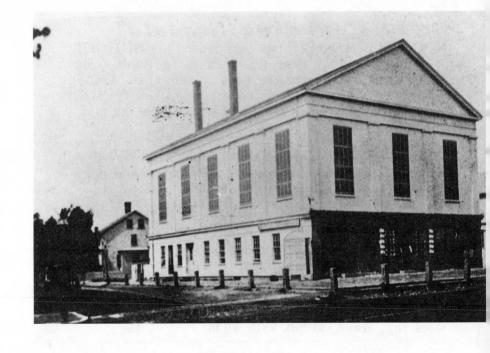

[2] Lyceum Hall, Lynn, Massachusetts, ca. 1850, where Mary Gove and other women were given an early opportunity to speak before mixed-sex audiences and where Mary delivered her first address on the evils of marriage. Lynn Museum.

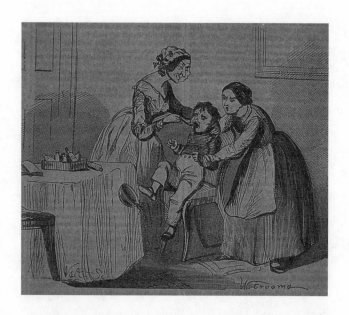

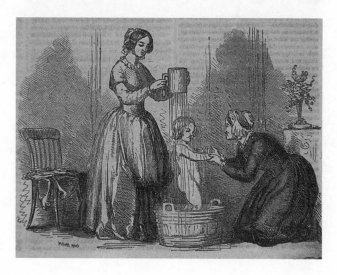

[3] Illustration in the *Water-Cure Journal* demonstrating the contrast between regular medicine's use of harsh drugs and hydrotherapy's reliance on pure water. *Water-Cure Journal,* April 1852.

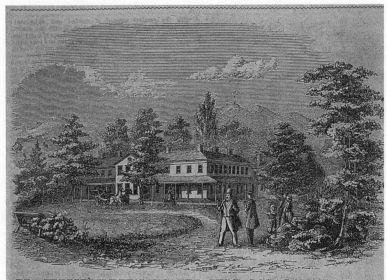

[4] Advertisement for Robert Wesselhœft's Water-Cure Establishment in Brattleboro, Vermont, where Mary first received training as a water-cure physician. *New Grafenberg Water-Cure Reporter,* January 1850.

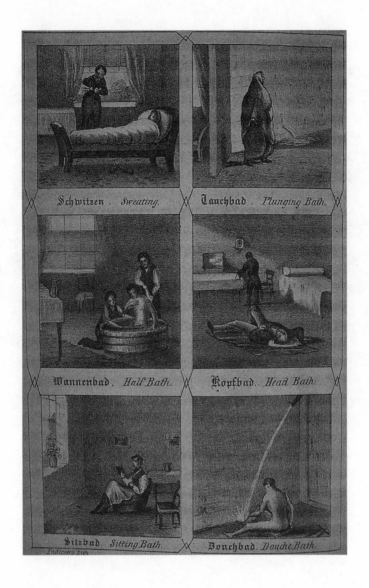

[5] Various water-cure techniques. Joel Shew's *Hydropathy, or, The Water-Cure*, Wiley & Putnam, 1845. Individually tailored for each patient, water-cure treatments involved a complex variety of baths, wraps, and douches as well as attention to diet, fresh air, and exercise. A leading practitioner, Mary described water cure as the "scientific application of the principles of nature in the cure of disease . . . never painful and seldom disagreeable."

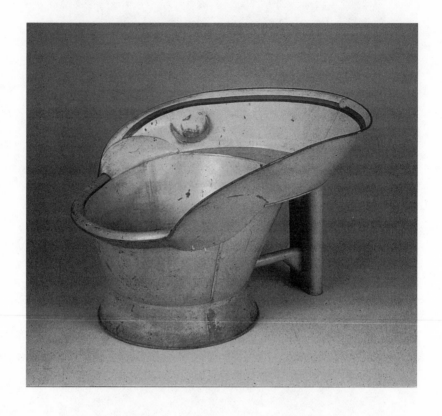

[6] A sitz bath, ca. 1875–1910, by John D. Hewitt Mfg. Co., Buffalo, New York. Filled with four inches of cold water, the "sitz" or "hip bath" was central to the water cure and was recommended for constipation, hemorrhoids, and "all the weaknesses, derangements, and disorders of the generative organs." Strong Museum, Rochester, N.Y.

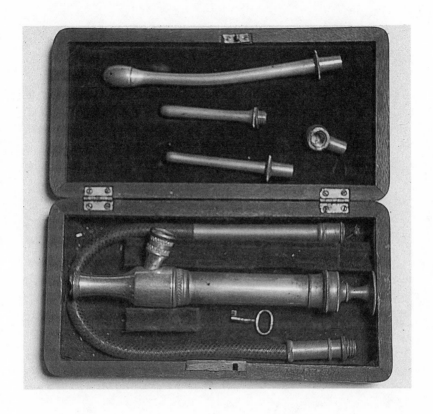

[7] A vaginal syringe kit. With immediately postpartum women, water-cure physicians regularly employed the syringe to "throw a pint of cold water upon the uterus"—a technique intended to facilitate contraction, diminish blood loss, and alleviate pain. College of Physicians of Philadelphia.

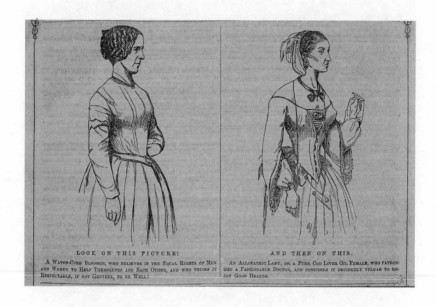

LOOK ON THIS PICTURE:

A WATER-CURE BLOOMER, WHO BELIEVES IN THE EQUAL RIGHTS OF MEN AND WOMEN TO HELP THEMSELVES AND EACH OTHER, AND WHO THINKS IT RESPECTABLE, IF NOT GENTEEL, TO BE WELL!

AND THEN ON THIS.

AN ALLOPATHIC LADY, OR A PURE COD LIVER OIL FEMALE, WHO PATRONIZES A FASHIONABLE DOCTOR, AND CONSIDERS IT DECIDEDLY VULGAR TO ENJOY GOOD HEALTH.

[8] Illustration emphasizing the relative health and confidence of the corset-free "Water-Cure Bloomer," who refuses to strangle her torso for the sake of fashion. *Water-Cure Journal*, November 1853.

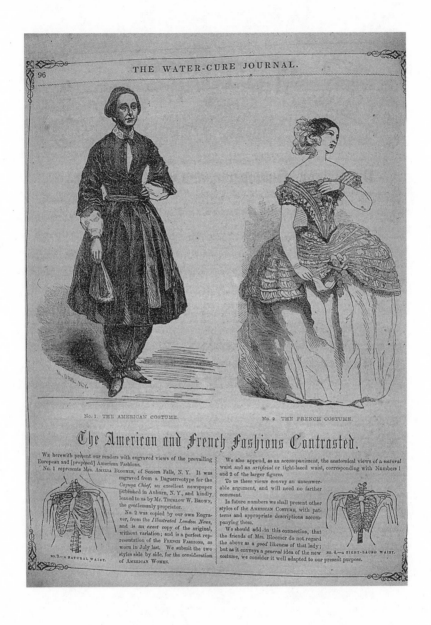

No. 1. THE AMERICAN COSTUME.   No. 2. THE FRENCH COSTUME.

The American and French Fashions Contrasted.

We herewith present our readers with engraved views of the prevailing European and [proposed] American Fashions.

No. 1 represents Mrs. AMELIA BLOOMER, of Seneca Falls, N. Y. It was engraved from a Daguerreotype for the *Cayuga Chief*, an excellent newspaper published in Auburn, N. Y., and kindly loaned to us by Mr. THURLOW W. BROWN, the gentlemanly proprietor.

No. 2 was copied by our own Engraver, from the *Illustrated London News*, and is an *exact* copy of the original, without variation; and is a perfect representation of the FRENCH FASHIONS, as worn in July last. We submit the two styles side by side, for the consideration of AMERICAN WOMEN.

We also append, as an accompaniment, the anatomical views of a *natural* waist and an *artificial* or tight-laced waist, corresponding with Numbers 1 and 2 of the larger figures.

To us these views convey an unanswerable argument, and will need no farther comment.

In future numbers we shall present other styles of the AMERICAN COSTUME, with patterns and appropriate descriptions accompanying them.

We should add in this connection, that the friends of Mrs. Bloomer do not regard the above as a *good* likeness of that lady; but as it conveys a *general* idea of the new costume, we consider it well adapted to our present purpose.

NO. 3.—A NATURAL WAIST.   NO. 4.—A TIGHT-LACED WAIST.

[9] Nineteenth-century health reformers also fought for women's dress reform. The scandalous "Bloomer Costume" allowed women relatively great freedom of movement. It also invited mockery, jeers, and sometimes physical abuse. *Water-Cure Journal*, 1851, 96.

[10] Advertisement for *Mary Lyndon; or, Revelations of a Life*, the autobiography that sealed Mary's reputation as a passionate defender of free love. From Stringer & Townsend's 1855 edition of the book.

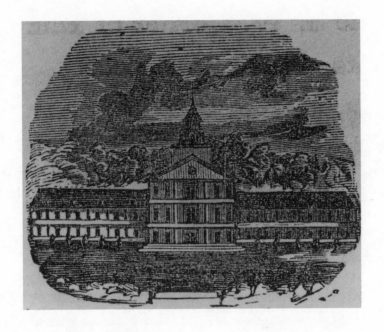

[11] Yellow Springs Water Cure, 1853. The Nicholses leased this property to the dismay of Horace Mann and other local residents who protested the infamous couple's plans to establish a "School of Life" in their town. Antiochiana Collection, Antioch College Archives.

instructive where he relates his own experience, and everywhere racy of the soil of which it treats."—*Spectator.*

"An interesting book, written with extraordinary vivacity, and full of amusement and instruction."—*Literary World.*

"Having read, we may say, all that has been written on American affairs since the war began, whether by English or Transatlantic pens, we can confidently affirm that Dr. Nichols is by far the most intelligent and trustworthy, because the most temperate, frank, and impartial of those writers."—*Dublin University Magazine.*

"Dr. Nichols' power lies in the force and truthfulness with which he recals the incidents of his past life, the manners and pursuits of the society with which he was familiar in his youth, the men whom he has known, the scenes he has visited. His book will give both pleasure and instruction to every intelligent person who consults it."—*Guardian.*

"We can scarcely recal a case since Washington Irving in which an American author has received a warmer or more unanimous welcome in England. When an author has satisfied the *Quarterly*, the *Examiner*, and the *Saturday Review*, he may well be content. In winning this English welcome, Dr. Nichols has yielded nothing to English prejudice. It is rare, indeed, that we bestow such unmingled praise, and for the reason that we rarely meet with a work that so nearly merits unqualified commendation."—*Index.*

DR. NICHOLS'
SANITARY AND PHILANTHROPIC INVENTIONS.

Besides writing and publishing books and periodicals and giving lectures on sanitary science, Dr. Nichols has endeavoured to give more practical efficacy to his work by supplying various dietetic articles and hydropathic appliances, which are sold at 23 Oxford Street, and also by agents in the principal towns of England.

DR. NICHOLS' WHEATEN GROATS, made from the best selected White Wheat, and specially prepared for the cure of inveterate constipation, piles, &c., are a delightful food for old or young, and are from the mode of preparation, superior in quality and flavour. Price 6d. per lb. in 1 lb. packages. Sold by Chemists and Grocers in all parts of the United Kingdom, and at the Central Sanitary Depot of NICHOLS & CO., 23 Oxford Street, London, W. Wholesale Agents—FRANKS & CO., 14 Little Tower Street, E.C.

DR. NICHOLS' SELF-RAISING WHOLE WHEAT MEAL, for instantly making light and delicious Brown Bread. This Meal is made of the finest selected White Wheat to be found in England, and contains all its nutritive and healthful properties, nitrogen, phosphorus, &c., accurately mingled with self-raising elements of perfect purity, so that a Loaf of light and beautiful Brown Bread can be made and put in the Oven in One Minute. 3 lb., 1s 10s. Packages Carriage free in London district. Orders to NICHOLS & CO., 23 Oxford Street, London, W.

HAND MILLS FOR GRINDING WHEAT, RICE, &c., so as to secure Economy in price, and freedom from adulterations, which fasten in a moment to shelf or table, are sold at 23 Oxford Street at 6s., 8s. 10s., 12s., 16s., and 20s., and a fine steel mill, hand-made for 30s. All sent by rail, but in ordering add one shilling for boxing.

DR. NICHOLS' SANITARY BREAD-RAISER, a perfectly pure and strong Baking Powder for all kinds of bread and pastry. In 6d., 1s., and 2s. cases.

DR. NICHOLS' FOOD OF HEALTH (*Registered Trade Mark*), a most nutritious and delicious food, prepared from the richest elements of the vegetable kingdom in the exact proportions required to form pure blood and give healthy nourishment to all the organs of the human body, is a preventive of and cure for dyspepsia, constipation, scrofula, and all the diseases of the nutritive system. No one who makes even one meal a-day upon this Food of Health will ever need aperients. Children thrive upon it in perfect health and vigour. One pound of Dr. Nichols' Food of Health contains more and better nutriment than 3½ pounds of beef or mutton. Price 8d. per lb., in ½ lb., 1 lb., and 3 lb. packets. Sold by Chemists and Grocers in all parts of the United Kingdom, and at the Central Sanitary Depot of Nichols & Co., 23 Oxford Street, London, W. Wholesale Agents—FRANKS & CO., 14 Little Tower Street, E.C.

COUNT RUMFORD'S SOUP, prepared and improved from the formulas of the celebrated Count Rumford, founder of the Royal Institution, &c., is a purely vegetable soup, very nutritious in quality and delightful in flavour. It is in a fine dry powder, and can be prepared by any one in a few minutes, and may be eaten by itself, or used as a stock for vegetable, rice, or maccaroni soups, and so infinitely varied. In packets to make a pint of soup, 1d. Trial sample package post free for 6d.

FILTERS FOR PURIFYING WATER, by the Best makers, and those expressly manufactured for Nichols & Co., 12s. 6d., 17s. 6d., 22s. 6d., may be seen at 23 Oxford Street, or will be carefully packed for rail on receipt of P.O.O. Add 1s. for packing.

HYDROPATHIC APPLIANCES.

DR. NICHOLS' PORTABLE FOUNTAIN BATH, OR RISING DOUCHE, is one of the most effective of all hydropathic appliances for the treatment of habitual constipation, piles, prolapsus, falling of the womb, and all the weaknesses and disorders of the generative organs in both sexes. Dr. Nichols has made this bath so portable that it may be used in every house, and at the bedside of every patient. With a powerful force pump, jets of two sizes, or a spray, are sent upward; and with a short hose and tube it can be used for injections or irrigations. Packed for transport 3s. extra. Price 35s.

DR. NICHOLS' PORTABLE TURCO-RUSSIAN HOT-AIR OR VAPOUR BATH cleanses the skin, opens the pores, quickens and equalises the circulation, removes common colds, congestions and inflammations, rheumatism, neuralgia, stimulates digestion, and is a preventive and cure of many diseases. It is especially useful in eruptive diseases—measles, scarlet fever, smallpox, &c.; also in quinsy, sore throat, mumps, bronchitis, pneumonia, pleurisy, dropsy, and liver and kidney diseases, nervous diseases, contagious diseases, blood poisoning, and is the only cure known for hydrophobia.

Dr. Nichols' Portable Turco-Russian Bath packs in a corner of a trunk; weighs under 12 lbs.; can be used anywhere, and made ready in five minutes. Price, complete for gas, 32s.; with spirit lamp, 29s. 6d.

[12] Advertisements for the inventions and supplies of Thomas L. Nichols. Promotional insert in Mary's 1874 book, *A Woman's Work in Water Cure and Sanitary Education*. The Nicholses believed health reform to be the "pivot" of all other social reform. As Thomas put it, "So long as people are diseased, nothing can be done for them."

Malvern, England, — —

Dear Pauline Davis;

I have your letter, reminding me that I was one of the first women in America who labored for the Rights of Woman, and inviting me to be present at your Convention.

I cannot come; but my interest in the freedom of Woman has not in the least abated during thirty years of labour or prayer for her emancipation. I claim one right for Woman which includes all human rights. It is that she be free to obey the Divine law of her own life—that she be not subjected to the lustful despotism of one man, or to the selfish or unwise legislation of many.

[13] Letter from Mary Gove Nichols to fellow health lecturer and women's rights activist Paulina Wright Davis, 1870, in which Mary reaffirms her unflagging commitment to the cause of women's rights. Vassar College Archives.

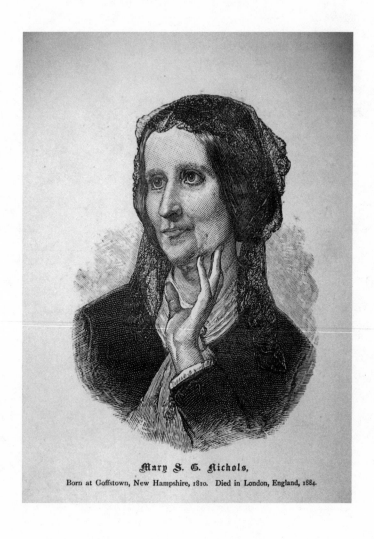

Mary S. G. Nichols,

Born at Goffstown, New Hampshire, 1810. Died in London, England, 1884.

[14] Engraving of Mary Gove Nichols (1810–84), based on a crayon portrait by her daughter, Elma Penn Gove. In 1846 Edgar Allan Poe described Mary as "rather below the medium height, somewhat thin, with dark hair and keen, intelligent black eyes." Frontispiece of the *Nichols' Health Manual: Being Also a Memorial of the Life and Work of Mrs. Mary S. Gove Nichols*, 1886.

Seminal Influence

ठ   ठ   ठ

THOMAS INTENDED TO join Mary in her work—but first he needed skills. With a sense of mission, he returned to medical school, this time finishing the professional training half-heartedly begun at Dartmouth sixteen years earlier. Early in March 1850, Thomas received his medical degree with honors from the University of the City of New York. He was thus the second husband whose medical training Mary had helped finance. Newly minted, Dr. Nichols was summoned into joint practice immediately; he and Mary abandoned the commencement-night party in response to an emergency house call. During this period, Mary was seeing enough patients to earn nearly one hundred dollars per week and was maintaining correspondence with John Neal and Alonzo Lewis, to whom she mentioned visits from her friend Herman Melville. She also wrote that she had not been "honoring any church with her presence."[1]

Over the next decade, the Nicholses' careers steadily merged, fulfilling Thomas's courting prophecy that "the time will come when I shall see you all day." Mary taught her husband the intricacies of water cure, which he eagerly adopted. He was beginning to see himself as a professional advocate of health reform as well as a licensed physician. During the summer after graduation, he even founded a Society of Public Health, whose constitution read: "Believing that disease and premature death are, in most cases, the results of ignorant violations of the laws of health, by individuals and communities; and that the amount of such sickness, and the extent of such mortality, demand of the intelligent and philanthropic some preventive action; we, whose names are hereunto annexed, form ourselves into an association."

The American Medical Association (AMA) had been founded three years earlier, in 1847, with a code of ethics that explicitly disenfranchised alternative practitioners—even from such hygiene-oriented posts as members of public health boards. A strong impetus for the founding of the AMA had been the 1844 repeal of New York State's medical licensing statutes, a reform that increased competition for "regular" physicians by expanding opportunities for medical sectarians. Unlike Mary, who lacked the legitimation of a medical degree, Thomas had the luxury of appending M.D. to his name. He envisioned his Public Health Society producing lectures, tracts, and books, while pressuring legislators to "abolish all destructive nuisances, and secure . . . cleanliness, pure air, [and] proper food." Everywhere, Thomas identified ways in which the city undermined healthy living. He wanted to make the world entirely clean, entirely wholesome, entirely salubrious. His wife, after all, was pregnant.[2]

On November 5, 1850, forty-year-old Mary gave birth to a second daughter. In that month's issue of the *Water-Cure Journal*, Thomas published a lengthy article entitled "The Curse Removed. A Statement of Facts Respecting the Efficacy of Water-Cure, in the Treatment of Uterine Diseases, and the Removal of the Pains and Perils of Pregnancy and Childbirth." "It is no egotism in me to say," he wrote, "that I have studied this subject with very peculiar advantages, and such as no physician in this country has probably ever enjoyed. I allude, of course, to the aid, counsel, and assistance of my wife, whose intimate acquaintance with this branch of medical science, and whose extensive and most successful practice, are widely known and appreciated. . . . She has taught me far more, in connection with this subject, than I could ever have learned in all our medical libraries or colleges; and to her is justly due the credit of some of the most important reforms connected with the hydropathic treatment." A brand new father, Thomas stood in awe of his wife's accomplishments. Mary's successful pregnancy seemed to prove her teachings. In "The Curse Removed," Thomas reassures women that childbirth can be easy:

> In the adaptation of Water Cure to . . . pregnancy and childbirth, its efficacy comes so near the miraculous, that I hardly expect to be believed. . . . We prevent the nausea and vomitings of a diseased nervous system; we continually strengthen the muscles of the abdomen; we daily give tone and energy to the organs of reproduction; and when we have produced that state of health which belongs to the woman of na-

ture, we trust nature to do her own work, giving all the aid she requires, and careful not to obstruct or derange her beneficent operations.[3]

Thomas had learned his lessons well.

The Nicholses named their daughter Mary Wilhelmina—perhaps after Mary's father, William Neal—and they called her Willie. Elma was eighteen years old. Before Mary gave birth, the family decided to leave their small house at 46 Lexington Avenue (their first home together for which Mary and Elma had left the group arrangement on Tenth Street) and move uptown to 89 West 22nd Street, where Willie was born. There they had rented a more spacious home within easy walking distance of Union, Madison, and Grammercy Parks and close to the stage lines that stopped on Seventh Avenue and Broadway. They bought new furniture and soon opened the house to patients, some of whom would take full board and treatment, while others came for the consultations that Mary and Thomas provided six days a week from ten A.M. to two P.M. Three downstairs parlors opened onto one another, giving the house an airy feel. The front parlor they decorated in rosewood and red velvet; the middle parlor with black walnut. The back parlor, decorated in red and full of hanging pictures, served as Elma's art studio.[4]

Mary and Thomas considered Willie an exceptionally beautiful baby. She weighed eight and a half pounds, and had blue eyes and golden hair. Her delivery had gone extraordinarily well, despite the "worn and wasted" quality of Mary's youth. During her pregnancy, Mary had also published authoritative (and wishful) descriptions of pain-free childbirth, detailing the tasks of a skilled hydropathic midwife by describing her own methods. Women reading Mary's columns would find reassurance both from testimonials and from learning exactly what to expect procedurally: "One young lady, who was really far from being strong . . . suffered slightly one quarter of an hour. Another, with a first child, and whose friends frightened her all in their power, took the cure under my care, and when she was delivered she could hardly be said to suffer at all. . . . I said, after the birth, 'Were these efforts painful?' She hesitated, and then said, '*Slightly*.'" To the rhetorical objection that natural childbirth reduced women to the condition of animals, Mary responded, "And why should not the human mother suffer as little as the animals?" To avoid "pangs worse than those of death," Mary advised women to follow a strict hydropathic regimen throughout their lives and especially throughout their pregnancies: to avoid medicines, alcohol, caffeine, spices, fatty foods, gluttony, sloth, overwork, stale air, tight clothing, dirtiness, anxiety, and sex (during pregnancy); and to seek exercise, relaxation, healthy foods, comfortable clothing, daily baths in cold water, fresh air, and encouraging companionship.

"The truth must be literally dinned in the ears of the people before they can believe it," Mary wrote. "All their experience contradicts it." After enjoying the painless delivery of a healthy child, a woman who had followed such a course would recover hydropathically:

> As soon as a lady is perfectly delivered, *I use the vagina syringe, with cold water, throwing a pint or more upon the uterus.* This causes the organ to contract immediately, and saves the patient from afterpains. . . . I then wash the patient with a sponge, or towel, in cold water, and put a long, cold, wet bandage closely around the abdomen. She then is dressed, goes into a clean bed, and generally sleeps five or six hours. When she wakes, she goes into a cold sitz bath for fifteen minutes, and is sponged over the whole surface, also; a fresh wet bandage is then applied, and she is allowed to sit up for a short time if she wishes. . . . All [my patients] get up the day after the birth.

It should be noted that today's standard of care in many obstetrics wards is to provide immediately postnatal women with ice packs. The importance of a woman's prenatal care was likewise recognized by water-cure physicians at a time when allopathic obstetricians concerned themselves most centrally with the baby's delivery. Before delivering Willie, Mary herself had yet to experience anything but torturous parturition of either sickly or stillborn children. During this sixth and final pregnancy, she surely followed her own advice.[5]

Mary returned to her medical practice one week after Willie's birth, scheduling her patients to allow for regular nursing. For three months, Willie nursed every two hours, and then every three. Allowing others to feed Willie when professional demands made such frequent feedings unmanageable, Mary continued to nurse Willie for seven months, on a regular schedule, without abandoning her career. At times Willie also required her medical attention. In the first month of her life, she suffered from whooping cough, which Mary successfully treated by packing her newborn in cool wet sheets twice a day. She also suffered for three months from frequent bouts of colic, during which she screamed violently. Mary and Thomas treated her with morning and evening baths, rubbing, daily enemas at 70° F., fasting, and occasional wet-sheet packing. Mary recalled that bathing Elma every day in cold water had helped her first baby survive despite what seemed a very fragile constitution.[6]

Articulating the principles of water cure had grown into a consuming professional commitment for Mary and Thomas. In 1850 Mary had published *Experience in Water-Cure*, which the *Democratic Review* favorably reviewed.[7] Soon after, Thomas published both *An Introduction to Water-Cure* and *The Curse Removed* (a pamphlet edition of his article in the *Water-Cure Journal*). Writing in the *Water-Cure Journal* on "The Diseases of Women," Thomas railed against the interventionist nature of allopathic obstetrics: "Their daily examinations, so utterly useless, cannot fail to outrage, and in time to blunt, every feeling of delicacy, while their scarifications, leechings, cauterizings, even the application of red hot iron to the mouth of the womb, produce the most deplorable results." It was not unusual for many allopathic physicians to rely on blood-letting, as they understood the cessation of menses during pregnancy to cause an excess of blood in the system, causing a harmful congestion. For treatment of menstrual disorders, Thomas recommended a "strengthening of the whole system," noting that "in the common practice of medicine, a local disease does not seem to be considered as a symptom of general disease. . . . In all cases where a local affection is not the effect of direct injury or poison, the disease is constitutional, and can only be cured by constitutional remedies." Thomas, who granted that it would probably surprise many readers, considered a menstrual period of "more than two day's continuance, or of more than one ounce, or even somewhat less" to be "a sign of disease." For prolapsed uterus (descent of the uterus into the vagina), Thomas recommended a local treatment intended to invigorate and tone the whole body: wet bandages around the lower abdomen, cold sitz-baths, and regular vaginal injections of cold water, self-administered as often as four times a day with a quart of cold water per application. Unlike allopathic physicians, hydrotherapists advocated a holistic approach to the body, viewing disease as constitutional in origin, and a localized disorder as evidence of a systemic problem.[8]

Their writings established the Nicholses as highly visible authorities on water cure. But other interests drew their attention as well. In 1849 Mary also completed her novel, *Agnes Morris; or, The Heroine of Domestic Life* and produced a new one: *The Two Loves; or Eros and Anteros.* That same year, Thomas published *Woman in all Ages and Nations,* an elaborate treatment of the political and social status of women throughout history and around the globe. There he defended women's history as being "of no less importance than men's." The 1854 edition of this work included a lengthy quotation from the 1848 Seneca Falls Declaration of Sentiments, which Thomas allowed to speak for itself, inserting only the comment that the document might "be of interest to the future historian."[9] Marriage had energized the Nicholses. Between their wedding in July 1848 and Thomas's graduation in May 1850, they wrote four books, contributed regularly to the *Water-Cure Journal,* treated hundreds of patients, and were expecting a child. Witness to suffering and strengthened in partnership, Mary and Thomas grew increasingly determined to bring about change in the emotional, political, and physical relationships between men and women.

THE AMERICAN HYDROPATHIC INSTITUTE

On September 15, 1851, Mary and Thomas opened the doors of the nation's first hydropathic medical school: the American Hydropathic Institute. For more than two years, Mary had felt the city needed a formal water-cure training institution. Quacks could prey on the water-cure community as well as on any other, and Mary saw danger in the haphazard use of hydropathic treatments. Cold water's potency required expert application. Thomas had at first argued against the establishment of a separate water-cure college, advising instead that those interested in becoming practitioners follow the course he had pursued: first graduating from a regular medical college and then procuring an apprenticeship with an experienced and trustworthy hydrotherapist at an established water-cure house. His advice grew not from respect for his own medical education, but rather from resistance to establishing a similar structure: "Again and again have I sat an hour, hearing a distinguished professor talking against time, and reeling off a ridiculous rodomontade because he was obliged to lecture an hour, when all he had to say could have been plainly stated in five minutes. . . . The truth is, this whole system of colleges, professors and lecturers comes down to us from the barbarous ages, with very little, and some think, no improvement."[10]

By the spring of 1851, however, Thomas had joined Mary in proposing a new school. With the exceptions of the New England Female Medical College, the Woman's Medical College of Pennsylvania, and Geneva Medical College, existing medical schools would not admit women and therefore could not meet the undeniable urban need for qualified female physicians. For a year, Thomas had been promising readers of the *Water-Cure Journal* that if the city's two medical schools would not accept women, then he, with assistance, would personally provide coeducational instruction in "all the necessary branches of a thorough medical course." Mary was already meeting privately with a group of women interested in becoming hydropathic practitioners.[11]

Once Thomas agreed to the plan for a new institution, he and Mary began to search for an appropriate site. They chose an elegant, spacious home at 91 Clinton Place, furnished with a gymnasium and all the necessary plumbing for a full hydropathic education. When they were not teaching, Mary and Thomas intended to continue their outpatient consultations. At the institute's inaugural ceremonies, Mary delivered an address entitled "Woman the Physician," in which she relied on common assumptions about female character to argue for the training of women as doctors. "Women are peculiarly fitted to practice the art of healing," she explained, as they have "tenderer love, . . . sublimer devotion, [and] . . . never to be wearied patience and kindness." But she went even further: "We want women who can break the bonds of custom, who are great enough to be emancipated from all that weakens, degrades, and destroys, and who will teach others . . . not to be independent of man, but that man and woman should be mutually dependent."[12]

Thomas also advocated medical education for women, writing in the *Water-Cure Journal:* "Women must become their own physicians, and the physicians of each other. They have leaned too long on a broken reed. Their diseases have been the subject of mercenary speculations, of mischievous medications, of torturing mechanical inventions, of nameless brutalities, and detestable charlatanism; but they have got little or no relief." By way of example, Thomas described an unnamed practitioner in New York City, a "libidinous wretch," who employed "manipulations and anointings, managed in such a way as to stimulate the passions, and produce a temporary excitement of the organs, which his deluded victims mistake for a beneficial result. These have to be repeated, until the effect is lost. . . . This has been the lamentable experience of thousands of women in this city; and as the practice is extremely lucrative, it has been taken up in other places. No words can add to the contempt and detestation every honest man and every pure-minded woman must feel for such shameful practices." Candidates who enrolled in the Nicholses' Institute understood from the start that their instructors had feminist aims.[13]

Despite his earlier objection to the lecture format, Thomas alone prepared and delivered 250 one-hour lectures during the school's first year of operation; he also contributed regular articles to the *American Vegetarian and Health Journal,* was elected secretary of the American Hygienic and Hydropathic Association of Physicians and Surgeons, and served as one of several vice presidents of the American Vegetarian Society. His life scarcely resembled the one he had known three years earlier before meeting Mary. "I believe that I look, and I am sure that I feel, ten years younger to-day, than I did three years ago," he wrote in February 1851. "I am at my highest point of weight, one hundred and forty pounds. I can carry a person as heavy as myself up a long flight of stairs; or undergo almost any amount of labor, bodily or mental, without permanent fatigue."[14]

Such energy was necessary for the ambitious curriculum the Nicholses designed. The complete course of instruction took three intensive months and covered anatomy, physiology, pathology, chemistry, natural philosophy, surgery, obstetrics, and hydrotherapeutics. In addition, students had access to a select medical library as well as to some of the city's hospitals, clinics, and anatomical museums. Wax and papier-mâché models, engravings, dissection, and various preparations supplemented anatomy lectures. Tuition totaled fifty dollars.[15]

Students attended three hours of morning lecture five days each week; on Saturdays they learned examination techniques. Occasional afternoons found the students studying anatomy and pathology in separate anatomical rooms. And in the evenings either the Nicholses or invited guest lecturers spoke on philosophy, morality, phrenology, and social science. During the fall of 1851, Mary delivered more than sixty lectures on "the principles of physiology and pathology, special diagnosis, the diseases of

women and children, . . . midwifery, and . . . special diseases." Thomas
spoke on natural philosophy, anatomy, physiology, pathology, and, with
special emphasis, diagnosis and therapeutics—two subjects he thought
lacking in the curricula of allopathic schools. Whenever possible he also
reinforced the advantages of vegetarianism.[16]

The first class of graduates included nine women and eleven men; the
second class, of about the same size, included an even larger proportion of
women. These students had come from places as far away as the deep
South, Ohio, and New England. Approximately half the first class—ranging in age from twenty-one to forty-one—had spouses. Some brought
their families with them to New York City, but most boarded in a group
house near Union Square that Mary and Thomas had arranged for their
students. The backgrounds of the students ranged considerably. Some had
practiced law or medicine; others had pursued the ministry, teaching, or
journalism; still others, the lecture circuit. Several simply sought to improve the quality of care they provided their own families, while others
later became practicing hydrotherapists. Several of these graduates went
on to found water-cure schools and practices of their own. The Nicholses'
school, of course, had no authority to confer professional medical degrees.
Instead, graduates received diplomas stating that they had completed the
full program of lectures and had "acquired such thorough knowledge of
the Principles and Practices of Medicine, Surgery, and Obstetrics," to ensure their competence "as water-cure physicians."[17]

Through their many columns in the *Water-Cure Journal and Herald of
Reforms,* Mary and Thomas further established their position of authority within the water-cure movement. Launched in 1844 under the editorship of Joel Shew, the *Water-Cure Journal* had attracted approximately
50,000 subscribers by the end of 1852. Russell Thatcher Trall took over
the role of editor in 1849. A large-featured man with full beard, high forehead, and stern brow, Trall, like Thomas Nichols, had earned a regular
medical degree before turning to hydrotherapy. The two men had a great
deal in common. Three years older than Thomas and also raised in New
England, Trall graduated in 1835 from Albany Medical College. (Had he
not left Dartmouth, Thomas would have earned his M.D. at the same
time.) Trall opened a water-cure house in Manhattan's west side in 1844,
only a year after Joel and Marie Louise Shew had established a similar
treatment facility in their home at 47 Bond Street. He soon moved his

"Hygieo-Therapeutic Cure" to 15 Laight Street, which remained its address into the 1860s and eventually came to occupy a double house and neighboring building, accommodating almost one hundred patients. Contributing regularly to the *Water-Cure Journal*, Trall advanced many of the same causes that inspired Mary and Thomas: dress reform, vegetarianism, temperance, the value of exercise, the importance of training women as physicians, and, of course, hydrotherapy.[18]

In 1852, Trall was serving with Thomas Nichols on the board of the American Vegetarian Society. Together with one Jonathan Wright, the two men also constituted the society's "Committee upon Resolutions," articulating the core purpose of the organization's 120 members. Their collaboration generated paragraphs of scientifically grounded defense for vegetarianism as well as calls for support from leaders of the Temperance Movement and from Sabbath school directors and teachers. Mary and Thomas Nichols, Russell Thatcher Trall, and Joel and Marie Louise Shew constituted the undisputed leadership of New York City's water-cure movement. For years, readers of the *Water-Cure Journal* received consistent advice from these encouraging advisers. But Trall and the Nicholses would soon become enemies.

In the spring of 1852, Mary and Thomas decided to move their school from New York City to the countryside. Leaving 91 Clinton Place, they purchased six acres of land in nearby Port Chester, New York, and began promoting the third term of the American Hydropathic Institute. At the same time, they kept an office in the city where on Wednesdays they continued to receive outpatient consultations and from which they could maintain ties with other water-cure professionals. William Alcott, the prominent health reformer who in 1838 had invited Mary to give her first lecture to the Ladies Physiological Society of Boston, helped to promote their efforts. Writing in the *American Vegetarian and Health Journal*, he declared, "If any body in this country, can succeed in carrying out the noble plan [they propose], it is our friends and fellow laborers at Prospect Hill, Port Chester. They are as free from humbuggery as seems possible . . . and as full of philanthropy. . . . We wish we could insert . . . the whole of the circular they have sent us. . . . In the name, and for the sake of bleeding, poisoned, dying humanity, it is impossible not to bid them God speed."[19]

ESOTERIC ANTHROPOLOGY

Thomas Low Nichols had finally found his footing. Thirty-seven years old, a physician, a writer, a husband, a father, a property-owner, and the proprietor of a school, this "fop" had come a long way. Mary had rescued him from a directionless existence of opportunistic journalism and bachelorhood. Her influence had sealed his commitment to health reform, to the principles of water cure, and to the rights of women. Thomas was ready for this cultivation. His early imprisonment in Buffalo provided him unusual empathy for anyone repressed by men of power. A lifelong affection for women and craving for audience likewise served his new focus. Mary encouraged his grandiose quests for praise and influence; they resembled her own. Therefore, Thomas did not have to divide his attention between his career and his wife. Devotion to one enriched the other.

Port Chester's fragrant air and expansive views inspired Thomas's work. Drawing together his mountain of lecture notes, Thomas threw himself into a project that would shape the rest of his career. In six weeks, he produced *Esoteric Anthropology; a Comprehensive and Confidential Treatise on the Structure, Functions, Passional Attractions and Perversions, True and False Physical and Social Conditions, and the Most Intimate Relations of Men and Women*. It was an outrageously sexual book. Lest authorship be confused, Mary assured her readers that she had not even read the book until it was "printed, bound, and laid upon my table."[20] She considered the work a masterpiece.

Describing *Esoteric Anthropology* (which he published himself), Thomas wrote,

> It is not a book for the centre-table, or the counter, but for the closet. All books of Physiology, so far as I have examined them, are dry, hard, mechanical, or chemical, without soul, or passion, or depth of intuition. The popular works are usually shallow in matter, and involved in method.
>
> For the most part, the books written upon the generative function have been false in science, absurd in philosophy, mischievous in morals, and mercenary in their motives.[21]

Thomas intended to hold his readers' interest. The text came to 482 pages and included 81 illustrations. From birth to death, from lust to sex,

Esoteric Anthropology balked at nothing. Practical as well as scientific, Thomas's book explained the processes of water cure; the gestation, delivery and management of infants; the methods of contraception; and the nature of many emotional disorders. It also covered anatomy, physiology, pathology, "the chemistry of man," and obstetrics. Thomas devoted chapters to the organs and diseases of "the general system," of respiration, of digestion, of the brain, and of the generative system. His unprecedented textbook merged the science of New York University Medical College with the hydropathic principles of Vincent Priessnitz, the dietetics of Sylvester Graham with the social theory of Charles Fourier. Intended to change the world, *Esoteric Anthropology* was an extremely thorough, broad-ranging, and sexually explicit work. It sold thousands of copies.

If one can believe the *Nichols' Journal, Esoteric Anthropology* appealed to married and single readers of both sexes and of widely differing backgrounds. One column on the "Opinions of Clergymen, Professors, Physicians, Ladies, and Others, of *Esoteric Anthropology*" presents a series of excerpts from effusive letters sent to the Nicholses in praise and appreciation of the book. "Your book . . . is a daguerreotype of Nature, undressed for the sitting," wrote "a physician from Georgia." A Philadelphia clergyman wrote to a friend that the book "ought to be possessed by every family throughout the . . . land, and universally read." Alonzo Lewis, "the celebrated bard and historian of Lynn," wrote to a friend: "My judgment is, that this is not only the best book on the subjects on which it treats, but the only true and satisfactory one ever written. It contains what every marriageable woman ought to know. A friend, to whom I loaned my copy, has kept it for his wife." An Ohio gentleman "would not exchange the ideas [he] had got from . . . *Esoteric Anthropology* for fifty dollars." And Isabel Pennel Stevens, who with her husband had graduated from the American Hydropathic Institute and opened a new water-cure establishment in Forest City, New York, wrote that the book "should be in the possession of all who desire their own or the world's welfare." Many other correspondents echoed these sentiments.[22]

Esoteric Anthropology, bound in flexible brown or black muslin with gilt lettering, cost one dollar and could be purchased through the mail. Promotional excerpts from the text appeared regularly in the *Nichols' Journal,* explaining the importance of exercise or the "reciprocity of influences" among the body's systems or the necessity of rest for the sick or the value of natural foods or the integral relationship between freedom and health. These relatively unobjectionable paragraphs may not have prepared purchasers of Thomas's work for the detailed anatomical engravings or for the unembarrassed descriptions that accompanied them. For example, illustrations of two erect penises literally framed the following text:

> Its shape is that of a cylinder, not perfectly regular, with a soft, delicate cushion, called the glans penis, at the end. This is the most sensitive portion of the organ, and in performing the sexual function, is the seat of exquisite pleasure. . . . In repose, it is small, soft, flabby, and easily compressible; but when in vigorous erection, it is distended, hard, and unbending. The change from one state to the other occurs in a moment, at a word, a thought, or a touch.

The visual representation of the female "organs of generation" was no less delicate. Rather than depict the female pelvis only in relatively modest cross section—a more traditional choice for popular health texts of the era—Thomas also selected an engraving that provided readers with a direct view of the female genitals, as if sketched by an artist positioned between a supine woman's spread legs. "The clitoris," explained the accompanying text, "placed about the opening of the urethra, is a miniature, imperfect penis, capable of erection, and, in the sexual congress, receiving, from the friction of the parts where it is situated, the most vivid excitement of pleasure." This ready willingness to discuss sexual pleasure sharply distinguished both Thomas and Mary from their medical peers— and they knew it.[23]

If the anatomical passages did not trouble prim readers, the unashamed descriptions of sex probably did. In a chapter deliberately titled "Miscellaneous," Thomas addressed such questions as "Is sexual enjoyment voluntary?" and "Can one love two or more persons at once?" Describing "the expressions of love antecedent to, and connected with its ultimation," Thomas wrote,

> The heart swells, and beats tumultuously; . . . a new delight pervades the sense of feeling . . . ; every touch, even of the hem of the garment, is a deep pleasure; the hands clasp each other with a thrill of delight;

the lips cling together in dewy kisses of inexpressible rapture; the bolder hands of man wander over the ravishing beauties of woman; he clasps her waist, he presses her soft bosom, and in a tumult of delirious ecstasy, each finds the central point of attraction and of pleasure, which increases until it is completed.[24]

Regarding orgasm, which he called "the most exquisite enjoyment of ... the human senses," Thomas explained that women, more so than men, had the power to control their own measure of sexual excitement. "Wives who do not love their husbands save all their amative feelings for their paramours," he wrote (a belief quite possibly based on personal experience). "There are thousands of women, however, who never experience the ecstasy of a sexual orgasm." He added:

> There are others in whom it can only be excited with great difficulty, and by various artifices. The more spontaneous the feeling, the less exhausting; the more difficult to excite, the more it tasks the vital energies. Men are naturally desirous that their partners should experience pleasure, as it adds to their own. To effect this, they resort to manipulations of the clitoris, with their fingers, etc., and to various novel, and, to a certain extent, unnatural methods and positions. Out of these grow terrible mischiefs, especially to women.[25]

Thomas explained that ovarian and uterine disease resulted from such contrived exertions. Some women, however, could easily enjoy "six or seven orgasms in rapid succession, each seeming to be more violent and ecstatic than the last" and sometimes "accompanied with screams, bitings, spasms, and end in a faint languor, that will last for many hours." Thomas likewise claimed to know a man who had nine orgasms a night. For health, however, he advised readers to seek no more than one orgasm per week on average—a recommendation that quadrupled the allotment suggested by Sylvester Graham twenty years earlier.[26]

The uncensored quality of Thomas's prose on this subject can best be appreciated when compared to contemporary medical work directed at a similar audience of readers. Consider the roundabout style of Dr. J. H. Pulte's *Woman's Medical Guide; Containing Essays on the Physical, Moral and Educational Development of Females and the Homeopathic Treatment of Their Diseases in All Periods of Life, Together with Directions for the Remedial Use of Water and Gymnastics:*

> The immediate effect of marriage on the well and fully developed female organism, consists in the greater vigor and increase of vitality and sensibility in all the organs influenced by the physical and moral changes which have taken place in her condition. . . . The enjoyment of the senses, so cautiously approached, but at the same time so rationally bestowed by matrimony, opens a new portal in the secret chambers of nature for another series of physical developments, different from what had taken place in the organism of the girl, during its preparation for womanhood, but based upon these proceedings, which are now brought to a higher and final perfection. . . . When in matrimony . . . the conditions of nature are fulfilled, this ovule becomes impregnated.

This text, like Thomas's, appeared in 1853. Yet by contrast, it included no illustrations, as those that would do justice to the subject "might be considered objectionable on the score of propriety and good taste." Pulte's work entirely avoided discussion of "healthy" sex, addressing the subject only in its diseased forms of nymphomania or anaphrodisy (the absence of erotic feeling). The first received consideration as a "criminal passion," and the second a delicate referral to a physician.[27]

Thomas, on the other hand, believed that the subject of sexual intercourse deserved serious and unflinching attention: "The strength of the attraction for sexual union, and the exquisite and delicious pleasure it brings, in a healthy state, to both sexes all point to other uses and ends than those of procreation. . . . It is folly to say that the exercise of such a faculty, and the enjoyment of such a pleasure, is a sin." Without shame, he discussed the nature and consequences of sexual arousal at a time when most people deemed even the critical discussion of marriage laws to be a radical pursuit. Resisting prudery, Thomas explicitly analyzed the complicated relationship between marriage and sex, judging these topics inseparable and vitally important. Though either might provide the deepest source of happiness, Thomas had no doubt that marital sex could also kill. "A cursed despotism under the name of legal marriage, compels a woman to receive the embraces of a man she loathes, or, if she loves him, at the peril of her life," he wrote, reminding readers of the dangers inherent to pregnancy. Men, too, found themselves trapped in bad marriages, and Thomas found their plight equally compelling:

> If a man moves into a bad house, he changes it for another; if he gets into a bad neighborhood, he moves out of it; if he falls into a quagmire, he scrabbles out. That two young persons, who have flirted, and danced, and simpered, and dawdled through a fashionable courtship, and then stood up before a parson, in white gloves, satin, and orange flowers, should be compelled to bore, and torment, and torture each other and every body about them, till one dies, or is sent to State prison, is a refinement of cruelty that only our absurd civilization could be guilty of.

Thomas was saucy but serious. The physical sequelae of bad marriages were often tragic. As a doctor, Thomas had encountered afflictions and injuries that would inform his candid discussion of reproduction—a discussion that addressed the responsibilities as well as the pleasures of sex.[28]

Thomas believed that woman, as "passional queen," should claim absolute control over her own body. Any lover should honor her wish that "'thus far shalt thou come, and no farther.'" Because women obviously bore the physical burdens of conception more severely than did men, Thomas argued not only for their undisputed right to decide when or whether to have sex but also when, or whether, to have children—and with whom. His book described a practical variety of contraceptive methods for use when abstinence was either undesirable or impossible. In addition to what is now known as the "rhythm method," Thomas explained the use of the condom, the vaginal sponge, the cold-water vaginal douche, and the techniques of withdrawal and of compressing the penis during ejaculation. One form of contraception he knew about but did not describe among the others was "male continence"—intercourse without male orgasm. Later in the text, Thomas acknowledged the possibility that "men with strong wills and moderate amativeness may obtain this control." Yet his wording suggests skepticism. He may also have felt that the method wrongly placed contraception under the control of men rather than women. However, the chief advocate for the practice of male continence, John Humphrey Noyes, shared Thomas's conviction that women should only have children at will. He preceded Thomas in boldly presenting his thoughts about the nature and politics of sexual intercourse.[29]

In 1848, Noyes published *The Bible Argument,* a brief pamphlet that explained and promoted the practice of male continence. Like Mary, Noyes's wife, Harriet, had suffered repeated stillbirths. In six years she had survived five births, four of which were premature and only one of which resulted in a living child. "After our last disappointment," wrote John, "I pledged my word to my wife that I would never again expose her to such fruitless suffering. I made up my mind to live apart from her, rather than break this promise." He made this decision in the summer of 1844. John and Harriet did not sleep apart for long, however. To find sexual fulfillment without risking conception, John learned to distinguish the "amative" from the "propagative" functions of sex. He considered his "discovery" a "great deliverance" and began to tell his friends about his newfound method of self-control. "The discharge of the semen, instead of being the main act of sexual intercourse, . . . is really the sequel and termination of it," he wrote. "Ordinary sexual intercourse (in which the amative and propagative functions are confounded) is a momentary affair, terminating in exhaustion and disgust. If it begins in the spirit, it soon ends in the flesh; i.e., the amative, which is spiritual, is drowned in the propagative, which is sensual. The exhaustion which follows naturally breeds self-reproach and shame."[30]

Noyes considered the amative properties of sex superior to the propagative, and described the practice of male continence as follows:

The situation may be compared to a stream in the three conditions of a fall, a course of rapids above the fall, and still water above the rapids. The skillful boatman may choose whether he will remain in the still water, or venture more or less down the rapids, or run his boat over the fall. But there is a point on the verge of the fall where he has no control over his course; and just above that there is a point where he will have to struggle with the current in a way which will give his nerves a severe trial, even though he may escape the fall. If he is willing to learn, experience will teach him the wisdom of confining his excursions to the region of easy rowing, unless he has an object in view that is worth the cost of going over the falls.[31]

In short, Noyes touted male continence as "natural, healthy, favorable to amativeness, and effectual." He also rejected the notion that men have a physiological need to discharge seed more often than they produce children: "Even if this were true, it would be no argument against Male Continence, but rather an argument in favor of masturbation; for it is obvious that before marriage men have no lawful method of discharge but masturbation; and after marriage it is as foolish and cruel to expend one's seed on a wife merely for the sake of getting rid of it, as it would be to fire a gun at one's best friend merely for the sake of unloading it."[32] Like Sylvester Graham and the Shakers, Noyes believed that semen should not be wasted, but this did not suggest to him the need for infrequent sex or celibacy.

Noyes employed these philosophies dramatically and rather publicly in the context of the Oneida Community, a highly controversial socialistic home in Utica, New York, which he and several of his family members established in 1848 and which thrived until 1881, when it became a joint-stock company known today for its quality silverware. As a Christian Perfectionist, Noyes believed that Christ's second coming had already occurred (in A.D. 70) and that it was therefore possible for a human being to live a morally perfect life—to be entirely free of sin. Through faith, argued Noyes, one could unite spiritually with the kingdom of saints in heaven; in fact, Noyes considered himself to be living a sinless life. His peers at the Yale Divinity School had found all of these claims heretical.

What most shocked the wider public about Noyes and his followers at Oneida, however, were their attitudes toward sex. Members of the Oneida Community considered sex to be a form of divine worship, reflecting the highest expression of spiritual love and not intended for monogamic relationships cloaked in privacy. Instead, they practiced "group marriage," a system by which all physically mature community members were (hetero)sexually available to one another. This began with early adolescence and depended upon male continence, which Noyes endorsed only for those who had achieved a "true faith and union with God"—i.e., members of Oneida. The use of male continence as a secular form of contraception was as abhorrent to Noyes as his own principles were to the general public. His religion led him to dismiss the health reform movement as misguided, believing that faith, not hygienic regimen or medication, cured disease. He even banished Graham bread from Oneida because it symbolized slavery to the physiologic laws preached by health reformers.[33]

With regard to a woman's right to control her own body, however, Thomas Nichols and John Humphrey Noyes were both radicals. No woman, they believed, should be asked or expected to bear a child against her wishes. The stillbirths suffered by Mary and Harriet led their husbands to write some of the nineteenth century's most forceful rhetoric in defense of women's physical self-ownership. That the two men had little else in common serves to underline the powerful influence of their wives' experiences. Noyes had written that "good sense and benevolence will *very soon* sanction and enforce the rule that women shall bear children only when they choose." Thomas echoed that "the ovum belongs to the mother," and he even went so far as to assert, "It is the same after pregnancy. [The ovum] still rests with the mother. . . . [Abortion] may be very wicked. But it is exclusively her own affair. The mother, and she alone, has the right to decide whether she will continue the being of the child she has begun. The wishes of the father should weigh with her—all obligations, moral, social, religious, should control her; but she alone has the supreme right to decide." No other nineteenth-century medical adviser had defended a woman's right to abortion with such categorical resolve.[34]

In his discussion of managing childbirth, Thomas likewise emphasized the importance of the mother's wishes. Even in later editions of *Esoteric Anthropology*, published when male doctors had in good measure displaced female midwives in the birthing chamber, Thomas argued that the presence of a male accoucheur was a question that "women should decide." Provided that the attendant possessed requisite skill, "the most proper man, I think, is the one a woman most wants," he wrote. "When called to a patient, my first object is to establish with her that degree of friendly and familiar confidence which will make my aid agreeable. This is very necessary; and the want of it may make the labor more protracted and severe." Such sensitivity to the woman's perspective encompassed more than token compassion for the awkward indelicacy of a man's assistance through childbirth. Thomas respected women's autonomy and women's bodies. In selecting engravings to illustrate his chapter on human anatomy, he even chose a drawing of a woman's body to depict "the Vital System": heart, lungs, liver, stomach, spleen, kidneys, and so forth. (The tendency of medical educators to rely on a male default model for the generic human became a late-twentieth-century issue of contention in American medical schools.) Writing that water cure "brings to women the strength and power of their natural condition," Thomas encouraged the realization of women's innate capacity with language that logically recommended the expansion of women's rights. At a time when society deemed women the "weaker" sex and denied them the vote, female "strength and power" attested to the need for political change. "I do not exaggerate the perfections of woman," wrote Thomas. "I think I know her character, and I demand her rights, not so much for her own sake as for the sake of all."[35]

Esoteric Anthropology challenged readers to abandon shame, propriety, and tradition. Its closest competitor was written by Frederick Hollick, an extremely popular writer and lecturer whose 1850 work *The Marriage Guide, or Natural History of Generation; A Private Instructor for Married Persons and Those About to Marry Both Male and Female* also treated its subject forthrightly. Hollick taught that a moderate amount of sexual activity was healthy; he also encouraged women as well as men to seek a thorough understanding of physiology and to consider the maintenance of health a moral issue. Likewise, Thomas was not the only widely read medical writer to address the pleasures of sex. Three years after the release of *Esoteric Anthropology*, William Alcott rhetorically asked thousands of readers whether God might have intended sex to be more than merely procreative: "Why should [women's] susceptibility to pleasure . . . continue beyond the age to which child bearing is limited?" He also noted that "the pleasures of love, no less than the strength of the orgasm, are enhanced by their infrequency."[36] However most medical prose of the era demurred from such conversation.

By emphasizing the connections between sexual physiology and politics, *Esoteric Anthropology* stood apart. "Nature has been very bountiful in the distribution of the sources of happiness," Thomas wrote in reference to sexual pleasure. "It is man alone that is niggard and perverse." Drawing on Fourier, Thomas reiterated the belief that God created no morbid passions. Rather, human society generated its own woes by condemning and suppressing desire. As Thomas put it, "No *natural* passion, no *healthy* attraction of any being is wrong. . . . We produce only discord, when we use our freedom to oppose them." Thomas did not advocate wild indulgence; he sought to modify rather than jettison the recurring emphasis on "self-denial" so apparent in contemporary hydropathic texts. Praise of temperance and disparagement of tobacco found their place in *Esoteric Anthropology* as well. Yet sexual love—with its extreme physical, spiritual, and social consequences—took analytical precedence: "The whole powers of the body and soul are engaged in [the sexual congress], which confers the greatest happiness upon the individual—which is the basis of social harmonies, or the source of social discords, and which is of absolute necessity to the life of the race." Nothing was more central than sexual well-being.[37]

When Thomas claimed at the end of his work that "I have not written a book on morals, but on science," readers were surely bemused. "Some of the most crushing sins against social laws, are acts of the simplest conformity to natural law," he argued. "What is more natural than that a healthful, passionate woman should give herself in love to a man whom she believes to be worthy of her? The stronger, and healthier, and better she is, the more she is impelled to such an act. . . . The women most likely to outrage society, in love relations, are the truest, the noblest, the greatest, and those we should most delight to honor."[38]

By June of 1853, the *Nichols' Journal* announced that demands for *Esoteric Anthropology* had required the release of six editions in less than four months and that the seventh and eighth editions would be printed and bound in two styles: "A FINE CABINET edition, superior paper, and extra full cloth binding . . . and the POCKET MAIL edition, in flexible muslin." In July, Thomas claimed to have sold over 10,000 copies. The large New York publishing house of Stringer and Townsend had also contracted for the wholesale distribution of the work.[39] Thomas and Mary were naturally encouraged by this enthusiastic reception of the book. But they faced disappointment as well: Russell Thatcher Trall—who shared much of the Nicholses' feminism and an equal devotion to water cure—despised it. Though for years a close colleague, Trall found Thomas's explicit and nontraditional treatment of sex an embarrassment to the water-cure community. As editor of the *Water-Cure Journal*, Trall did not even acknowledge the book's existence.

PROSPECT HILL

Russell Trall's refusal to promote *Esoteric Anthropology* in the pages of the *Water-Cure Journal* infuriated Thomas. When Thomas made brief reference to the book in columns devoted to other subjects, Trall eliminated these lines before sending the proofs to press. As Thomas later wrote, "neither love nor money" could persuade the editor of the journal to recognize his work.[40] Thomas was even denied the purchase of advertising space. Trall wanted no association between his *Water-Cure Journal* and the scandalous book. But *Esoteric Anthropology* did more than offend Trall. It also competed with Trall's own new book, *The Hydropathic Encyclopedia: A System of Hydropathy and Hygiene,* which the reform-oriented publishing house of Fowlers and Wells had brought to press in 1850 and which Thomas heartily recommended in the opening pages of *Esoteric Anthropology.*

Trall's two-volume, 972-page text overlapped considerably with Thomas's briefer work. In fact, when discussing childbirth, Trall quoted at length from Thomas's pamphlet *The Curse Removed,* as well as from Mary's *Lectures to Ladies. Esoteric Anthropology* and *The Hydropathic Encyclopedia* even shared many of the same engravings, though not the racy ones. (In 1853, copyright laws did not prevent free reproduction of published illustrations, even without credit to the original source.) Both works covered the topics of anatomy, physiology, obstetrics, water cure, diet, and hygiene. And yet the works differed. Trall devoted many more pages to the history of medicine, to descriptions of particular diseases, and to hydropathic cookery than did Thomas, in addition to including more than a hundred pages on surgical procedures, a subject Thomas did not address. Likewise, *Esoteric Anthropology* explored territory untouched by Trall. Some index headings that appear in Thomas's work but not in the index of the *Hydropathic Encyclopedia* include: amativeness, bosom, clitoris, coition, food (amatory), impregnation, jealousy, love (eight listings), polyandry, polygamy, sexual congress, and sexual morality. To an allopathic physician, Thomas Nichols and Russell Trall might have appeared indistinguishable—but they were not.

As a follower of Fourier, Thomas sought to restructure society on a grand scale. His devotion to health reform and specifically to the self-help nature of water cure had as much to do with freedom as with physiology. The condition of the body reflected the condition of the soul. False social conditions induced the "dis-ease" and unhappiness that parents passed to their children. Both Russell Trall and Thomas Nichols considered the balanced expression of passions integral to health, but Trall's medical advice reinforced traditional mores, whereas *Esoteric Anthropology* sought social reform. "All the propensities with which we are endowed were intended to be exercised actively and vigorously," wrote Trall, "but if one or several 'grow mutinous and rave,' the whole physiological and psychological nature experiences a deterioration proportional to the time and degree in which ungoverned passion is in the ascendant." Thomas would agree with this generalization. But where Trall advised readers to "cultivate the 'better passions'" and "study to acquire self-government," Thomas directed those suffering from "passional diseases" to "energize the mind, and purify it of false ideas." He specifically recommended the writings of Charles Fourier and the tract *Science of Society* by Stephen Pearl Andrews.[41]

Clothing his arguments in a consistent tone of rational empiricism, Thomas braided his radical political opinions with accepted science. "No essay on the function of generation can be complete, if it leaves out of view the phenomenon of prostitution," he wrote, presenting opinion as fact.

> The common prostitute is, in some respects, worse off than the victim of marriage. She earns her living by the prostitution of her body, as the other does, but without legal sanction and respectability. . . . [Yet] she has more freedom; and though she may be compelled to submit to the embraces of some man, she has, to a certain extent, the power to refuse those who are especially repulsive to her. She is liable to venereal diseases, but these are not much worse than falling of the womb, whites, and involuntary pregnancies and childbirths. Besides, wives do not always escape gonorrhea and syphilis. . . . Bad as [prostitution] is, many a married woman is worse off than the average of prostitutes.[42]

Russell Trall, in contrast, considered his discussion of reproduction complete without a full page of text comparing wives to whores. *Esoteric Anthropology* was full of such passages. Thomas chose to notice what others preferred to mask.

"[Masturbation] prevails to about an equal extent in both sexes, and probably not more than one person in ten, of either sex, entirely escapes it," Thomas calmly explained, unruffled by the idea that 90 percent of the population practiced "self-pollution." Regarding homosexuality, he wrote, "I see no reason for punishing a man for an act which begins and ends with himself, or with a consenting party. . . . Sodomy . . . has been practiced from the remotest ages, and is still so common in Eastern and tropical countries, as not to excite remark." He noted the arbitrary nature of modesty, observing: "A delicate lady, who would blush to show her leg to the knee, thinks nothing of . . . showing half her bosom." With a "facts are facts" attitude, Thomas even addressed the morally loaded subject of monogamy as if it were a question of elementary mathematics:

> Can One Love Two Or More Persons At Once? This is simply a question of capacity. One man is stronger than another; one has far greater versatility. . . . I knew one woman who slept with two men on alternate nights, and she declared that she loved them both, and could not endure the thought of parting with either. They were two respectable business men in New York, satisfied with her, and not jealous of each other. . . . Over three quarters of the world polygamy is tolerated, and more or less practiced. It is absurd to suppose that no man ever loves more than one wife; as absurd as to suppose that European and American women, as long as they love their husbands, can love nobody else. . . . The monogamic idea is . . . the parent of jealousy and all its tyrannies.

These were no minor claims. In a book that also explained how to bathe, what to eat, and how to manage illness, Thomas Nichols advocated free love, free divorce, free thought—and inviolable self-ownership. "Our bodies change, our opinions change, our feelings change," he wrote persuasively. "No exclusive love can possibly last that does not satisfy."[43]

Like Thomas Nichols, Russell Trall believed himself strongly committed to the honest presentation of scientific fact and unfettered by the "false delicacy" of small-minded moralists or misguided allopaths. His *Hydropathic Encyclopedia* defended the education of women as physicians, explained the physiology of conception, and, despite its controversial nature, taught the contraceptive practice of the rhythm method: "There are thousands of married persons . . . whose circumstances . . . render many children a source of regret to the parents and misery to the offspring. . . . And who shall say that a knowledge of the origin of life is not as legitimately to be sought and understood as a knowledge of the growth, development, education, and preservation of it?" Though Trall's description of "sexual connection" consisted of no more than those two words, his straightforward explanation of the menstrual cycle's "safe" periods for intercourse reflected no squeamishness. And his subsequent defense of the passage sounded like something Thomas Nichols might have written: "I have no sympathy with the advocate for ignorance in relation to this or any other physiological law ordained for man's government. If God has made the law, it is man's privilege to learn it, and his duty to obey it; and, further, if there are such persons in existence as the objection supposes, they are themselves the strongest argument I can adduce in favor of my position. *They* should never be parents." Though a zealous advocate of health reform, Trall discovered his conservatism in reading *Esoteric Anthropology*.[44]

As with more famous rifts among philosophical peers, it is generally those most dedicated to an intellectual course who find any deviation intolerable. Freud's split with Jung stands as one of history's most famous examples. To those outside the water-cure movement, the Nicholses' dispute with Trall surely seemed "a tempest in a teapot." Yet for Mary and Thomas the situation proved to be life altering. In response to Trall's censure, they initiated the *Nichols' Journal of Health, Water-Cure, and Human Progress*. The monthly journal cost twenty-five cents per year for an individual subscriber and thirteen to sixteen cents per year for clubs of one hundred, depending on location. Its first number, printed in April 1853, devoted nearly a full page to Thomas's version of the couple's break with the *Water-Cure Journal*. "We continued to write, according to our promise, until our articles were first expurgated, and then declined; and we felt that we were absolved from our engagement." In other words, Trall had closed the door in Thomas's face. "It would have been strange," Thomas explained, "if my wife had consented to write for a paper from which her husband was thus excluded." Earlier in the same article, Thomas had described the feeling of this rejection: "It was like being turned out of a railway-train, in which our friends had taken passage. We were at liberty to take another train and lose our good company, or build a new railroad." Given the choice between submitting materials to the editor of some other journal and claiming the editorial chair for themselves, the Nicholses chose the latter. Thomas had considerable experience in journalism, and both wanted to convey their undiluted messages to the widest possible audience. It is also likely that they hoped to take some of "their readers" with them, as rebuke to Trall.[45]

In their new and unconstrained journal, the Nicholses described their "School of Life" at Prospect Hill in Port Chester, New York, a coastal town situated on the border between New York and Connecticut. For Thomas, the move from New York City to a breezy, green hillside overlooking Long Island Sound fulfilled a craving for the lost countryside of his youth. Living exclusively in cities for twenty years had enriched his romantic fantasies of the bucolic life, which were strong from the start. "What a picture of city life is this," Thomas had written as a young man, "when those who eat, drink and sleep, separated from us only by a brick wall four inches thick, neither know nor care, whether we are happy or miserable, dead or alive! The bride couch and the death-bed, may be separated by a thin partition. . . . Wherever we live, let us die in the country!" He dreamed often of a farm by the water, a small place of five or so acres, equipped with a boat—and not too far from a major city. Port Chester seemed to answer his dreams. Only an hour's ride from New York City on the New Haven Railroad and served by six trains each day, Port Chester made it possible for the Nicholses to begin building their utopian vision in earnest. The peace of mind and restful surroundings recommended by the Nicholses for many hydropathic cures was finally available to the prescribers. Time seemed to slow down. Surrounding apple orchards sweetened the air. From their two verandas, Thomas guessed they could gaze across two hundred square miles. Remembering life in the city, Thomas wrote, "Time is in a hurry, and at every pause we hear the ring of his scythe behind us." On Prospect Hill, with long views of sea and valleys, the days felt long.[46]

During the academic semesters, Mary and Thomas continued the curriculum of the American Hydropathic Institute. Their vision of the role they could play as educators had steadily broadened. During the first summer of 1852, Mary and Thomas had even begun to experiment with the establishment of a new "School of Integral Education," distinct in scope from their hydropathic medical college. Though ultimately envisioning a coeducational institution, they commenced with a class of about twenty girls and women, ages twelve to forty, and six teachers, including Elma. Brothers of some of the students lived with the Nicholses as well. Their presence convinced Mary and Thomas that coeducation would not hinder students' progress. In fact, Thomas asserted years later that "there are real evils in the separation of the sexes, which are possibly greater than would be likely to arise from their education together in well-ordered and properly regulated institutions, while there are considerable advantages to manners, morals, and intellectual development, in the influence which each sex has upon the other." From Prospect Hill, Mary wrote that she and Thomas no longer "consider ourselves doctors in the common understanding of the word . . . , but we consider ourselves educators—set apart by Providence for the work." By the end of the school's third term, Thomas estimated that between January and April of 1853, he and Mary received approximately four thousand letters, at the rate of three to four hundred per week, from all over the country. After the second summer, Thomas published a detailed description of the evolving school.[47]

At six o'clock every morning a bell awakened the community of students and teachers. Everyone was expected to take a full morning bath, using fresh water supplied daily to the bedrooms. The days followed a regular pattern of family-like communal living. The group breakfasted regularly at seven A.M. on coarse cream of wheat flavored with sugar and milk; "stewed potatoes; oatmeal; brown and white bread, butter, applesauce, milk, and water." After breakfast, everyone enjoyed free time until the day's first lecture at 10 A.M. Some used the mornings to study, others to exercise; some to play the piano, and others to relax or go into town. The morning lecture, drawn from a broad syllabus that sought to cover "nearly the whole range of science and expression," lasted for two hours. Such comprehensive lectures were followed by an hour of gymnasium exercise and then dinner at 1 P.M. (consisting of vegetables, eggs, puddings, and sometimes fish). After dinner, students' time was their own. Among other activities, the girls rowed boats on Long Island Sound, swam at the beach, collected rocks and plants, made use of private art studios, or participated in French or German classes. At 3 P.M. a second lecture, "equally comprehensive," demanded the group's focused attention. Many lectures took place outside, under the trees or at the beach. Supper at 7 P.M. included only bread, butter, and fruit. Evenings were devoted to music, dancing, and the rehearsal of plays (which Mary and Thomas felt compelled to defend as "lessons in elocution, and manners"). Everyone observed a strict lights-out at ten o'clock.[48] In many ways, days at Prospect Hill's "School of Integral Education" resembled those of students at today's liberal arts colleges.

Writing in April 1853 before this lovely summer schedule began, Thomas outlined the program of their new institution. He envisioned two four-month terms, beginning on the first of May and the first of November, leaving two two-month vacations. Students of all ages, both sexes,

single or married, would study together, each exerting a "refining influence" and sharing "harmonious sympathies," as in a large family. The
school would foster both physical and intellectual development, seeking
to create strong and graceful students as well as moral philosophers. To
this end, all students would bathe and exercise daily, partake of a plain
diet, and attend classes ranging from elocution to logic, from ancient
Greek to math, and—of course—from anatomy to physiology. Two
months later, the *Nichols' Journal* enthusiastically noticed that three former graduates of the American Hydropathic Institute, Dr. and Mrs.
Stephens (the latter of whom had served as their assistant in the summer
of 1852) and Miss Caroline E. Youngs, had initiated on May 1, 1853, "a
school of physical and mental education . . . modelled upon our own at
Port Chester." Despite their troubles with Russell Trall, the Nicholses' influence continued to spread.[49]

By the mid-1850s, hygienic doctrines preached by the water-cure movement had gained general acceptance. Even writers who did not consider
themselves health reformers were starting to emphasize the importance
of clean skin. As Jane G. Swisshelm put it in her popular book, *Letters to
Country Girls:*

> You good-for-nothing, baking, boiling, washing, scrubbing, scouring,
> saucy jades, how can you be so dirty? . . . Your body is perpetually de-
> caying and being renewed. . . . The way for these little dead particles
> to get away is through these thousands of curious little doors [pores]
> in your skin, and if you let them stick fast until the doors get closed
> up, . . . they must stay where they are not wanted, and load the fresh
> young blood with impurity, rottenness, and disease, just as if people
> were left in the house after they were dead and decaying. When you
> do not wash yourselves . . . no matter how much floor-scrubbing or tin-
> scouring you have done; no matter how many clean clothes you have
> on, you are dirty.[50]

Who today would argue? Most Americans feel less than wholly clean without a daily shower. We take for granted the importance of exercise and
fresh air, the dangers of alcohol and tobacco, and the desirability of comfortable clothing. We have even given women legal ownership of their
own bodies. Medical science and gender politics have come to vindicate
the radical hydrotherapists of antebellum America.

SIX

The Costs of Conviction

ભ્ર   ભ્ર   ભ્ર

MARY AND THOMAS looked around at their thriving school, their independent journal, the success of their graduates, and their happiness together and took confidence in their ability to succeed. Their vision began to expand. Why should their school turn away so many worthy applicants for want of space and funding? Why not build an enormous home for those who wished to learn and work in harmonious attraction? And then they picked up the morning paper. There they read the headline: "Dr. Nichols' Water Cure Establishment—A General Stampede Among The Female Pupils—The Supposed Cause—The Establishment For Sale." It was July 21, 1853, and the Nicholses had a scandal on their hands.

The article, which consisted of a letter signed by "Villager," had appeared first in the *New York Tribune*, but other papers reprinted it verbatim. The letter began with a suspicious tone, accurately summarizing the "ostensible" educational aims of the Port Chester Water-Cure Establishment: "the instruction of young ladies in the truths of physiology as more particularly relating to their own organization and in the principles of Hydropathy, &c." It went on to list the unusual textbooks relied upon by lecturers, notably *Esoteric Anthropology* and Stephen Pearl Andrews's *Love, Marriage, and Divorce*, a document that elaborated the theory of "individual sovereignty" in matters of love and passion. The letter continued:

> It seems that for some time past, [the young women] had been plied
> pretty freely with communications, both oral and epistolary, in which
> the doctrines respecting woman and her sexual functions, duties and
> privileges as inculcated [in these texts] . . . were insisted on, and given

a personal direction and application to the parties addressed. . . .
Whether the practical application was sought among the pupils, I cannot say from personal knowledge; there is, however, every reason to believe that it was.[1]

Attention had been drawn to these circumstances, according to the author,
by a veritable "stampede" of students from the school. Once she fully understood the messages reinforced in her classes, one of the girls took flight
"in a state of alarm" and sought refuge with protective friends in New
York City. Soon all the others but one "decamped," returning to the safety
of their homes and parents. The writer concluded by declaring that "the
'American Hydropathic Institute' may now be considered among the
things that were."[2] Thomas and Mary had indeed put the property on the
market that summer, planning for relocation and growth. They had no
choice but to challenge this widely disseminated slander.

The September 1853 issue of the *Nichols' Journal* reprinted the *Tribune*'s
letter along with the reply Thomas submitted to the paper the following
day. "For my opinions, read my published works," Thomas wrote. "For my
conduct, in all the relations of my life, as husband, parent, teacher, physician and man of business, ask those who know me. I court the most searching investigation. I have violated no trust, and there lives not the man or
woman who can truly charge me with immoral conduct. . . . Any assertion
to the contrary, is false, and if made in an actionable form, by a responsible person, I will bring it before a Court of Justice for legal investigation."[3] This reporting of the exchange was followed by six columns of additional response from Thomas and Mary, each writing separately on the
affair.

According to the Nicholses, Russell Trall was behind the calumny.
Thomas accused Trall of spreading poisonous lies in a disgraceful expression of professional jealousy. One girl, Thomas granted, had left the
school and returned to Trall's house. Rather than consult Thomas, Trall
used the girl's claims as a pretext to initiate a conspiracy against the
Nicholses, seeking to disband their school. Thomas quoted a letter pur-
portedly written him by a former student:

They told me that you were banished from New York, because of your
baseness; that you claimed to be reformers only as a device to obtain

notoriety; and that you were rejected and cast out by all *true* reformers, who understood your motives. They said that your marriage was not real, but was assumed only as a cloak to your deep and darker designs. I cannot tell you of all the horrible details—of your baseness in former years, and of all which I heard; *and all this Dr. Trall confirmed with added relations!*[4]

Indeed, Russell Trall had recently issued the prospectus for his own proposed hydropathic college, and the *Nichols' Journal* had attained a wide circulation in competition with the *Water-Cure Journal.* In retaliation for the "Villager" disaster, Thomas used the *Nicholas' Journal* to question the character of Trall's own proposed school, which advertised "a department for the special management of those female diseases which are incurable without peculiar mechanical and surgical treatment." Thomas called these methods "obscene quackeries," and suggested that no "decent" woman would ever perform such procedures. "It can only be done by men," he asserted, "and this 'peculiar' treatment requires men of an equally 'peculiar' character."[5]

The former colleagues were at war. Trall could not tolerate the Nicholses' leadership role in the water-cure movement. In February 1856, he attempted to rewrite history: "The *Buffalo Medical Journal* insinuates that a notorious advocate of free love, anti-marriage, and various other isms and antics and heresies, is a Water-Cure doctor; whereas, she is no doctor at all; has never had a medical education in any school, is not recognized at all by the hydropathic fraternity, and does not practice the system." For Thomas, he had this description: "This doctor, whatever he may do, say, profess, or possess, has never had a hydropathic education; nor does he practice Water-Cure, except as thousands of "picked-up" or self-constituted doctors may practice any system . . . nor are his doctrines, book-writings, or teachings, admitted into the hydropathic school."[6] Trall neglected to explain that no hydropathic school existed before the Nicholses founded the American Hydropathic Institute, and that the inaugural address of their school had appeared as the *Water-Cure Journal*'s lead article in October 1851 when Trall himself was the journal's editor. Even if he were not the anonymous "Villager," Trall likely deserved the Nicholses' suspicion.[7]

As if this negative publicity were not headache enough, in 1853 Charles

Wilkins Webber published the novel *Yieger's Cabinet. Spiritual Vampirism: The History of Etherial Softdown, and Her Friends of the "New Light."* The Tenth Street housemate whose engagement to Elma had been squelched by Mary sought his revenge publicly. His novel referred to Mary as "Etherial" and to Thomas as "Mr. Narcissus." Webber wrote, "Did Etherial care that [her "lusty and good-looking young Quaker" husband's] spiritual death must be her life? She laughed and screamed with the joy of unutterable ferocity! Eureka! Eureka! They shall all be my slaves! They taunt me with being born without a soul, with being underwitted! I shall devour souls hereafter by the hundreds! . . . Ah, glorious!"[8] This work depicted Mary as a monster who could self-induce revolting attacks of lung hemorrhage at will. To readers of the *Nichols' Journal,* Mary described Thomas's response to *Spiritual Vampirism* as follows: "My husband read it, and asked me and my daughter to promise never to read it, or allow any one to tell us what was in it. He characterized it as infernal—and it is this book which has been circulated at Dr. Trall's establishment, with my name and that of my daughter, written in, in place of those of the fictitious characters." Mary then described Webber's family's history of insanity and reminded readers that while in "a sane state," Webber had testified under oath in defense of her good character when Hiram had brought suit against the man who had returned Elma to Mary.[9] Business at the American Hydropathic Institute suffered as a result of the *Tribune's* letter and perhaps from Webber's book as well, but the Nicholses remained eager to expand their school.

By September 1853, Mary and Thomas had begun promoting Desarrollo, which was to be "an Educational and Industrial Institute, such as does not now exist, but such as the world needs more than any other."[10] Its name, of Spanish origin and pronounced "Des-a-roh-yo," means "development." Located on one hundred acres of land directly adjacent to the experimental community of Modern Times on Long Island, New York, the main residence hall for Desarrollo was to stand four stories high, with a sixty-foot tower serving as a reservoir and housing bath rooms. It would accommodate one hundred students. A library, lecture hall, gymnasium, dining room, art studios, and more were planned for future perpendicular wings. Ultimately, the Nicholses envisioned a complete quad, with the final building housing a printing office, "stereotype foundry, power presses, and book bindery, model kitchen, bakery, and laundry, with an engine-house in the center, with steam to carry all the machinery, raise the water, cook, wash, and warm the whole range of buildings, and supply warmth to the winter garden in the central square." Their ambitious plan adorned this central square with fountains and statuary. Students would follow that schedule already proven delightful at Port Chester: meals, lectures, work, exercise, entertainment, and rest in refreshing interchange. A separate department would offer medical training.[11] Readers of the *Nichols' Journal* were invited to contribute all they could afford to this magnificent Long Island project.

In the *Nichols' Journal*, Mary and Thomas had taken frequent notice of doings at Modern Times, a community of "individual sovereigns" founded on Long Island in March of 1851 by their friend Josiah Warren and his radical associate Stephen Pearl Andrews, a patient at the Port Chester Water Cure. Andrews believed in universal human equality and liked to hold forth on his views. Though he may not have been a member of the Nicholses' faculty, it is likely that many of the students perceived him as an instructor. It was no surprise, then, when the Nicholses proposed to build their new school on property adjacent to Modern Times.

Two laws only governed those who settled plots of land at Modern Times: "sovereignty of the individual" and "cost the limit of price." Both principles had originated in the anarchist thought of Josiah Warren. To Warren and his followers, individual sovereignty implied the right to live however one wished, so long as it did not infringe upon the right of another individual to do likewise. The slogan "cost the limit of price" summarized an original economic philosophy put into practice at Modern Times that was intended to render trade cooperative, not competitive. It eliminated profit in all transactions involving goods and services, which were instead exchanged precisely at the cost of the materials and labor, without a mark-up for capital gain. Warren called the combination of individual sovereignty and cost the limit of price "Equitable Commerce." Among others, the plan appealed to *New York Tribune* editor Horace Greeley, who showed support by quietly purchasing seven plots at Modern Times, though he did not live there. Like Modern Times, Desarrollo would depend on each member respecting and tolerating the freedom of everyone else. At their advanced school, free of arbitrary compulsion, the only measure of wrong would be injurious consequence" to someone else.[12]

Mary and Thomas moved to a small house at Modern Times in July

1853. They would stay there for a little over two years before defaulting on both their $2,000 property mortgage and on the $400 house mortgage.[13] Like the other members of Modern Times, Mary and Thomas had bought a cottage within the community: lot 77 at Fifth Street and Third Avenue. In October, they published an extended description of their planned Institute of Desarrollo, soliciting contributions that never came. They simply proposed the impossible: an Eden, a society of perfect harmony. Desarrollo's members would enjoy shared intellectual pursuits as well as constructive work. Living in a healthful environment, surrounded by fulfilled peers, and endowed with the same natural rights as everyone else, students of Desarrollo would rarely fall ill. The sickening miseries brought on by society's arbitrary despotisms would find no place among the fountains. If it had come to pass, Desarrollo would have combined the antigovernment principles of Modern Times with productive association. Yet Mary and Thomas pleaded in vain for financial support. Bitterly they reflected that they had been "abused with the vilest slanders . . . from persons ostensibly engaged in the same cause. . . . Well may reformers say, 'Save us from our friends.' Enemies everybody is prepared for."[14] The grand foundation of Desarrollo—already dug on Long Island—would ultimately remain a large, expensive hole in the ground.

USEFUL LEGS

In June of 1853, a month before the *Tribune*'s letter undercut their momentum, Mary published one of her clearest and most hopeful explanations of the relationship between society and physiology. Entitled "A Word to the Believers in the Sovereignty of the Individual," her brief column forged links between the anatomy she taught and the liberation she preached. It also revealed her growing spiritualism.[15]

Offered as a plea for the right of self-government, Mary's column related natural law to political law. Using explanations of the body's mechanism to argue for particular social practices was not an original rhetorical approach. Indeed, most antebellum physicians and health reformers relied on their understandings of anatomy and physiology to advocate the moral pursuit of a healthy life. This pursuit involved behavioral choice. Detailed manuals advised readers to seek cleanliness, temperance, regimen, piety, and self-control. To be healthy was to evidence morality and virtue. Health teachers reasoned that an understanding of the intricacies of God's material creation—the human body—would illuminate the laws by which God intended us to live.[16] Mary shared this logic with her medical contemporaries. But unlike many whose physiological exploration yielded only justification for the status quo, Mary found physical argument for social revolution.

"We must learn the truth for every passion of the soul, for every function of the body, and bring all into harmony with this truth," she wrote. In other words, physical needs and inborn passions should prescribe behavior: we should derive our lifestyles from the dictates of our bodies and the cravings of our souls. What others had applied rhetorically—not imagining the same logic being used to assault accepted morality—Mary tenaciously pursued to its natural limit. The difficulty came in regard to passion. Where others saw cause for repression and self-denial, Mary saw an additional aspect of healthy physiology. Denying passion was akin to denying hunger or fatigue. Mary was writing against a cultural mindset that perceived erotic feeling as a contaminant of spiritual love.[17]

For Mary, the word *passion,* like *purity,* carried a positive connotation. There is some inconsistency between her acceptance of passionate attraction and her portrayal of masturbation as a terrible disorder. Passion she clearly associated with love, a holy and social emotion; while "onanism" lacked such legitimation. Passion did not imply lust or licentiousness. But Mary also recognized that there were destructive extremes. Of these exceptional cases she wrote, "The man who cannot govern himself, without bringing evil upon himself and others, must be governed, as whoso has broken legs must have crutches—and yet all men have the natural right of unbroken, useful legs." Though Mary left no record of having made the connection herself, she had adopted her mother's language of the need for "usefulness," language she had once found oppressive. According to Rebecca Neal's daughter, those with "useful legs" would walk a five-step path: first, they would gain understanding of the body's needs and passions; second, they would live according to that knowledge; third, they would thereby achieve both purity and happiness; fourth, they would effortlessly magnetize others towards the True Life; and fifth, they would thus perfect society. Mary campaigned for every person's inalienable right to pursue this path. Her philosophy reflected devout optimism for the race.

Like other health reformers, Mary saw human destiny shaped by personal constitutions. Physiological knowledge could teach people how to maximize individual strengths and compensate for inborn limitations. Mary recognized that everyone does not possess an equal capacity for health. She shared the widespread belief that children inherited their parents' tendencies toward physical or moral disease.[18] In her theoretical understanding of predispositions, Mary generally reflected the mainstream; doctors also praised her grasp of anatomy and physiology. Yet it was her radical application of this knowledge that led to professional isolation. It was also her integration of medicine with spiritualism.

No one claimed to understand the vital force that animated the physical matter of a living human body. It was presumed to come from God. To strengthen the life force through healthy behavior was to obey and please God. Mary believed that this life essence circulated among people. "The life spirit of the race . . . carries with it, as does the blood, disease and death, or love, purity and life," she explained. "Our life does not stop with us, whether it be good, or evil, any more than the blood stops in the heart, or the arm."[19] One would err in reading these words as mere metaphor. To Mary, one person's influence over another had a literal, physiologic explanation. She may not have recognized the airborne bacterium of tuberculosis, but for Mary the state of the soul was clearly contagious. "If I have a true bravery for God," she wrote, "I magnetize those who are most my own with my spirit. If I am mean, craven and worldly, others who depend on my magnetic life, become so. If I love an evil, those who love me are likely to love it. If I love purity, my love is living, and gives life to those who can receive life from me, and this is true of all men and women."[20] Every individual had enormous power and responsibility. The life one led could contaminate or purify an ever-widening circle. By this reasoning, all constraining social institutions inflicted a form of biological warfare on innocent millions. If one were trapped in a loveless marriage, for example, deprived of legal escape and forced to submit to the lusts of a repulsive partner, then untold numbers would suffer through magnetic transference. "Freedom, with individual enlightenment" was the only solution.[21]

What had started as a brief series of anatomical lectures fifteen years earlier had evolved into a crusade for individual happiness. Where Mary's early lectures had presented biologic information against the backdrop of culture, *Desarrollo* reflected the Nicholses' hope for a political world in which such knowledge could thrive. Still in Port Chester, Mary and Thomas already seemed to be catching the refreshing spray of Desarrollo's fountains. But the *Tribune*'s destructive letter shifted the winds.

FREE LOVE AT MODERN TIMES

Forty miles east of New York City and four miles inland of Great South Bay, Modern Times did not command the invigorating panoramic view available from Port Chester's Prospect Hill. Small brick cottages lined short, straight avenues. Overrun with scrub oak, the colony offered garden loam and quiet. In this revolutionary yet calm village, the Nicholses spent most of their time writing. Between July 1853, when they moved to Modern Times, and October 1855, when they left, Mary and Thomas published thousands of pages in addition to maintaining their voluminous correspondence. By April of 1853 they were actively discouraging readers of their journal from writing letters asking for medical consultation before reading their published works. In January 1854, Thomas estimated that he and Mary often received one hundred letters a day, which took several hours simply to read. A handful of these letters found publication in the *Nichols' Journal*, which by its fifth number claimed to have nearly thirty thousand subscribers. The majority of readers lived in New York, Indiana, Ohio, and Illinois. One small Ohio town had amassed a subscription club of 150 people, while two unnamed villages had more subscribers than they had houses.[22]

Long Island's easy rail access to New York City simplified the task of printing the *Nichols' Journal* and sustained the Nicholses' connection with a wider community. At No. 65 Walker Street, the journal's city office, Thomas also established a reform bookstore that offered mail-order delivery of both texts and hydropathic instruments. With special enthusiasm, Thomas promoted a ten-ounce syringe of his own invention. Made of "fine white metal," this device involved the basic cylinder and piston, along with four attachments: "a short straight tube for giving enemas to the sick, or to children; a long curved tube; a short tube, which screws on this for self-injection; and a perforated bulb, which also screws on the curved tube, for vaginal injections, by which nine-tenths of all female complaints may be cured." The entire apparatus cost two dollars. An additional dollar would buy a copy of *Esoteric Anthropology*. With *Esoteric*

Anthropology and this instrument, wrote Thomas, "no woman need ever require a doctor or drugs for any purpose."[23] In the spring of 1854, he relocated both the bookstore and the office to the very busy corner of Anthony Street, in the second-story front room of No. 333 Broadway, nearly opposite the Broadway theater. Elma, established as a successful crayon artist, opened a new studio only a few doors away within a year.

Mary and Thomas relied heavily on the *Nichols' Journal* to promote sales of their books, along with those of Stephen Pearl Andrews, Josiah Warren, and Marx Edgeworth Lazarus. Meanwhile, back at Modern Times, they were collaborating on a new work: *Marriage: Its History, Character, and Results; Its Sanctities, and Its Profanities; Its Science and Its Facts. Demonstrating Its Influence, as a Civilized Institution, on the Happiness of the Individual and the Progress of the Race.* Its publication in 1854, followed by *Mary Lyndon, or Revelations of a Life. An Autobiography* in 1855, established Mary and Thomas as leaders of the free-love movement. But by the time they moved to Long Island, the Nicholses were already devotedly wed to antimarriage philosophy, and Modern Times seemed an ideal home.

Of over one hundred experimental colonies established during the nineteenth century, Modern Times made itself exceptional by refusing collective government. Its founders had assured prospective members that "no pledges are required, and no understanding, implied or expressed, is had with the settlers, that they are to live . . . *in any given way.*"[24] This anarchical framework thoroughly distinguished Modern Times from other utopian designs and was what had attracted Mary and Thomas. Ironically, it was precisely this "live and let live" expectation that created problems for the Nicholses, who had very specific ideas about how other people should conduct themselves: the "True, Physiological Life" *required* free love. Others at Modern Times—particularly Josiah Warren—quickly came to resent the Nicholses' *requiring* anything.

This tension came to a head only two months after Mary and Thomas moved to Modern Times. Still reeling from Trall's betrayal, the *Tribune*'s slander regarding Port Chester, and the demands of producing their own journal, Mary and Thomas wasted no time in promoting their new home in the *Nichols' Journal.* Enthusiastically, they endorsed the principle of individual sovereignty in relation to love. "There is the most absolute freedom and toleration," wrote Thomas. "People who need the restraining force of law, or custom, or public opinion—people who wish to govern their neighbors, or who require to be governed themselves; people who have no confidence in themselves and no faith in humanity, should not go to Modern Times. And no person ought to go there who is not willing to mind his own business."[25] Thomas had used the words *should* and *ought*. But Mary, perhaps unwittingly, used the word *must*. By drifting into the language of mandates, she undermined the very freedom her writing sought to celebrate: "Each person who wishes to go to Modern Times, must answer readily and affirmatively such questions as the following: . . . Have I the honesty and heroism to become of no reputation for the truth's sake? . . . Am I willing to be considered licentious by the world, because of my obedience to a law, higher than worldlings can conceive of?"[26] Josiah Warren wasted no time drafting a public reply, which he posted on a village bulletin board for signatures.

Entitled "Positions Defined," Warren's letter rejected the notion that any one individual could speak for the other individual sovereigns at Modern Times. "I wish it to be distinctly borne in mind, that *no person* in his or her deportment of conversation, writings or lecturing, is to be understood as my representative . . . and that no newspaper or journal is to be understood as an organ for me, excepting so far as it may have my signature to the articles it may contain," he wrote. "Positions Defined" also asserted each individual's right to refrain from discussion of any topic at all, including free love. "I decline even entertaining the subject, either for controversy or for conversation. I have a right to be the maker of my own reputation." Warren had founded Modern Times on the broad principles of equitable commerce, not sexual freedom. While he did not believe in restricting others from experimenting at their own cost, he did resent the growing public association between free love and Modern Times. Thus, his letter also sought to distance the village from the risk of perceived licentiousness: "For myself, so far from proposing or wishing to see any sudden, unprepared changes in the sexual relations, I am satisfied that they would be attended with more embarrassments and more disastrous consequences than their advocates or even the public generally are aware of."[27] Josiah Warren saw Modern Times, his equity experiment, under siege. In defense, he declared the freedom of sovereign individuals to choose traditional marriage as well as any other arrangement.

The *Nichols' Journal* reprinted Warren's letter in its October issue. In

response, Mary and Thomas granted that their calls for "real and vital
change in . . . domestic relations" would meet with contempt and scandal.
Mary had said as much in the column that Warren challenged. The bulk
of their October reply simply reiterated the need for social reform. "Truth
in love relations brings health, vigor, long life, and happiness," they wrote.
"There is a true, genuine, God-ordained relation of the sexes, in mutual
love, which is the real marriage; but all civilization is full of counterfeits,
abuses, perversions and [falsities], and not less filled with their consequences—satiety, disgust, misery; sickly and short-lived, bodily-deformed,
or soul-perverted offspring." In about one hundred words, they summarized their incentive for writing *Marriage:* "Mr. Warren may refuse to discuss this subject; we cannot refuse. . . . The world wants light on this more
than on all other subjects, and it shall have what light we can give it. *Are
we right or wrong?*"[28] Writing unapologetically as "we," the Nicholses
noted that Josiah Warren "scarcely ever uses the personal pronoun plu-
ral." Their observation implied social isolation on the part of their critic.
To the charge of falsely representing themselves as the authorized voices
of Modern Times, Mary and Thomas did not directly respond.

Despite this rocky initiation into the neighborhood, the Nicholses remained at Modern Times for nearly two years and continued their effusive promotion of Josiah Warren. In the August 1854 issue of the *Nichols'
Journal,* Mary wrote a lengthy description of Warren, in which she
claimed to share a "sympathy" with him: "I am not surprised that Mr.
Warren feels at this time great anxiety and fear for the results of our
promulgation of truth. . . . It is an honor to his delicate, sensitive, and most
benevolent organization." She also claimed to have first "known" Warren
through her "psychometric examination" of a sealed manuscript he had
written. "When I hold in my hand a letter, and know by its impression on
my spirit, the personal form and appearance of the writer, his character
and disposition, his general condition and particular motive in writing the
letter, the subject, and perhaps the words of the writer, and all this without opening the letter, but by merely holding it in my hand, the information is not obtained by any ordinary perception of the senses. . . . Such
facts or phenomena are termed psychometric." (Mary's claims to clairvoyance broadened during an era committed to spiritualism and later
played a role in her ability to heal.)[29]

The Nicholses were unlikely to find an environment more conducive to social reform initiatives, convenient to New York City, and respectful of individual freedom than Josiah Warren's colony. At Modern Times a common nursery kept Willie safe and occupied through her toddlerhood, which freed her parents to write. And despite Warren's reluctance to join in a crusade for free love, others at Modern Times shared the Nicholses' perspective. Stephen Pearl Andrews had published lengthy defenses of free love, and years later he would go on to support the candidacy of free-lover Victoria Woodhull for president of the United States. "I ask for the complete emancipation and self-ownership of woman," he wrote in 1853. "*Sexual purity*, I will say, *is that kind of relation, whatever it be, between the sexes which contributes in the highest degree to their mutual health and happiness, taking into account the remote as well as the immediate results.*"[30] Even earlier he had reiterated the Fourierist belief that "the condition of woman in any given state of society is the true measure and gauge of the degree of advancement of the society towards its own normal, perfect and harmonious condition."[31] More than anywhere they had yet found, Modern Times enabled women to live on an equal footing with men.

SPEAKING OF CLOTHES, SPEAKING OF CUSTOM

Modern Times eventually came to occupy ninety acres of Suffolk County. Always at risk for brush fires ignited by the sparks of passing trains, the region also offered relatively poor soil. The male settlers of Modern Times included a lithographer, a harness maker, farmers, carpenters, and former pastors. Women (of whom there were an approximately equal number) worked side by side with these men to build log cabins or brick cottages, dig gardens, and find work. Many of their basic household needs were supplied by the village "time store," a nonprofit shop operated on the principles of equitable commerce. The proprietor charged customers only for the price of the materials purchased as well as for the time (labor) involved in the transaction. A clock over the counter was reset for each shopper. Customers paid cash for the *materials* so the store could replenish its supplies from outside the village; yet to minimize contact with money, they reimbursed *labor* with homemade onionskin certificates called "labor notes." These notes, which approximated today's dollar bills in size, promised a fixed amount of labor in the customer's area of expertise or a fixed amount of corn. A typical labor note read, "TWO HOURS LABOR IN SIGN

PAINTING OR 16 POUNDS OF CORN; OR, with the consent of the holder, 20 cents."[32]

By the time Mary, Thomas, and Willie arrived at Modern Times, they were joining the company of more than sixty settlers—enough to sustain regular discussion groups, a library, and social dances.[33] A reporter for the *New York Weekly Leader* attended one of these dances in the summer of 1854 and found to his surprise that all the women wore Bloomers—and, as often as not, they asked the men to dance. As if to underline their commitment to "progress," noted the observer, the women wore their hair short and the men let theirs grow. The mockery women faced for challenging traditional femininity in the mid-1850s could deter even the strong-hearted. A fair comparison might be drawn to the courage required today of American feminists who opt to stop shaving their legs. After the 1852 National Women's Rights Convention in Syracuse, New York, the *New York Tribune* had asked:

> Who are these women? what do they want? . . . Some of them are old maids, whose personal charms were never very attractive, and who have been sadly slighted by the masculine gender in general; some of them women who have been badly mated . . . and they are therefore down upon the whole of the opposite sex; some, having so much of the virago in their disposition, that nature seems to have made a mistake in their gender—mannish women, like hens that crow; some of boundless vanity and egotism, who believe that they are superior in intellectual ability to "all the world and the rest of mankind."[34]

Those at Modern Times remained figuratively as well as literally unruffled. At one point in the evening, reported the journalist at the summer dance, everyone joined in singing a popular ode to "The Bloomer," sung to the tune of "O! Susanna." Its last verse proclaimed:

> I'll never mind the scoff or hiss
> Of senseless fop or belle,
> For they have sorrow, I have bliss;
> They're sick, but I am well.
> My garments e'er shall indicate
> Thought, purity of mind.

My form shall be elastic, straight,
Attractive and refined!
O the Bloomer! that's the dress for me!
Soon may its beauty, freedom, health appreciated be![35]

Mary could finally, without harassment, wear the clothes she liked.

In 1852, when she began wearing a short dress and Turkish trousers, Mary faced ridicule in the New York streets. In Connecticut, she had even been hit by a rock thrown by a woman. As Mary explained, "I am no *ite*, and believe in no *ism*, in this matter; I only wear the so called Bloomer dress, because it combines more advantages than any other that we poor serfs of women have liberty to wear."[36] At Modern Times, Mary was one of many women who chose to wear comfortable, practical, unfeminine clothing. Woman's long garments "mark her as a thing owned," Mary wrote. "To be healthy, and enterprising, and self-sustaining as man is, women must dress more like men," she argued. "The public puts its mold upon us, and we come out as nearly alike as peas. Our waists and feet just so small and 'delicate,' our minds just so dull and stupid, our bodies *bagged*, and our whole lives belittled."[37]

One month after Mary published this plea, Elizabeth Cady Stanton wrote a letter to her cousin, Elizabeth Smith Miller, describing the wonder of Bloomers: "I love what I suffer for, and I have suffered a good deal for this [short] dress. . . . It has been such a boon to me this past winter . . . running from cradle to writing-desk, from kitchen to drawing-room, singing lullabies at one moment in the nursery and dear old Tom Moore's ditties the next moment on the piano-stool. If I had on long skirts, how could I accomplish all this? God only knows." A month later, however, even the courageous Stanton had ceased to wear the short dress in public. In another letter to her cousin she explained, "How could you ask me if I would not visit in a bloomer? You know I gave up the short dress not because I did not like it, but because others allowed me no peace so long as I wore it."[38]

It was as much the restriction of clothing choice as the absurdly restraining fashions themselves that galled Mary. "I loathe and abhor prescription and proscription," she declared (even as Josiah Warren faulted her for prescribing free love and proscribing convention). "What we want is, not the liberty to wear a particular form of clothing like the Quakers, or the Bloomers; but freedom to dress as fancy or use may dictate."³⁹ Excursion to New York City still required traditional clothing if a woman wanted to go in peace, but at Modern Times, women wore trousers.

Thomas and Mary enjoyed working together during their brief stay on Long Island. Mary began publishing her autobiography in serialized form; Thomas spent hours poring over the Old and New Testaments, the Koran, the Book of Mormon, and a multitude of other sources, collecting notes for a series on comparative religion that would ultimately be published as a book in 1855. Thomas's earlier research for *Woman in all Ages and Nations* had introduced him to hundreds of narratives describing the historically harsh and unjust treatment of women throughout the world and across faiths. At home, the Nicholses strove to do better. Thomas, full of affection for his wife and daughter, had taken to praising Mary in the pages of the *Nichols' Journal*. He once grew so effusive that Mary felt forced to defend herself against charges of egotism, explaining that she had not seen her husband's remarks until they were in print. She wrote that badgering him to cease the practice had proven useless, which she asserted was rare evidence of "bad taste" on Thomas's part. But clearly Mary enjoyed the public flirtation with her spouse, whose admiration of her talents continued to offset the abuses of her first marriage.⁴⁰

In addition to this mutual appreciation, the *Nichols' Journal* included chapters from *Mary Lyndon*, a book that powerfully underlined the differences between Hiram and Thomas. Mary intended to convert her years of suffering into something constructive. Over and over, she described to her readers how the respectful love of a nonpossessive man had saved her life. Redundantly and defiantly she preached what she had practiced: "Do I live with my husband because we are married according to law? No more than I refrain from stealing or murder on account of law. If a legal decision . . . had not freed me from my first husband, I should still have been just as much the wife of Dr. Nichols. . . . And no law could make us live as husband and wife a day after we felt that the Divinity of our marriage was destroyed." In this *Journal* series, entitled "Human Culture," Mary carefully articulated her understanding of God's will regarding marriage: "My thought of impurity has nothing to do with the human law. Those 'whom God has joined, let not man put asunder.'" Mary's use of Christ's words to defend free-love doctrine reflected a scandalous reinterpretation of the very Bible verse priests used to justify indissoluble marriage. "I can commit no adultery," she continued, brazenly redefining the term. "The church and the world have yet largely to learn that union without love is adultery . . . that an unloving maternity is a sin against God." What the courts considered illegal union of the sexes might well be a holy union in love. It was simple: "I do not need law," she wrote.[41]

Mary saw bonds loosening all around her in 1854. Elma, twenty-two years old, was preparing to leave for three years in Italy, where she would study art. It would be their first extended separation since the summer Hiram had taken Elma away. It was also around this time that Mary's mother, Rebecca Neal, died. Only recently had she come to take a supportive interest in her daughter's life work. After years of distance, Mary and her mother had finally grown close. In the face of these losses, Mary struggled to keep herself busy. She finished writing the story of her life, which she promised readers would reveal "the golden chain of the Divine Providence by which I have been drawn upward."[42] It was a powerful attempt to bring coherence to her own sense of identity, but in 1854 Mary did not know where she was headed. In May, forty-four years old, she suffered a breakdown. For a five-month period, she tried to avoid overtaxing intellectual projects and primarily sought rest. As autumn gained color, Mary felt herself recovering.[43]

THE QUESTION OF DIVORCE

Mary's rejection of "civilization's" laws reflected her Fourierism. Fourier's beliefs on love had received a new burst of attention in 1852 when Mary's friend and former housemate Marx Edgeworth Lazarus published *Love vs. Marriage*, which drew a distinction between true love and traditional marriage, arguing that marriage constitutes "the tomb of love." Lazarus opened his book with two quotes from Scripture: "For in heaven they neither marry nor are given in marriage, but are as the angels of God" and "Thy kingdom come, Thy will be done, on earth as it is done in heaven." God, he believed, did not intend for people to form indissoluble unions with individual others—or, consequently, to isolate themselves in separate households that inherently multiply drudgery, reduce variety, and extinguish happiness for all. "Marriage converts lovers into owners of personal

property, and often renders the most charming love relations at last in-
different or odious by the meannesses, monotony, and exclusiveness of the
isolated household," he wrote.[44]

A restructured society could change all of that. Because "love, like the
other faculties of the soul, requires for its vigor and permanence in action,
the charm of variety, [and] the alternation of its objects," monogamy
would represent only one legitimate choice among many alternative relationships within the Fourierist communities, called phalanxes. Traditional families—sources of misery and frustration—would naturally fade
away, replaced by more favorable arrangements. Young children would
find nurture in collective nurseries; women would be freed from mind-
numbing, thankless routine. "The phalanx emancipates love from the two
principal arbitrary causes of exclusiveness in marriage; to wit, the civil
law, and the personal obligation to the support of their children in the isolated household," Lazarus explained.[45] Three years earlier, Thomas had
likewise insisted that God "never could have intended . . . woman, for a
long life of roasting over kitchen fires, of menial labors, and the anxious
cares of our petty family establishments. Her nature cannot endure the
stupid monotony and harassing fatigues of such a life."[46] Lazarus claimed
that not only Albert Brisbane but also John S. Dwight (of Brook Farm)
and Henry James Sr. agreed with his opinions, even if "considerations entirely personal may prevent them from taking openly the same grounds
as myself."[47]

In 1849, Henry James Sr. anonymously translated Victor Hennequin's
work, *Love in the Phalanstery,* a text that Lazarus endorsed and that the
Presbyterian *New York Observer* vehemently condemned. James, increasingly cautious, reviewed *Love vs. Marriage* in the *New York Tribune* on
September 18, 1852. While granting that marriage was indeed "badly administered," James compared Lazarus to the "insatiate ape" for his attacks
on what most considered to be divine marriage.[48] Nonetheless, the *Observer* continued to lump James with those who advocated polygamy, free
divorce, or Fourierist freedom. In response to this characterization, James
sent a lengthy, defensive letter to the *Observer* and a second copy to the
New York Tribune, which published it. "I have invariably aimed to advance the honor of marriage by seeking to free it from certain purely arbitrary and conventional obstructions in reference to divorce," explained
James. "[Marriage] is not administered livingly, or with reference to the

present need of society, but only traditionally, or with reference to some wholly past state of society." Unlike Lazarus, James did not seek to overthrow marriage, but only to soften laws that permanently bound even those living in "the reciprocal relation of dog and cat."[49]

To the *Tribune's* irascible and often self-contradictory editor Horace Greeley, even this expressed too great a tolerance for marriage reform—too loose a reading of Christ's teachings. Arguing that freer divorce would result in "a general profligacy and corruption such as this country has never known," he portrayed marriage laws as most conducive to the expression of honorable affection. "Our own conviction and argument decidedly favor 'indissoluble marriage,'" he wrote. "But for the express words of Christ, which seem to admit adultery as a valid ground of divorce, we should stand distinctly on the Roman Catholic ground of no divorce except by death.... We *should* oppose even *that*, if it did not seem to be upheld by the personal authority of Christ. Beyond it we are inflexible."[50] (It is obviously difficult to reconcile this perspective with Greeley's financial support of Modern Times.)

In addition to his own response, Greeley published a critical letter from the Nicholses' friend and fellow reformer Stephen Pearl Andrews. Thus began, in November of 1852, a public debate in the *New York Tribune* that Andrews ultimately collected and published as a separate book the following year, titled *Love, Marriage, and Divorce, and The Sovereignty of the Individual. A Discussion Between Henry James, Horace Greeley, and Stephen Pearl Andrews.*[51] Though all three men had been inspired by the writings of Charles Fourier, each voiced a distinct perspective regarding the question of marriage. Greeley expressed the ultraconservative view; James took a middle ground; and Andrews advocated the radical doctrine of individual sovereignty, which was shared by Mary and Thomas Nichols.

Andrews also took by far the most liberal position regarding the equality of women. "*Human beings do not need to be taken care of,*" he wrote. "What they do need is such conditions of justice and freedom and friendly co-operation *that they can take care of themselves.*... Our whole existing marital system is the house of bondage and the slaughter-house of the female sex." With individual sovereignty, he argued, "woman shall be placed upon a footing of entire pecuniary independence of man and installed in the actual *possession*, as well as admitted to the *right*, of being an individual."[52] It was only as recently as 1848 that the married women of New York State had won the right to own their own property. With the exception of adultery as legitimate grounds, no New Yorker had the right to sue for divorce—and divorce was the only type of lawsuit that a married woman was allowed to bring in her own name.[53] Andrews was arguing for more than women's financial independence or the right to divorce, however. As an advocate of individual sovereignty, he was concerned with sex. Like the Nicholses, Andrews defined adultery as any sexual union motivated by feelings other than mutual love, and he defined as pure any loving union at all, marital status notwithstanding.

James and Greeley each took issue with the philosophical doctrine of individual sovereignty, both asserting the fundamental need for certain checks on individual freedom. Greeley explained his faith in state power unambiguously: "Men who roll vice as a sweet morsel under their tongues are yet desirous that virtue shall be generally prevalent," he observed, arguing that the state "not only does, but should, judge and deal with offenders against sexual purity and the public well-being." In response, Andrews rejected the idea that "somebody else, or everybody else" has the jurisdiction to declare any particular action immoral. "Who is the umpire, or standard of right and truth?" he demanded to know. James, a transcendentalist Swedenborgian, presented his case less clearly and managed to misrepresent the doctrine of individual sovereignty. Characterizing individual sovereignty as the right of all people to do what they please so long as each accepts the consequences of those actions, James omitted the important clause that the proposed freedom did *not* allow a person to burden anyone else with the consequences of his or her actions. "I have uniformly viewed man as under a threefold subjection, first to nature, then to society, and finally to God," he wrote. "What kind of sovereignty is that which is known only by its limitations, which is exercised only in subjection to something else?" After rebuking James for overlooking individual sovereignty's requisite regard for others, Andrews replied to the assertion that every person lives under a partial subjection to society: "Does the fact that man must ever remain under a necessary or appropriate subjection to society—that is, under a certain limitation of the sphere of his activity by the legitimate extension of the spheres of other individuals—does it follow, I say, that it is an absurdity to inquire and fix scientifically what that limit is?"[54] When collected, the exchanges among these men filled more than sixty pages.

Mary attempted to contribute to the *Tribune* debate by writing a statement that Andrews included in one of his submissions. However, Horace Greeley, Mary's old friend from Tenth Street, refused to publish any part of the submission. This rejection may have motivated Andrews to print the full debate as a separate text, published under his own name, with his own introduction, and including his and Mary's rejected words. In that particular submission, Andrews had introduced Mary's quotation by describing her as "a noble and pure-minded American woman, one to whom the world owes more than to any other man or woman, living or dead, for thorough investigation and appreciation of the causes of disease and the laws of health, especially in all that concerns the sexual relations and the reproduction of the race." In a footnote, he added, "She is a lady who couples the most wonderful intuitions—the spiritual 'sphere of woman'—with a truly masculine strength and comprehension of general principles, such as characterizes the highest order of scientific mind." Mary had written:

> The woman who is truly emancipate . . . has a heaven-conferred right to choose the father of her babe. If she is fixed in indissoluble marriage with a man she must abhor—a selfish, sensual tyrant—who makes her his victim, and perpetuates in her children his lust of the flesh and of gain, with all the deep damnation of his nature, must woman lie prone under all this, suffering and transmitting the disease and crime which are its ordained product, because it is according to law?
>
> In the Medical College at Albany there is an exposition of indissoluble marriage, which should be studied by all those who begin to see that a legalized union may be a most impure, unholy, and consequently, unhealthy thing. In glass vases, ranged in a large cabinet in this medical museum, are uterine tumors, weighing from half a pound to twenty-four pounds. A viscus that in its ordinary state weighs a few ounces is brought, by the disease caused by amative excess—in other words, licentiousness and impurity—to weigh more than twenty pounds. Be it remembered, these monstrosities were produced in lawful and indissoluble wedlock.[55]

Horace Greeley had considered these sentiments unfit for publication. "I utterly abhor what you term 'the right of woman to choose the father of her own child,'" he had earlier written in response to Andrews. For his part, Andrews considered Mary's paragraphs an "unanswerable" protest. "In five years more," he anticipated, "the voice of that woman will be the voice of thousands."[56]

Andrews was right. The following year, Elizabeth Cady Stanton wrote to Susan B. Anthony:

> The right idea of marriage is at the foundation of all reforms. . . . I ask for no laws on marriage. I say . . . remove law and a false public sentiment, and woman will no more live as wife with a cruel, bestial drunkard than a servant, in this free country, will stay with a pettish, unjust mistress. . . . Man in his lust has regulated long enough this whole question of sexual intercourse. Now let the mother of mankind, whose prerogative it is to set bounds to his indulgence, rouse up and give this whole matter a thorough, fearless examination. . . . I feel, as never before, that this whole question of woman's rights turns on the pivot of the marriage relation, and, mark my word, sooner or later it will be the topic for discussion. I would not hurry on it, nor would I avoid it.[57]

SANCTITIES AND PROFANITIES, SCIENCE AND FACTS

Mary responded to Horace Greeley's censorship as a fire responds to wind. In 1854, she and Thomas jointly published their own dissertation on marriage—a heavy tome excoriating the injustices of past and present. Calling marriage a "penalty" for sexual attraction, Mary and Thomas described husbands smothered in droning lives as "money-making machines" and wives reduced to slaves.[58] Because marriage encouraged the spirit of narrow acquisitiveness, they wrote, it concentrated wealth in the hands of the few and impoverished the many. Married men, looking out for their own families, were less inclined toward charity; they were also more likely, given the "exhaustion, monotony, and disgust" bred by indissoluble marriage, to turn to drink.

And why should the law suppress harmless sexual pleasure? "What the law calls fornication, when it is the union of mutual love, may be the holiest action two human beings can engage in," declared Thomas. "One of the hideous evils of our marriage system is the unnatural celibacy that it forces upon vast numbers [of single people]," he wrote. "Love, with its ultimations, enjoyments, and results, is the right, as it is the function, of every human being. Physical and mental diseases and miseries are the consequences of a deprivation of this right." Mary had begun her career with the recognition that emotional distress could cause physical sickness; with the publication of *Marriage,* she and Thomas had come to argue that even the *absence of pleasure* could do the same. Advancing the doctrine of individual sovereignty, Mary asserted: "The liberty to do wrong can be had in marriage and out of it. The freedom to do right is what we seek."[59] This freedom would yield happiness, for Mary yet believed that "God is paid when man receives; T'enjoy is to obey."

In their collaborative writing, Thomas generally assumed the role of anthropologist, historian, or philosopher, while Mary spoke to the reader's heart. The organization of *Marriage* reflects this division. Thomas contributed the first and third parts of the text's 430 pages—titled "Historical and Critical" and "Theoretical and Scientific"—while Mary wrote the shorter middle section, "Narrative and Illustrative." His words seem literally to shield hers from both sides. "In this work, we appeal to the deepest sympathies and highest aspirations of our common nature," they wrote. The more strident Thomas and Mary became in their repudiation of marriage, the more powerful their own bond. Together, they worked to compose an exhaustive attack: "The writers of this work know something, by personal experience of this subject. They have lived for six years in a marriage of ever-increasing love and uninterrupted happiness; as blessed a union, probably, as now exists, or ever existed, upon this earth; and it is in all the sanctity and all the happiness of this union of mutual love, that they write this book on marriage. If, therefore, they could have any prejudices, on personal grounds, they would be favorable to the institution. . . . The slaveholder's condemnation of slavery may be less pathetic than that of the slave, but it is not likely to be less effectual."[60] With no further comment on the irony of their position, Mary and Thomas condemned marriage from all sides.

At great length, the Nicholses expressed views that after paragraphs of example and detail invariably skidded to sharp conclusions: "For a human being to surrender up all right of choice and will, during her whole life, to another; to merge her legal, political, and to a great extent, her social existence in his; to have no separate individuality or sphere of action; to be during his life a meek, mild, submissive adjunct, a housekeeper, nurse, and slave, and after his death a *relict*—is a sad lot for any being whom God has endowed with a human soul." That any individual should be inescapably bound to so unjust and potentially abusive an arrangement led the Nicholses to recommend more than the liberaliza- tion of divorce laws. Like Stephen Pearl Andrews, Mary and Thomas sought to abolish marriage altogether. The right to divorce they consid- ered "nothing less than the abrogation of marriage itself. . . . It is the pre- tense of freedom without its actualization." Because the civil law of in- dissoluble marriage found its origin in Christian doctrine, the Nicholses yanked at this root as well. "Church and State may insist upon [life-long "imprisonment"], but the Church is unmerciful, and the State unjust. . . . How can I truly promise what I will do, or whom I will love, ten years hence? All that God requires is that we live our own lives truly; and *there is no truth but in freedom, and no freedom but in truth!*" A political mani- festo, *Marriage* preached revolutionary measures. This elaborate work defined the outer limit of feminist radicalism. "Ladies of the Woman's Rights movement, you must look this question full in the face," wrote Thomas.

> You cannot dodge it much longer. When you demand Woman's Rights, you demand the abrogation of the civilized marriage. . . . You can have no right until you assert your right to yourselves. You think that all you require is a concession here, a privilege there, permission to be better educated, and to have a wider sphere of action. You are like the colonies, petitioning your monarch and avowing your loyalty. What you want, and the only thing, and that which includes everything else, is INDEPENDENCE. You want freedom in all the relations of life, and above all, in the highest and purest—the realm of the affections.[61]

But Thomas, an experienced and persuasive writer, did not open the book at so commanding a pitch.

Wishing to treat the subject of marriage "scientifically," Thomas began his discussion by establishing clear definitions for potentially ambiguous terms. *Adultery* he defined as "sexual commerce unsanctified by mutual love"; *right*, as "in harmony or accordance with the laws of nature, or, what is the same thing, the laws of God"; *law*, as "the written expression of the governing power, whatever that power may be"; and *marriage*, as "the form of the sexual relation, having the sanction of custom or law." Mary, in contrast, adopted a highly personal voice. "I suppose the lot of man is really as hard and bitter as that of woman," she wrote, "but I know woman's life of suffering and endurance better than I do man's." Her pages described intimate details of life with Hiram, of consultations with female patients, and of talks she shared with students and servants. "It may seem strange," she noted, "that I can so well recollect conversations. . . . I remember remarks made to me thirty years since . . . as if the words had just been uttered in my hearing."[62] Preferring the specific case to the theoretical example, Mary told stories. She used life as her text. Thomas, in balance, literally quoted Scripture and verse.

The opening sections of *Marriage,* written by Thomas, collected every explicit reference to marriage found in the Old and New Testaments. Rather than remark on each quotation in turn, Thomas arrayed the passages without interruption, reminding readers that the patriarchs had practiced bigamy, had kept mistresses, had commanded their men to take virginal women as war booty, and had encouraged murder of the enemy's nonvirginal women. St. Paul had established man as the head of woman and had declared: "I suffer not a woman to teach, nor to usurp authority over the man, but to be in silence." Thomas reserved all comment on these many pages until considerable evidence had been displayed. He then concluded: "We have seen in this whole History the servitude of woman, the want of all recognition of any right over her person or actions. Polygamy and concubinage, violence and rapine, are sanctioned by the highest authority and examples. The right of property in woman is rigidly guarded by the severest laws; but the equality of woman with man, from first to last, is nowhere admitted, but rather everywhere denied."[63] By foregrounding the unsavory aspects of Judeo-Christian treatment of women, Thomas made it more difficult for Christian readers to adopt a holier-than-thou attitude toward the practices of other religions and cultures subsequently described.

These examples were drawn from the research notes Thomas had collected for *Woman, in all Ages and Nations* and ranged, in Thomas's view, from the horrifying to the admirable. In Tonquin, he wrote, "women convicted of adultery are killed by an elephant, trained to the office." Yet "in Congo, the negroes take their wives a year on trial; at the end of this time the relation may cease at the requirement of either party. . . . O mothers of civilization! how many bitter tears might be spared . . . if you had the sense of a Congo negress in this one particular," he wrote. Thomas challenged his readers to question the presumed superiority of men to women and to recognize the universal sense of male entitlement that shaped pagan, Jewish, and Christian cultures. Advocating a critical approach to received wisdom, he wrote, "The time has come when a clear-minded, honest man, may examine any doctrine, even if it come prefaced by 'THUS SAITH THE LORD.'"[64]

Extending the analysis to the nineteenth century, Thomas quoted at length from the 1848 Seneca Falls Declaration of Sentiments delivered at the first National Woman's Rights Convention, emphasizing that the momentous document also assailed marriage. Mary reinforced the attack:

When she is owned by a man who can maintain her, though he is loathsome almost as death to her; when her health is utterly lost in bearing his children, and in being the legal victim of his lust; when her children are not hers, but his, according to inexorable law; when she has no power to work, and no means of sustenance but from this owner; when public opinion will brand her with shame, most probably, if she leaves her husband, and most certainly if she enter upon ever so true and loving relations with another man—what is such a woman to do but to live a false and unholy life? . . . A new thought has dawned upon the world—that of fidelity to one's self.[65]

Thomas elaborated on the physical oppression of wives: "She has married a husband, perhaps she finds a tyrant; she thought to be united to a tender lover, and finds in him a monster of lust, who profanes her life with disgusting debaucheries. She is his slave, his victim, his tool. Her duty is submission." Thomas intended to be taken literally. "Thousands of women suffer where one complains. The minister, the physician, or sometimes an intimate friend, hears of these things; but there is a deep *hush!* . . . The physicians of this city could testify to bruises, and even broken bones, which wives have received from their husbands, in the 'most respectable families.'" Even death, Thomas wrote, was inflicted on wives by husbands—"oftener than slaves are killed by their masters."[66]

At the time of their writing, subjects like domestic violence had not yet become part of mainstream American discourse. Neither had the assumption that normal women craved sexual pleasure. Yet without embarrassment, the Nicholses argued that marriage sanctioned male violence and squelched female libido. They sought to reveal the naked truth. "A healthy and loving woman is impelled to material union as surely, often as strongly, as man," Mary argued. "Would it not be great injustice in our Heavenly Father to so constitute woman as to suffer the pangs of childbirth with no enjoyment of the union that gives her a babe? The truth is that healthy nerves give pleasure in the ultimates of love with no respect to sex; and the same exhausted and diseased nerves, that deny to woman the pleasures of love, give her the dreadful pangs of childbirth."[67] Contrast her words with those of William Alcott: "Woman, as is well known, in a natural state—unperverted, unseduced, and healthy—seldom, if ever, makes any of those advances, which clearly indicate sexual desire; and for this very plain reason that she does not feel them."[68] Nonsense, argued the Nicholses. Women who lacked sexual desire also lacked freedom and health. Both Mary and Thomas agreed that this was *not* God's intention.

What Mary considered her most powerful argument against marriage was not the wife's deprivation or suffering, however. It was the effect of hateful unions on children. Beyond injuries, she charged, unhappy marriage caused an enormous range of disorders that parents would inevitably pass to their offspring. The "polluted hot-bed of a sensual and unloving marriage" would induce masturbation in children, for example, especially if sex had been forced during pregnancy or nursing. "People are constantly asking the question, What would become of children if married persons were allowed to separate?" wrote Mary. "*Let me tell conservatism that nine-tenths of the children that now burden the world would never be born.*" Those who would be born would be wanted, healthy, and "pure." They would be delivered without agony into peaceful homes. The narrative of her own experience revealed the source of this fantasy: "I have borne children in torture that the rack could no more than equal. I have had abortions and miscarriages that were as truly murders as if my infants had been strangled, or had had their brains beaten out, by a brutal father. I have had my life drained away by uterine hemorrhage, and worse than all, I have had the canker of utter loathing and abhorrence forever eating in my heart, and for one who was ... sharing my bedroom and spoiling my food."[69] The Nicholses condemned state and church alike for sanctioning such tyranny.

Even if readers sympathized with the social critique posed by *Marriage*, few could easily endorse the book's far-reaching defense of free love. As Mary wrote: "If a woman marries seven husbands in succession, and has a child by each, you do not complain of her, provided she was seven times legally married, and seven times a widow. Suppose these men were each dead to her, or suppose she loved them all in turn, and continued to love them, what harm is it to you? Does the fact of her great love hurt you? . . . Mark me. I am not pleading for a plurality of love relations, but for freedom, and truth." Mary and Thomas were asking their readers to make a giant philosophical leap—to risk censure and ostracization—to challenge their governments and their churches. "The age has dawned in which woman shall stand between God and man, the arbiter of her own fate and the medium of inspiration, not to an owner, but to another self," declared Mary.[70]

The publication of *Marriage* unequivocally established Mary and Thomas as leaders of the growing antimarriage movement. While they were not the only medical writers to view sex as natural and healthy, they distinguished themselves by suggesting that the happiest and therefore the healthiest sex might be had outside the bonds of matrimony. Marriage, they argued, was simply more dangerous to society than sexual freedom. In the September issue of the *Nichols' Journal,* Thomas claimed that two thousand copies of the book had been sold in a few months and that the second edition had been exhausted. Advertisements asserted that "no person, in any manner *interested in its subject,* should fail to read this radical and revolutionary volume."[71] Even Dr. Harriot Hunt, Mary's former friend and ally in the fight for women's medical education, trembled at what Mary had become. In 1838, when she was still teaching school in Lynn, Mary had welcomed Harriot Hunt into her home one or two days each month when Dr. Hunt was making professional calls in town. In her memoir, Hunt (who preached herbal medicine and never earned a formal medical degree) expressed admiration for Mary's original lecturing to ladies. It had been Mary's "deep interest in anatomy and physiology" that had brought the women together in the first place. But this attachment did not weather time and change. "With regard to Mrs. Nichols," she wrote, "I must regret that the discipline of her life has resulted in her present convictions. As a lecturer on physiology she was excellent. . . . Doing full justice to her talents, and recognizing the good she has done, I cannot look with leniency on the peculiar doctrines she has embraced in later life. I not only cannot sympathize with them, but I shudder at their character, and would remove myself from *every influence* tending to favor them. My sympathies are with their deluded followers, many of whom know misery as a result of their conversion."[72] The incendiary beliefs espoused in *Marriage* brought special attention to Mary's autobiography when it reached the public in 1855.

MARY LYNDON

On August 17, 1855, the *New York Daily Times* devoted nearly four full columns of text to denouncing *Mary Lyndon; or, Revelations of a Life. An Autobiography.* The reviewer, *Times* editor Henry J. Raymond, admitted that such extended attention to a single work was rare, but he felt the length justified.[73] Entitled "A Bad Book Gibbeted," the review meticulously addressed a litany of dangers posed by Mary's advocacy of a "true life." But first it attacked Mary. Accusing the anonymous author of engaging in a "public crying spell, garnished with spasms and hysterical shrieks," Raymond had barely warmed up. "She is thoroughly and completely a sensual woman" he continued, "the slave of the coarsest lust;— and all her attempts to dignify this by giving it fine names, and claiming for it the sanctions of nature and of religion . . . cannot conceal her real character, nor disguise or excuse the infamous immorality of her conduct and her creed." Desire for principled literature did not motivate this venom; after all, other novels of the day depicted any variety of immoral actions. It was the same year that Walt Whitman's sexual poetry, *Leaves of Grass,* reached the public, averring that "Sex contains all, bodies, souls," that "Without shame the man I like knows and avows the deliciousness of his sex, / Without shame the woman I like knows and avows hers."[74] No, this reviewer paid special attention to *Mary Lyndon* as a radical work of social reform. As strongly as Mary had attempted to rally troops for freedom, this reviewer summoned the opposition forces of conservatism.

Rightly grouping *Mary Lyndon* with works devoted to Fourierism and defense of passional attractions, the review reduced this entire class of books to one central and alarming tenet: "[Their] fundamental idea is . . . that the passions are the lawgivers for mankind—that the instincts of nature, the impulses and cravings of appetite, should be indulged and obeyed as the highest revelations of divinity—as the true voice of God in the human heart."[75] Mary did, in fact, believe that God intended physical passion in mutual love—that the disease and misery resulting from a loveless union proved the sinfulness of such mating. She had consistently argued for a woman's right to love *or not love* whom she wished. Indeed, the right *not* to love took precedence for Mary and constituted, above all, a woman's "right to herself." But it was also the clause that her detractors consistently overlooked, scandalized instead by the demand for freedom of affections.

The idea that personal happiness and physical well-being could serve as a compass to the laws of nature—to God's laws—opened up a Pandora's box. The *Times* review condenses the many cultural anxieties aggravated by the writings of Mary and her radical peers. What about duty? What about law? What about social order? By column four, Raymond had begun to demand answers: "If a wife or a husband may be abandoned at the convenience of either, why not a child or a parent or a friend? Why should *any* obligation continue binding, after it becomes irksome? Why should the sexual passions enjoy an immunity from restraints of law, and not the passions of revenge, of avarice and of ambition, as well?"[76] Many who read Mary's writing balked at the magnitude of change she envisioned. To most, sexual freedom and divorce-on-demand spelled nothing less than social chaos: men would abandon their middle-aged wives in pursuit of younger women; children would go fatherless; mothers and babies would sink into poverty. The reviewer of *Mary Lyndon* offered that if a woefully unhappy spouse chose to forgo only the sexual aspects of the marriage obligation, society could grudgingly cast the abstinence as praiseworthy self-denial. It would be tolerable. But it was precisely Mary's sense of entitlement to a satisfying sex life that crossed all boundaries. Not only did the author crave the right to drive a detested husband from her bedroom; she also craved sexual happiness. This was simply too much. In his review, Raymond entirely avoided the book's treatment of what we would today call marital rape.

That Mary challenged cultural assumptions so publicly, so persistently, and at such great cost to her own reputation led the reviewer to charge Mary with "unbounded self-conceit" and to conclude that "her experience of life has sharpened her intellect, exasperated her temper, inflamed her sensual appetites, augmented vastly her self-esteem, and made her ten fold more the 'child of hell' than she was before."[77] The *Norton Literary Gazette* and the *New York Daily Tribune,* although far kinder in their reviews of the work, likewise warned readers of the questionable political views of its author. Despite his conservative views on indissoluble marriage, Horace Greeley printed a lengthy advertisement for *Mary Lyndon* on the first page of the *Tribune,* asserting that the book would be "more read and talked about than any other novel of the time" and quoting favorable advance reviews from four other periodicals.[78] Though it never became the *Uncle Tom's Cabin* of the marriage institution as Mary and Thomas had hoped, *Mary Lyndon* found an audience. The prominent *Times* attack most likely increased its sales.

SEVEN

Spirited Encounters

ớ⃗   ớ⃗   ớ⃗

IN THE *Nichols' Journal*, Mary serialized chapters of *Mary Lyndon* and solicited advance subscriptions for the completed volume—one dollar for the bound edition (with portrait of the author, drawn by Elma) and fifty cents for the "cheap mail edition."[1] The book concluded with rousing pleas for women's independence and free love. As letters of encouragement and subscriptions to the *Journal* came from many parts of the country, it was clear that although Desarrollo foundered, Mary and Thomas could still harbor realistic hopes for establishing a "harmonic home," the germ of a new society.

In the early summer of 1855, the Nicholses took a trip from Long Island to Ohio and Michigan and found themselves drawn to the Midwest. Cincinnati, one of the largest and most intellectually thriving cities of the West, was only thirty miles from Josiah Warren's previous experimental "equity village" called Utopia; from him they likely learned much about the area. Optimistically, Mary and Thomas wrote that the tenor of the West seemed, "like its soil, more open to culture and more productive than the [East]."[2] Stranger factors influenced them as well: in June, the Nicholses reported that spirits had advised them to establish their harmonic home far from Modern Times. They decided to move to Cincinnati, a city well populated by active spiritualists.

By the early 1850s two million Americans believed that departed souls regularly communicated, through "mediums," with the living. Ever since 1848, when two adolescent girls in Hydesville, New York, first reported the sound of mysterious "rappings" in their bedroom, belief in spiritual manifestations had surged. What had begun as an isolated incident quickly led to innumerable reports of bizarre encounters with the spirits of the dead. Hundreds of individuals, women and men alike, discovered in themselves the uncanny power to convey messages from the deceased to the living. These mediums drew huge audiences, and soon there were millions of believers. Thomas, who considered himself "a man of science, and a philosopher of the most positive school," could not dismiss the extraordinary evidence before his own eyes. He had attended a séance conducted by one of the famous Fox sisters of Hydesville, New York, and could not account for the effects produced. Inexplicable "percussive poundings" had signaled the medium to recite the alphabet, which new raps interrupted to indicate chosen letters, ultimately forming sentences. "Each professed spirit had its own characteristic rap," remembered Thomas. "The raps which purported to come from the spirits of children were slight and infantile. . . . I failed to detect the slightest sign of deception, collusion, machinery, sleight of hand, or anything of the sort." Other educated men found themselves equally convinced. Congressmen Nathaniel P. Tallmadge of Wisconsin and Robert Dale Owen of Indiana became avowed spiritualists, as did James Fenimore Cooper, William Cullen Bryant, William Lloyd Garrison, Horace Greeley, and New York State Supreme Court Justice John Worth Edmonds.[3]

In his new work, *Religions of the World. An Impartial History of Religious Creeds, Forms of Worship, Sects, Controversies, and Manifestations,* Thomas described the various means by which human spirits made themselves known to mediums. These methods included "rappings," "explosive noises," "tipping or moving . . . tables," "ringing bells," "playing upon musical instruments," "the forcible raising and carrying of light or heavy bodies," "writings, either by the hand of an unconscious medium or without such aid," "the contact of invisible hands," and, most remarkably, the conveying of "intelligence as is commonly supposed to belong to disembodied spirits." There were writing mediums, whose hands were controlled by spirits to write in different handwriting or in foreign languages. There were speaking mediums, whose voices changed under the influence of spirits. There were "impressional" mediums, who had both words and ideas imparted to their minds by spirits. There were tipping, rapping, and drawing mediums. There were even healing mediums, who, by laying on of hands or by "magnetizing" an article of clothing to be held or worn by the afflicted, could cure disease. Mary became an impressional and healing medium.[4]

People often received highly personal communications from departed loved ones, including information seemingly impossible for the medium to acquire independently or through guesswork. Summarizing the doctrines "most widely taught by the spirits," Thomas listed:

The immortality of the soul
Eternal progress
The untruth of nearly all the dogmas of theological systems
The authoritative character of the commonly received Scriptures
The falsity of the commonly-received doctrines of the Fall of Man,
    the Atonement, Hell, and Resurrection, as usually taught in the
    Christian Church.

He also noted that "the ideas of God, and of the Universe, appear to be nearly as vague, with most spirits, as with most men. They are no longer in fear of Hell, and they find their state very different from the Heaven of their previous imaginings."[5] As one convert put it: "The Bible is a book to conjure by, but it is a poor book to die by."[6] Given her mother's belief in universal salvation and her father's religious skepticism, Mary must have found spiritualism's portrait of the afterlife less alien than did many other converts, taught from early childhood to fear damnation. Not surprisingly, the most severe criticism of spiritualism came from the clergy. Religious leaders watched with dismay as the more liberal members of their congregations gravitated toward a movement that directly undermined the teachings of organized religion.

Séances became a widespread form of entertainment in the 1850s. By 1857 there were sixty-seven spiritualist periodicals. A variety of earlier influences fed the nation's sudden enchantment with spiritualism. In 1844 the telegraph was first demonstrated in the United States, establishing communication between Baltimore and Washington, D.C. Within two years, the major cities of the east coast had all been connected by telegraph. Significantly, the first spiritualist journal was titled *The Spiritualist Telegraph*. The 1840s also witnessed the popular growth of gothic literature, with writers like Edgar Allan Poe blurring the distinction between life and death.

A growing interest in "animal magnetism" likewise contributed to the spiritualist movement. Anton Mesmer had first asserted the presence of a mysterious "fluid," akin to gravity, that surrounded and suffused all bodies; his subsequent demonstrations of hypnotic trance enthralled Europe in the 1780s. By the 1840s "mesmerism" had become a familiar term in America. One of the most prominent American spiritualists and an active participant in most of the social reform movements of his day, Andrew Jackson Davis considered himself clairvoyant after experiencing his first trance state in December 1843. Thereafter, he gave philosophical lectures while in a trance, which he published in 1847 as an 800-page book, entitled *The Principles of Nature, Her Divine Revelation, and a Voice to Mankind.* The spiritualist movement drew its highest concentrations of adherents from the Northeast and from Ohio. In moving to Cincinnati, Mary and Thomas had chosen to trade one like-minded region for another.[7]

Before moving west, the Nicholses grew increasingly ambitious to consolidate their followers under clearly defined principles and under their own leadership. They claimed that influences from the spirit world guided them in this direction. To this end, Thomas wrote a prospectus for "The Progressive Union: A Society for Mutual Protection in Right." There he outlined the union's principles, vision, and strategy for growth as well as a plan by which every member of the fledgling organization might be made known to one another. Thomas claimed to have written the entire pamphlet in one inspired sitting—"given as the direct impression of a society of spirits."[8] He considered the Progressive Union a natural outgrowth of spiritualism.

Those who had witnessed strange and unsettling yet convincing superhuman phenomena necessarily had to rethink their sense of the world and the afterlife. Old formulas would not suffice to explain levitating tables or the magical power to heal. Both shaken and thrilled by the implications of these occurrences, thousands of intelligent people abandoned their former religions and sought out other spiritualists. "Spiritualism everywhere tends to Socialism," wrote Thomas. "Its first action is the sundering of old ties, the bursting of old bondages. Set free from existing religious and conventional relations, people are drawn together, by the desire of more truthful ones. They are forming now little groups, and these groups will soon join in larger societies."[9]

By July of 1855, Thomas and Mary were actively promoting the Progressive Union. Together they envisioned an ever-expanding society, comparable to a religious order in its missionary aspirations. A list of the names and addresses of all those who had expressly endorsed the union's principles—or the "Laws of Progress in Passional Harmony"—would be forwarded to each member. Those who did not wish to have their identities revealed would be enrolled on a private list and would not receive the names of other members. They would, however, receive the Nicholses' publications and, "in case of any need," would have the name of a particular member sent to them so they might seek assistance. "This may be of use to women, now in the bondage of unhappy domestic relations," explained the *Nichols' Monthly*. The arrangement thus constituted a primitive emergency hotline for victims of spousal abuse.[10]

Mary and Thomas listed their new address—No. 14, East Fourth Street, Cincinnati—as the "Central Bureau" of the Progressive Union. They solicited no dues, only voluntary contributions. The Central Bureau, they wrote, "claims no right of dictation or direction," but "will receive and transmit intelligence or suggestions." They hoped that union members, once known to one another, might arrange local meetings. "Let some wise man, or, still better, some wise woman, be the center of such an organization," they wrote. "Let the meetings be more social than formal; and . . . let other advanced persons be invited and indoctrinated."[11] From these gatherings, the Nicholses hoped to recruit a subgroup of followers who explicitly pledged to live by the union's strictest rules. Though entirely voluntary and wholly retractable, this commitment would establish its adherents as the "germinal group of the Harmonic Society." For a limited probationary period intended to cleanse members of sensual habits, these most determined participants agreed to "be chaste in thought, word and deed"; to devote themselves "spirit, soul, body and estate" to personal and group development; and to be "as far as possible pure in spirit; pure in person; . . . [and] pure in diet." They also agreed to give notice as soon as they felt any impulse to break the rules. Articulating the union's broadest goals, Thomas wrote: "We aim at a true SOCIAL HARMONY, in which there shall be the equilibrium of an exact equality, and a real justice; and in which the use of freedom is the pursuit of happiness, and its limitation the encroachment upon the rights of others."[12] By definition, whatever increased personal happiness without constraining others was inherently good. Thomas's ten-page description of the Progressive Union firmly asserted the Nicholses' commitment to individual sovereignty.

Four years later a *New York Times* writer claimed that "the spirits, be-sides being unmistakable blockheads, . . . were not in the field five years till they sought a 'fusion' with the Free-Lovers, began to assail the mar-riage relation, invent new causes of difference between man and wife, and find excuses to satisfy the consciences of bigamists, and adulterers and for-nicators."[13] Prudish critics disapproved of "séances" in which men and women sat holding hands in the dark. In this regard, the Nicholses' as-sertion that they were not making war on society but were claiming "the individual right to progress out of its corruptions" did not soften moral-izing critics.[14] Still, Thomas spent tremendous energy trying to clarify his views. On December 22, 1855, he delivered a lecture in Cincinnati's Fos-ter Hall titled "Free Love: A Doctrine of Spiritualism." Having learned, perhaps, from the squabble at Modern Times, Thomas prefaced his re-marks with the caveat "I only speak for myself."

Thus qualified, Thomas declared free love—rightly understood—to be the "Great Central Doctrine of Spiritualism," as obvious as the fact that "two and two make four." Spiritualists were highly divided over the issue of free love. Some legitimately felt that discussion of the subject gave spir-itualism a bad name and hurt the movement. To the general public, the term *free love* evoked "free lust" and promiscuity. The Nicholses had struggled against this widespread impression for years, countering with the snipe that "men look into their own hearts and lives for the motives of others." Only a few months had passed since they had settled into their new home, when Thomas, who claimed he felt "commissioned" to artic-ulate the sins of society, found a podium from which to declare: "There is no *true* love anywhere, but in freedom." Often, when writing on this subject, Thomas relied on comparisons to "state prison"—a clue from his past as to the origin of his passion: "We have no right . . . to send a man to state prison because he does not love as we do. Belief is an involuntary act of the mind accompanying evidence; love is just as involuntary an at-traction of the mind towards what is lovable and what is lovely."[15]

The belief that "God has not mocked man with desires never to be ful-filled" undergirded all of the Nicholses' reform initiatives. "That which we can conceive of and desire, must be possible to us," insisted Thomas:

FREE LOVE, I repeat, is the teaching of all High Intelligences.
Free Love is the Central Doctrine of Spiritualism.

Free Love is the necessary condition of moral purity.

Free Love is the hope of Social Harmony.

Free Love makes possible the realization of "Attractions proportional to Destinies."

Free Love is the absolute condition of a True Life on the Earth and in the Heavens.[16]

One month after Thomas delivered this lecture, he appeared as the keynote speaker in Cincinnati's celebration of the 119th anniversary of the birthday of Thomas Paine, hero of the American Revolution. Music of the United States' Military Band from the Government Barracks at Newport, Kentucky, welcomed the hundreds of people who pressed down the aisles of Greenwood Hall, the auditorium of the Ohio Mechanics' Institute. To honor Paine's devotion to liberty, the event's organizing committee had placed no restrictions on the content of the presentations. Thomas drew hearty applause as he declared Paine an "uncompromising foe of all despotisms, and the unwavering friend of Freedom and Humanity." He then went on to portray Paine as a philosophic mirror-image of himself.

Thomas placed his intellectual mentor in the camp of Fourier: "Paine understood the true basis of Human Society . . . in the affections or attractions of the Human Soul. . . . It was not enough for him that America was free—he asked the freedom of universal man."[17] The hundreds who gathered to commemorate Paine constituted the most sympathetic mainstream audience Thomas had addressed since adopting spiritualism and free love. For nearly an hour he artfully wound his own doctrines into those the masses had gathered to cheer. "Thomas Paine was a religious man," declared Thomas. "In our day he would be called a Spiritualist— he would be claimed as a MEDIUM." To defend this claim, Thomas quoted from Paine's *Age of Reason*: "There are two distinct classes of what are called thoughts; those that we produce in ourselves by reflection and the act of thinking, and those that bolt into the mind of their own accord. . . . [I]t is from ["these voluntary visitors"] that I have acquired about all the knowledge I possess." A relative newcomer to Cincinnati, Thomas had made a formidable impression. With great personal hope he concluded: "The time is coming when the true reformers of mankind shall be honored as they deserve. America will repent of her ingratitude. She will rise above the mists of error that have obscured her vision."[18]

Thomas saw spiritual communications as a veritable technological advance for humanity. Fellow spiritualist Andrew Jackson Davis successfully established "Harmonial Brotherhoods" throughout the country, as well as the Children's Progressive Lyceum, a spiritualist version of Sunday school. By 1871 this lyceum had branches in seventeen states and in England. Davis, with the Nicholses, believed that spiritualism, like science, provided insight that was crucial to the elevating reform of humanity. Associationism, Swedenborgianism, and spiritualism all advanced the cause of universal harmony. At a time when railroads, steam mills, and telegraphs were reconfiguring the physical and social landscape of America, thousands of soul-searching individuals turned to these intellectual movements for reassurance and hope. In the context of impersonalizing technological growth, these belief systems emphasized human individuality and mutual connection: Fourier with his 810 personality types, Swedenborg with his unique matches of conjugial love, and spiritualism with its promise of social life after death (based elsewhere than heaven or hell). Like the industrialists financing westward expansion, leaders of these movements spoke the optimistic language of "progress." Reflecting on human nature, Thomas had written that "the most terrible punishment that can be inflicted on a human being, is to be utterly and forever alone."[19] As if in a coffin, one might say. By preaching against isolated households, by endorsing free love, and by adopting a faith that liberated its adherents from the terror of death, the Nicholses and thousands of others fought off the possibility of this terrible aloneness.[20]

Writing years later, Thomas recalled that Mary initially "had a strong repugnance to what became known as Spiritualism, in spite of her own second-sight experiences." She had been converted to spiritualism around 1850 in New York City, when an obscure medium named James B. Conklin—"a simple common sailor, who had a room in Canal Street, open free to all comers"—had presented to Mary convincing messages from the spirit world. Since then, Conklin had acquired national fame as a physical and writing medium whose regular communications with departed spirits had convinced even the most ardent skeptics. Mary and Thomas invited him to Cincinnati, where he held séances that brought about the inexplicable movement of heavy tables and the delivery of a message from a dead father to his living son. The evidence was irrefutable to the Nicholses. "We became satisfied, by careful examination . . . of the objective reality of spirit manifestations," wrote Thomas. "The one thing proved beyond all doubt by the facts of Spiritualism, is that the individual man survives the death of the body. *It is certain that we live on—it is rendered probable that we shall live for ever.*" By doubting the reality of hell, as Thomas explained to readers of the *Nichols' Monthly*, spiritualism had "taken from the pulpit its great engine of terror, and the means of governing men by their fears."[21]

Spiritualism called for no churches and required no pledges of faith to doctrine. It simply appealed to Americans' individualist impulse to believe that which one personally witnessed. Evidence of the spirit world was treated as scientific evidence, honored by many who considered themselves dispassionate observers of the natural world. Not least, women were as likely as men to become mediums—an equity virtually unknown among other religions. By 1856, Mary was impressing others with an apparently clairvoyant ability to describe "the size, position, and condition of the abscesses as they formed, opened, and discharged" in her own lungs. Thomas called her a "seeress," who could detect subtleties of character and foresee distant events.[22]

For twenty-first-century readers, jaded by the deceptive power of airbrushed photographs, computer-generated images, and films' diverse special effects (not to mention television, cell phones, and the internet), it is difficult to believe that so many truly intelligent Americans accepted the phenomena of spiritualism as generated by the spirit world. These effects were often silly: trumpets flying through the air, for example, or table legs rising and falling. I must confess that initially, at the point of their immersion into spiritualism, the Nicholses "lost" me. The language with which they described the Progressive Union and the cause of "harmonialism" only distanced me further. And yet it was clear that Mary and Thomas had in no way lost their minds; their critiques of society remained sharp and shockingly modern. Thomas Nichols spoke directly to my anxiety when he wrote in 1864,

> But a philosopher would like to know what kind of a delusion can have led astray some millions of "the most intelligent people on the earth." . . . If so many people, from senators, governors, and judges, down to the great mass of ordinary observers . . . have been deceived, befooled, and humbugged—one might wish to understand what deceived

them.... Now I flatter myself that I am as shrewd as my neighbours, and as learned as most of them; and I frankly confess, that ... I can offer no reasonable explanation of the facts.... I cannot tell what made the heavy thumps or percussions in the case of the Fox lady, and I can no more tell what moved the table in the case of Conklin.... A movement, sound, or motion, indicates force. A movement that gives information, true or false ... indicates intelligence acting by force. Question this invisible intelligence, which moves tables or pounds on them, and it declares itself to be the spirit of your grandfather, your friend, or acquaintance. You cannot easily credit this; but it ... submits to a cross-examination, and tells you things known only to you and the pretended spirit.

If you say Spiritualism is absurd, I agree with you.... What can be more absurd than for the spirits of Shakespeare or Bacon, Napoleon or Wellington, Washington or Franklin, answering the questions of every rude and vulgar person who chooses to call for them? And the answers and communications of these alleged spirits are commonly absurdly different from what we expect from them. Furthermore, these pretended spirits often lie.... Of course this does not disprove a communicating intelligence.

In retrospect, Thomas considered the primary effects of spiritualism on American culture to have been threefold: first, that it acted as a "segregating and scattering force" by driving thousands of people away from their prior religions and into no organized alternative; second, that it brought many who had lacked all faith to believe in the immortality of the soul; and third, that it provided deep solace to those grieving the loss of loved ones. Thomas also noted that in many cases spiritualism encouraged a tendency to insanity, an effect he compared to that induced by the century's earlier religious revivals.[23]

Despite their fascination with the spirits, all was not mystical with the Nicholses, who still had to earn a living in a new city. In 1856 Mary and Thomas self-published *Nichols' Medical Miscellanies: A Familiar Guide to the Preservation of Health, and the Hydropathic Home Treatment of the Most Formidable Diseases*. A compilation of their many previously published medical columns, this work was intended as a convenient handbook for a wide readership. The same year, Thomas contracted for the publication of his two new general-interest works, *Religions of the World. An Impartial History of Religious Creeds, Forms of Worship, Sects, Controversies, and Manifestations* and *The Illustrated Manners Book*. The latter, which ran to several hundred pages, was first published anonymously in New York in 1855 but later appeared under the name "Robert DeValcourt."[24] *The Illustrated Manners Book* adopted the frisky tone of Thomas's earlier journalism. Though it treated most subjects likely to be found in comparable manners books of the day, it also offered the spice of free love: "First love is never last love, unless the soul is crushed under some despotism," wrote Thomas. "I have known a whole series of light fancies, which might have been mistaken for loves, to be followed by the earnest passion of a life." Few other mid-century guides to "polite accomplishments" would advise that

> a gentleman should scorn to put any constraint upon the lady of his love; the constraint of jealousy or fear—of a promise or an obligation. He should say, "My blessed one, be free. Love me if you can; be mine if you love me; but I ask no promises, no vows." . . . And a lady should say, "To-day I love you, or I think I do. Let to-morrow tell its own story. I must do ever what my heart tells me to do. As long as I love you, I am yours." No honest man can ask for more. The true woman of civilization is not a Circassian slave, to be bought and sold and made property.[25]

Judging by the title of this work, a casual purchaser might well have been shocked to discover the philosophies it endorsed. Thomas and Mary also continued to publish the *Nichols' Monthly*, the organ of the Central Bureau of the Progressive Union.

MEMNONIA

After seven years of marriage and the forging of a shared professional life, Mary and Thomas still sought a secure community among friends. Cincinnati did not answer. Once again, Willie watched her parents prepare to move. She was five years old and had already lived in four different homes. During that time, her parents had trained scores of people and treated hundreds more with dripping sheets and cold baths, sponges and wraps. They had also written and published six books and an independent journal. In Cincinnati their first order of business had been to establish ties with new publishers. Their second had been to search the region for an ideal home. Mary and Thomas leased a water-cure resort in the small town of Yellow Springs, Ohio, seventy-four miles northeast of Cincinnati in Greene County. Mary was forty-five; Thomas was forty. Again, they planned to intertwine work with home.

Richly saturated with iron, the waters of Yellow Springs produced a golden glow along the limestone banks of the Little Miami River. Shawanoe Indians had long enjoyed healing qualities in the yellow water that flowed from the deep springs between two of their settlements: Mad River Village, south of Springfield, and Oldtown, north of Xenia. In the 1830s their trails to the springs were worn as deep as buffalo paths. But the birth of the town called Yellow Springs awaited a more formidable thoroughfare. In 1843 a man hired to help build the Springfield-Xenia road described Yellow Springs as "unnoticeable." Seeking work, he had trekked east from Dayton, through Byron, and on to Frogtown, where a sign indicated "Yellow Springs—1 mile." In that last densely wooded mile, he encountered only one structure: an old Methodist Church. Reaching the central springs above the union of two creeks, he found a small cabin that served as the village post office.[26]

Three years later the finished Springfield-Xenia road began to carry settlers to the banks of the Little Miami tributary. By 1855, when Mary and Thomas were shopping for land, Yellow Springs had achieved regional notoriety for two of its institutions: a popular water-cure establishment (complete with two large bowling alleys); and Antioch College, a two-year-old progressive institution led by the celebrated educational reformer Horace Mann.

Mann, a tall and captivating Massachusetts legislator, had devoted the bulk of his career to public education. He had accepted the presidency of Antioch College at its inception, attracted especially by the founders' commitment to nonsectarian "Bible Christianity." Liberal in its educational philosophy and seeking a stature commensurate with Harvard's, Antioch accepted black students as well as white and hired female as well as male instructors. Many luminaries visited the campus, including Horace Greeley, Charles Sumner, Theodore Parker, and Wendell Phillips.[27] The school adopted daring social policies, and its president vigilantly guarded against scandal of any kind.

Dedicated to coeducation, the founders of Antioch College still maintained grave concerns over the mingling of sexes on campus. To prevent even the temptation of misconduct, strict rules segregated male and female students: literary societies were to have only single-sex membership; students were permitted in the rooms of only same-sex peers; male and female students were forbidden from visiting the creek's glen together; no student could board with families accommodating boarders of the opposite sex; and any student who married was expected to leave the institution. At the same time, all Antioch students were given abundant opportunity to interact with each other under faculty supervision, to reduce the need for private meetings.[28]

Long before completion of the Springfield-Xenia road and the founding of Antioch College, Yellow Springs had welcomed social experimentation. In 1825 followers of utopian socialist Robert Owen established a short-lived community along the west bank of Yellow Springs Creek. There they built a single-story structure of upright split logs, filling the gaps with plaster. This long house provided private rooms for a number of families as well as a group kitchen and dining room. But the communalists could not meet their debt on the land, and by January of 1827 they had resigned all claims to the property, which later became part of Antioch's campus. In 1840 Daniel Webster, Henry Clay, and Martin Van Buren all included Yellow Springs in their campaign routes. By 1855, with a road and a college, approximately four hundred residents occupied the lovely and historically progressive town.[29] To Mary and Thomas, Yellow Springs seemed perfect.

In February of 1856, Thomas published a three-page circular advertising the "Memnonia Institute," due to open on the first of April. The institute was named for a mystic statue on the Nile, said to greet each sunrise with music. On April 7, in celebration of Charles Fourier's birthday, the Nicholses would invite the public to a formal dedication.[30] "MEM-NONIA will be a School of Health; a School of Progress; a School of Life. We wish to gather here, as in a carefully cultured nursery, the germs of a new society," declared the pamphlet.

Rather than envisioning a utopian community—society abruptly transformed—the Nicholses intended to establish a place of preparation, a training ground. Memnonia would provide a calm, salubrious, and beautiful setting for individual progress in a group context. Desarrollo may have miscarried, but Mary and Thomas still expected to welcome "a New Era for Humanity." This hope led them to recruit three classes of people to Yellow Springs: members of the Progressive Union seeking a "Purer and Truer Life"; invalids seeking treatment; and students of either sex and of any age seeking "integral education." At the same time, they took pains to deter other company, specifically "legal or illegal experimentists or sensualists." Modern Times had shown Mary and Thomas the dangers of an open-door policy. They wanted no nudists, no women attempting to live solely on beans and water, and, most to the point: no one challenging their purpose. Memnonia's advertising circular thus expressed the Nicholses' terms without equivocation: "It is to be understood that, taking all responsibility, we shall exercise the right to reject any application, or to dismiss any inmate of our home. MEMNONIA will be, provisionally and necessarily, a despotism, as wise and benevolent as circumstances will admit. It is to be neither a community nor a house of refuge, but, as far as possible, a refined and beautiful Harmonic Home." Those who joined this home would be expected to keep a vegetarian diet, to bathe daily, to abstain from tobacco, and to maintain neat attire and a courteous demeanor. They were also to be chaste. To those who accepted these terms, the Nicholses explained, "You are Harmonists. This is your world designation. You are now distincted [sic] from the Experimentists. You have no battle to fight." Memnonia's motto? "Freedom, Fraternity, Chastity."[31]

Despite the sound of it, Mary and Thomas had not simply abandoned the doctrine of free love. They still believed that physical passion should enjoy the same freedom as every other passion—but they had come to believe that such freedom would actually result in a *stricter* chastity than that required by the most restrictive state laws. In the harmonic future they sought, a perfected society would set all passions free. Health would be restored, and lusty over-indulgence, like all disease, would be purged. Mary and Thomas continued to place sexual fulfillment in the wider context of Harmonial Progress. "The law of Progression in Harmony gives us this law of sexual relations," they wrote:

"Material Union is only to be had, when the wisdom of the Harmony demands a child." The wisdom of our Harmony teaches us that birth, under existing conditions, is seldom and exceptionally a good; and not to be sought contrary to the laws of the society and State in which we live. We, therefore, not only require the chastity which the civil law demands, but we repudiate the sensual license it permits. We ask the far purer chastity of a higher law, which commands us to garner our lives, and avoid the waste of all the evils of sensuality. . . . [W]e will not assume any responsibility, either as teachers or healers, toward any person who can not cordially accept and live to the spirit of this law.[32]

In the Nicholses' view, concern for the welfare of children surpassed every other consideration in importance. While the probationary requirement of chastity prevented the waste of vital energy expended in orgasm, it more significantly prevented the reproduction of inharmonic adults into an inharmonic society. "We by no means condemn birth, even in our progress from the discordant to the unitary," wrote the Nicholses, "but in our transition work, when the passions are excessive and inharmonic in their action, we would have men and women thoughtfully wise—we would have them understand their rights, and know very certainly whether they are dominated by diseased amativeness, or by a desire to give a worthful Life to a child, who shall be worthy of the gift."[33]

The Nicholses would not have their mission perverted once again. As if they had not expressed the case clearly enough, their promotional circular reiterated Memnonia's policy regarding sexual freedom: "Citizens of the State, and members of a civil society, we shall require of all the inmates of our home, conformity to the civil law respecting Marriage and Paternity." The words *free love* do not appear anywhere in the pamphlet.

The Yellow Springs Water-Cure, which the Nicholses leased for a period of five years, had thrived under a string of managers. Its grounds stretched east up a gentle hill from the banks of Shelden Glen, just downstream of the fork that defined two branches of Yellow Springs Creek. The central building, painted white, stood several stories high and overlooked a plateau of lawn surrounded by a forest of sycamore, oak, walnut, and basswood. It comfortably housed one hundred people. A winding path connected the main house with a small brick station of the Little Miami Railroad, built on the west bank of Shelden Glen expressly for use of the Cure. After descending toward the creek and crossing a bridge, visitors followed an uphill path toward the main house, passing wide circular fountains sparkling with goldfish and lilies. A cement conduit fed these fountains at good pressure, drawing water from an elevated spring. An even higher spring on the opposite bank of the creek supplied water to the buildings via a lengthy connection of wood pipes, each about twenty feet long and three inches in diameter.[34]

Despite local physicians' skepticism of hydrotherapy, the Yellow Springs Water-Cure had once been so popular that weekend and summer guests from Cincinnati and Dayton had been forced to sleep on cots in the halls. In 1852 the managing physicians advertised treatment for "Rheumatism, Nervous Affections, Spinal Diseases, Dyspepsia, Chronic Diarrhea, Chills and Fevers, Insipient Consumptions [*sic*]" and a variety of other chronic disorders.[35] The Nicholses, in turn, advertised to "the wearied, exhausted, and diseased, who have yet a recuperative vitality." In addition to the diverse baths, packs, douches, exercise, relaxation, fresh air, and pure water fundamental to hydropathic treatment, Mary and Thomas also intended to provide "when required, Clairvoyant examinations, and Magnetic and Spiritual Ministrations." They hoped, with "proper Mediums, and a Harmonious Circle . . . to develop a corresponding power of healing."[36] In 1856, however, it was neither hydropathy nor spiritualism that kindled fierce local resistance to the Nicholses. It was, once again, free love.

STAKING CLAIMS

On Friday evening, March 7, 1856, readers of the *Daily Springfield Nonpareil* encountered the following notice: "We are informed that the citizens of Yellow Springs held a meeting a few days since for the purpose of quashing an attempt made by certain persons to inaugurate 'a free-love association' in their midst, that they are determined to prevent the formation of such an institution in their beautiful locality. That is the way to do, begin at early dawn, nip it in the bud, and if possible prevent every movement calculated to corrupt society."[37] The following night a second, even larger gathering convened in Yellow Springs to hear details of the proposed Memnonia. There, Thomas Nichols attempted to defend himself against the invective of a formidable antagonist: Horace Mann. As president of Antioch College, Mann considered his institution enormously threatened by any possible association with the infamous Nicholses. He called their theories "the superfoetation of diabolism upon polygamy."[38] Already some of the college students had begun distributing their works. Mann could not tolerate such an influence—not on paper, and certainly not half a mile down the creek. Not only did he despise the seeming licentiousness of their teachings, but he also had an immediate crisis on his hands. To Mary and Thomas Nichols, April 1, 1856, marked the start of a five-year lease; to Horace Mann, that same date marked the final deadline by which Antioch would have to raise $120,000 to meet its debts.[39]

Worried about the very survival of his school, Mann proceeded to rally the town against Mary and Thomas before their lease even took effect. He feared that the Nicholses' proximity to Antioch would both discourage prospective students and frighten away current students, especially women. Thomas's protestations that he was a law-abiding citizen with every right to develop Memnonia in peace did not warm the crowd, who had only grudgingly allowed him to speak in the first place. Mann and others had read recent issues of the *Nichols' Monthly,* whose contents seemed to belie the Nicholses' declared respect for the marital laws of the state. Columns of particular concern included excerpts of *Esperanza: My Journey Thither, and What I Found There,* an unfinished utopian novel Thomas was writing, which, in his own words, captured "the actual working and daily expression of a Harmonic Society."[40]

In *Esperanza,* a "Land of Hope," people lived much as they might have in Desarrollo: attending optional lectures on science and art; sharing stimulating conversation; bathing daily; laboring from attraction rather than compulsion; rehearsing plays; racing sailboats; and eating corn, rice, peas, potatoes, and fruit. Drawing on the bureaucratic language of Stephen Pearl Andrews and Charles Fourier, Thomas created for Esperanza an "Order of Recreation" and an "Order of Industry." Happy workers wore badges suited to their particular tasks and received "Orders of the Day" from a fictional leader who bore a remarkable similarity to Thomas Low Nichols. Inhabitants of this Edenic world enjoyed the benefits of a unitary kitchen; a centralized laundry, bakery, and nursery; a library; shops; and a Festive Hall.

Thomas's Yellow Springs adversaries perceived danger in a separate aspect of Esperanza, however. In the fictional, Fourierist world Thomas described—an earthly world that sought to emulate the spirit world—sexual reproduction would be determined by the "demands of harmony," not by monogamy. The *women* of Esperanza would exclusively determine when "Harmony" favored reproduction. Free love, if not licentiousness, would prevail. Naturally readers of the *Monthly* drew a connection between the love imagined for Esperanza and the potential incarnation of Memnonia. "Did ever the cloven foot expose itself more openly, or did ever the stench of the pit offend more grievously the nostrils of the people?" demanded the newspaper. At the height of this controversy, Mary suffered another severe pulmonary attack.[41] Though acutely aware that he was unwelcome and very concerned about his wife, Thomas publicly refused to break his lease.

The property owner, a homeopathic physician from Cincinnati named Ehrmann, likewise rejected pleas to reconsider the Nicholses as tenants. On March 19, 1856, Ehrmann and a friend visited the property with intent to reclaim it from its current tenants, Dr. and Mrs. Hoyt. Mrs. Hoyt, who happened to be at home alone, argued with Ehrmann that her lease still had several months remaining. After their unrecorded discussion, Ehrmann proceeded into town to declare that he was granting immediate possession of the Cure to the Nicholses. Meanwhile, Mrs. Hoyt undertook to lock Ehrmann's companion in an empty room and begin boarding up the house against intruders. When Ehrmann returned to find his own property barricaded, he attempted to break down the door. Forty men rushed to defend Mrs. Hoyt, with the result that Ehrmann dropped his keys and fled along eight miles of railroad track to Xenia. Later that night authorities returned Ehrmann to Yellow Springs to face charges for housebreaking.[42]

Mary and Thomas were unable to occupy the property before the first week of July, three months later than planned. In the interim, they used their *Monthly* to condemn Horace Mann as the murderer of any whose lives might be lost for want of Memnonia's treatment. Thomas claimed that Mann had threatened to resign if the Nicholses settled in Yellow Springs. At the same time, they happily noted that the excitement over Memnonia had provided the Progressive Union more publicity than it could otherwise have achieved in the same period. In August, Horace Mann wrote to his wife that "Nichols . . . boasts that he has overcome all opposition, and is fluttering his wings proudly." But it required more than the passage of time to ease tensions. In June, the former sailor and current seer James B. Conklin came to Yellow Springs.[43]

Mary and Thomas had known Conklin for more than five years. Back in New York City, he had replaced Mary's initial aversion to spiritualism with utter faith. Conklin later conducted séances with the Nicholses at

Port Chester and traveled to Cincinnati at their invitation and expense. Mary and Thomas had been profiling his experiences in the *Nichols' Monthly* since June of the previous year. Conklin's summer visit to Yellow Springs revealed dramatic and convincing manifestations of the spirit world. In short order, he converted many respectable citizens, including an elder of the First Presbyterian Church, as well as members of Antioch's faculty and student body; he thereby also helped his besieged friends.[44]

That summer Horace Mann took a trip to the Great Lakes and returned to find the Nicholses firmly established across the creek. Perhaps in retaliation for his attacks on Memnonia, the *Nichols' Monthly* criticized Antioch's severe restriction of contact between its male and female students. While Mary and Thomas advocated warm and unrestrained friendship between the sexes, Mann had written to a friend, "I have seen enough of young men to satisfy me, that in our present state of society there is not any great majority who would not yield to the temptation of ruining a girl if he could." In short order, Mann was forced to contend with ardent Nichols sympathizers in his own school.[45]

One student in particular, Jared Gage, had distressed him ever since Mary and Thomas had distributed the Memnonia circular. Gage had enrolled in Antioch's large preparatory school one year before the trouble began. On the night of the first closed meeting regarding the Nicholses' proposed lease, Gage had approached President Mann on campus and asked if the meeting were to be open. Mann said no, and as the two walked toward the bookstore, Mann asked Jared whether he knew Thomas Nichols. Gage explained that he not only had read many of his writings but that he had also lived with Nichols a few years earlier while suffering very poor health. "What do you think of him?" asked Mann. "He is a man for whom I have the highest respect and the most unbounded esteem," replied Jared. "Mr. Gage," Mann answered, "I shall have to alter my opinion very *much,* either of *him,* OR OF YOU." The conversation thus ended at the bookstore.

Dr. W. N. Hambleton, the student who ran the bookstore, had that very day put up notices advertising the Nicholses' works for sale and declaring that "error alone fears investigation." Hambleton had attended the American Hydropathic Institute. The Nicholses described him as one of their "most zealous and thorough graduates" and a "very skillful and reliable man." The day after posting his notices, Hambleton was given the choice of ceasing to sell the Nicholses' books or of leaving Antioch. Outraged, he chose to leave.[46] Horace Mann also sent a letter to Jared Gage's father, expressing continued concern over Jared's endorsement of the Nicholses:

> *Dear Sir,*—I have just returned home . . . and have found Mrs. Gage's letter and yours awaiting my arrival. . . . Mrs. Gage says she is acquainted with the writings of Mr. and Mrs. Nichols, and that if they are "honest," they have "her warmest sympathies." I do not think it is possible she can have read all their writings. In their book on "Marriage," he says expressly that what the law calls "fornication," may be the "holiest relation" . . . ; he calls "adultery" a "virtue," and she details . . . a conversation which she had with . . . a married woman—to persuade her to commit adultery. . . .
>
> We want nothing to do with him, unless we could reform him. We must disconnect ourselves from every body who upholds him. . . . With entire good feeling towards your son, and with friendship to you, we must request you to restrain him from advocating these doctrines and circulating these books, and introducing the advocates of them to our students, (as he has done,) or we must request him to leave.

Jared received a similar ultimatum directly. Outraged at what he considered the limitation of his constitutional freedom, he attended the public meeting at which Thomas Nichols sought unsuccessfully to diffuse the community's wrath. Near the start of the summer vacation, Jared posted a notice that he had for sale a variety of works on spiritualism and social reform. He also began to board with the Nicholses down at the Water-Cure and to use their baths. He considered Mary and Thomas old friends.

A few days after Jared posted his advertisement, President Mann came to his room to inspect the collection of books, which included work by the Nicholses. Jared's was a clear act of defiance. When Mann attempted to forbid Jared's sale of any books on free love, Jared "refused to acknowledge the right of the 'faculty' to prohibit any lawful business." He told the college president that he did not consider their conversation conclusive.

Jared was soon expelled. The technical issue for which the faculty voted him home to his parents ultimately did not involve the sale of books; it related to Jared's decision to board with the Nicholses. The thirty-sixth rule of the college declared that "without permission of the Faculty, students will not be allowed to board with families in the village, who take boarders of the other sex." There followed a dispute over both the spirit and wording of this rule. Jared contended that all students had taken the rule to imply prohibition of living in families with "*student* boarders of the opposite sex." Because no female Antioch students boarded with the Nicholses, he did not consider that he had broken any rule. In fact, he knew many other students who had similar living arrangements elsewhere. When President Mann attempted to enforce the letter of the rule, denying any awareness of such a limited interpretation, Jared replied in kind, pointing out that the rule only applied to families "*in the village,*" which the Nicholses, half a mile down the stream, technically were not. Mann replied that the Water-Cure had always been considered subject to the rule. Not surprisingly, a faculty vote after a full hearing decided the case in favor of President Mann's interpretation. Jared Gage left Antioch at the end of September.

Two months later, Antioch's Adelphian Union Literary Society voted to return to a recent anonymous donor copies of *Marriage* and *Mary Lyndon*. Notes from their meeting show that the society rejected the gifts for "their tendency to oppose the marriage system as now existing." For good measure, the group then voted also to expel *Esoteric Anthropology* from their collections as well as "books presented by J. D. Gage."[47]

An uneasy coexistence thereafter ensued between Antioch and Memnonia. One Yellow Springs woman recalled that "no one in the place or vicinity associated with [the Nicholses]. They would drive into town for business or for mail, then drive back to the Cure."[48] Though Mary did not record her feelings regarding this social isolation, she surely suffered. Only one year earlier, she had described the pain associated with her previous shunning by Quakers in New Hampshire. "There are wounds that never gape or bleed to human eyes," she had written. "There may be opposition and violence that can suffocate and kill, and yet no word may be spoken, no hand raised apparently. Often had I gone to Quaker meetings, when in the stillness of absolute rest and perfect quiet[,] eyes like spears had pierced me. A wall of adamant had been built up against me, and I could hardly have been more crushed had the ceiling been made to descend upon me."[49] Elsewhere in autobiographical prose, Mary had described herself as "deficient in self-esteem from my birth. . . . I longed for approval with limitless longing, and my parents starved the desire from a sense of duty."[50] Mary's adult strivings reflected this desperate wish for acceptance and community. All her grand, idealistic plans for social reform involved the quest for sympathetic friends with shared vision. Mary and Thomas may have received much supportive mail on their trips into town, but letters hardly could have satisfied their enormous craving for human connection.

In the August issue of the *Nichols' Monthly*, Thomas—never a man to lose face—asserted that Horace Mann alone was treating members of Memnonia with less than "uniform respect and kindness."[51] Yet even Thomas might have preferred bad press to no press. By January 1857, the *Daily Springfield Nonpareil* had changed the tone of its abuse: "Dr. Nichols, of the Yellow Springs Water Cure, is a good deal worse in theory than in practice. The prospective evil effects of his doctrines find no fulfillment. . . . His fanaticism, like other species of the same genius, will be harmless if let alone."[52] The paper spoke truth. By the end of March 1857, Memnonia had disbanded on its own.

Three years later a visitor to Yellow Springs happened to meet a beautiful, intellectual woman who had lived at Memnonia. This woman described the majority of its members—of whom there were never more than about twenty—as Eastern and English transplants. Most, she recalled, were "persons who had met with disappointments and grief in the life of the affections—the unrequited or the divorced."[53]

EIGHT

Unsettling Departures

ᘒ ᘒ ᘒ

THE TWO BRANCHES of Yellow Springs Creek merged just below Meditation Point, a jut of land situated in the middle of this river-fork, south of the town's famous mineral spring. From Meditation Point, one could see grand oaks and cedars capping the yellow-tinged rock formation known as Indian Mound. Each stream had carved a deep ravine in its soft mineral bed, creating high limestone bluffs and spraying falls. The two gorges met at the top of Shelden Glen, spilling their creeks together into a small, smooth-bottomed pool before proceeding another mile south, past Antioch College and the Water Cure, to join the Little Miami River. Antioch students used this pool as a swimming hole when it was not doing service in baptisms conducted along its gently sloping floor.[1]

Yellow Springs—rich with mineral waters, preequipped with a relatively new hydropathic establishment, serviced by both rail and coach lines, and surrounded by fragrant forests—had seemed to Mary and Thomas worth the fight. Though deeply influenced by Fourier's visions of the phalanstery, the Nicholses did not expect Memnonia to produce spontaneous harmony. Instead, Mary and Thomas saw it as a preharmonic place of stringent reformation. Whereas Fourier had anticipated sudden Harmonic Balance from the structured association of diverse personality types, Mary and Thomas advertised a home of slow preparation—a chaste home, free of civilization's excesses. They defended the evolution of their own thinking: "They say this is a very different freedom from that advocated in the *Anthropology*. Suppose it is. What then? Are we bound never to grow wiser, because we have stated our best wisdom at a given time or times?"[2]

To recruit new members, Mary and Thomas had welcomed the public for Sunday-afternoon discussions on human progress. In addition to these open meetings, residents of Memnonia met for private discussion circles— that is, spiritualist séances—every morning at 7:30 as well as on Friday and Sunday evenings. Willie, who was six years old and surrounded by intellectual endeavors, did not attend school. Instead, she adopted her parents' library and claimed at once to be reading Plutarch's *Lives* and the Koran, and comparing different Christian Bibles. Thomas marveled at the speed of his daughter's reading and at her ability to memorize paragraphs in a glance. He wondered if she might be gifted with the skill of "mental photography."[3]

Though no formal classes or lectures structured Memnonia's days, many members took lessons in various fine arts, elocution, and composition. Daily group confessions, the exchange of criticism, and the assignment of penances further ensured mutual involvement, if also an unfortunate measure of resentment and jealousy. Financial insecurity loomed as well. Maintaining group cohesion required constant vigilance. As shepherds who had abandoned the license of Modern Times, Mary and Thomas sought to guide their enlisted family with firm authority. The free love they now endorsed cast aside all sensualism and instead expressed "the sum total of our spiritual affinities for other beings."[4] This philosophical combination of free love and chastity dissatisfied both conservatives and radicals. "When we proclaimed the great law of freedom in all relations, conservatism charged us with licentiousness," wrote Thomas. "When, in the exercise of that freedom, we proclaimed . . . '*Material union is only to be had when the wisdom of harmony demands a child,*' selfists, individualists, and experimentists denounced us as tyrants and ascetics."[5] Still, the Nicholses had preached, fought, and prayed for Memnonia. By the early months of 1857, they were struggling to make it work.

CONVERSION

Thomas recalled that during those first years in Ohio, he and Mary "were Spiritualists, with not merely a faith in immortality, but an assurance based upon observation."[6] In séances, they had regularly encountered spirits of the dead, many of whom offered advice and opinions. During one such circle, early in 1856, an apparition appeared to Mary that initiated a climactic, permanent transformation in their lives. For many who read of their bizarre experience, the story yielded nothing short of stupefied amazement. Mary and Thomas could scarcely explain it themselves.

Thomas related his version of the events in a column entitled "Letter to Our Friends and Co-Workers," published in the *Catholic Telegraph and Advocate* on May 23, 1857. It all started, he explained, when Mary was approached during a séance by an unfamiliar spirit who claimed to be a Jesuit. This Jesuit apparition advised Mary to study the history of the Society of Jesus, whose goals overlapped with her own. Skeptical of this unknown spirit—who had received no introduction from Mary's "guardian spirit"—Mary ignored the mysterious advice.

Six months later a second apparition appeared and chastised Mary for her indifference to the prior counsel. Wearing Jesuit garments, he announced that his name was Gonzales. "Justice! Justice to the Society of Jesus!" he declared. Confused and perhaps a bit shaken by this encounter, Mary wrote a descriptive letter to Archbishop John B. Purcell of Cincinnati, who referred her to Father Oakley, rector of the Jesuit-managed St. Xavier College, also in Cincinnati. While Mary and Thomas waited for earthly guidance, the spirit of St. Ignatius Loyola himself appeared to Mary and offered what he called "a method of reduction," or "directions for an order of life." Intrigued enough by this string of visits to read a biography of St. Ignatius Loyola, the Nicholses nevertheless did not immerse themselves, as directed, in the study of Catholic dogma.

Then another spirit visited. Calling himself "Frances Xavier," this last apparition took it upon himself to instruct Mary in church doctrine. His teachings covered "the incarnation and redemptive sacrifice of Christ, His formation of the church, the mystical body of Christ, the sacraments, miracles, the communion of saints, and the apostolic succession." From her trance-like state, Mary relayed these lessons while Thomas transcribed. Later he sent the transcripts to a Catholic acquaintance in Virginia for verification, since Yellow Springs was not a Catholic town. This friend submitted the papers to a local priest, who confirmed their accuracy. Both Thomas and Mary professed to have read no works on Catholic doctrine during this period. (Given his prior research for the comparative textbook, *Religions of the World*, however, one might question Thomas's claim of utter ignorance regarding Catholic doctrine outside these spirit visitations.) Finally, the spirit of St. Xavier instructed Mary and Thomas to appeal for "oral instruction of the Church" and to seek conversion.[7]

On Sunday, March 29, 1857, Mary, age forty-seven; Thomas, age forty-two; Willie, age six; and one Franstina Hopkins, who lived at Memnonia and had been with the Nicholses in Port Chester, were converted to Roman Catholicism at Saint Xavier Church in Cincinnati. Reverend Oakley performed the baptisms. Three other members of Memnonia—Mr. and Mrs. Gardiner Waters and their son—had been baptized nearly two months earlier.[8] The secular, spiritualist, and Catholic presses all took note, astounded by the Nicholses' humble recantations. The *New York Daily Tribune,* in an article entitled "Free Lovers Converted to Catholicism," quoted from the 1857 letter Thomas sent to Archbishop Purcell, who then published it in the *Catholic Telegraph and Advocate:* "In deep humility and contrition, we submit ourselves to [the Church's] divine order; we accept what she teaches, and we repudiate and condemn what she condemns. Whatever, in our writings and teachings, and in our lives, has been contrary to the doctrines, morality and discipline of the holy Catholic Church, we wish to retract and repudiate, and were it possible, to atone for."[9]

The *New England Spiritualist,* a paper in which Thomas had previously expressed his views on free love, offered different excerpts from Thomas's letter to Archbishop Purcell:

> We have been . . . Socialists of the school of Fourier, and have believed in, and earnestly labored for, the establishment of a unitary, or harmonic society. Our studies and efforts . . . brought us to the conviction that such social regeneration could be possible only in an orderly and holy life. . . . [I]t pleased God to bring us . . . acceptance of his holy Church. In that Church . . . we see the order, the devotion, the consecration, the faith and obedience, necessary for the great work of human redemption.

Former allies now struck Thomas as sadly confused. At Memnonia, the group had been "vainly trying to make a harmony," blind to the "Great Harmony already established," reflected Thomas. "If the Infidels and Socialists, the Reformers and Spiritualists, with whom we have labored in sincere, zealous, but misguided efforts for the good of our race, could see, as it had been revealed to us, that the holy Catholic Church is the divinely established society for the regeneration of man, . . . they would fly to her bosom for rest and peace. . . . I have found already, in my first experiences, inexpressible peace."[10] It was an astounding reorientation.

The editor of the *New England Spiritualist* noted that because the Nicholses were "possessed of minds capable of resisting any amount of external pressure," their abrupt conversion warranted thoughtful consideration. It was not the only example of "intelligent, strong-minded people" abandoning Protestantism for Roman Catholicism, despite the latter's much-maligned status. "The more progressive the tendencies of an individual," speculated the editor, "the greater the probability that [the demands of one's religious nature] will be felt in this life. "Such philanthropic souls generally devote themselves to the various reform causes of their day," he noted. And yet, "having completed the circuit, and yearning for a yet unattained something, the religious nature begins at length to assert its demands." Fourier and his followers had not adequately "provided for these *religious* wants of the soul."[11]

John Humphrey Noyes, founder of the religious Oneida Community and scholar of American socialist experiments, came to a similar conclusion years later, when reflecting on the relative failure of Fourierist efforts compared to those of the Shakers and of other more enduring initiatives: "The one feature which distinguishes these [successful] Communities from the transitory sort, is their religion; which in every case is of the earnest kind which comes by recognized afflatus [divine impulse], and controls all external arrangements."[12] The editor of the *Spiritualist,* who viewed Catholicism as just one among many despotic religions, explained that Spiritualists find "THE CHRIST not so much in the historic records of the past as in the *Divine in Man*—the *God manifest in the flesh,* of the present." Still, he may have come very close to understanding the true impulse behind the Nicholses' pull toward "Rome" when he wrote: "Protestantism, in itself, is but a *negation*—a protest against certain dogmas and assumptions. Whatever of *positive* religious truth may have been incorporated into any of its numerous creeds, belongs to . . . true Catholicity. . . . [N]either the intellect nor the soul can long subsist on *negations.*"[13] This passage recalls Mary's characterization of her own father: "He said *No,* to every one's proposition in medicine and religion, but he had no *Yes* to utter."[14]

The first response of twenty-first-century feminists to the Nicholses' conversion may be one of disappointment. We do not often associate the Catholic Church with progressive gender politics. How could such forward-looking radicals embrace the patriarchal and rigid doctrines of

Catholicism? What about women's rights? What about personal freedom? When considered from the perspective of 1857, however, the choice of Catholicism seems less paradoxical. Against the backdrop of America's secular patriarchy, Catholic patriarchy did not seem such a political step backward. On the contrary, Catholic schools and convents encouraged female education in harmonious enclaves akin to those the Nicholses had attempted to found. They offered positions of leadership and relative self-government; the latter also provided women room to live and work without sexual pressures. Within the church, women were honored as saints. And three years before the Jesuit spirits visited Mary, Pope Pius IX had initiated an unprecedented emphasis within the Catholic Church on the importance of the Virgin Mary, whom he believed had cured his epilepsy. On December 8, 1854, the pope issued a bull, *Ineffabilis Deus,* which declared: "The most Blessed Virgin Mary was, from the first moment of her conception, by a singular grace and privilege of almighty God and by virtue of the merits of Jesus Christ, Savior of the human race, preserved immune from all stain of original sin." This doctrine of the Immaculate Conception elevated Christ's mother to a position above the human race and preserved her from committing any sin in her life. For the subsequent century, Catholic theologians would pursue a branch of study known as "Mariology." Thomas's 1857 letter to Archbishop Purcell expressed the Nicholses' devotion to the Virgin Mary, in whose honor they imagined creating "a religious order of chaste birth"—a plan that never materialized.[15]

Mary's sudden conversion and immediate interest in founding a religious order devoted to the Virgin Mary invite speculation about her own psychology. The hateful marriage to Hiram Gove made Mary extremely reflective about sexual attractions. After years of being raped, she devoted the rest of her life to bathing, to the cause of women's self-ownership, to a quest for harmonious relations, and to an ultimate defense of chastity. "I had obeyed [Hiram], even as a machine obeys the hand that guides it," she wrote.[16] Her own virginity could not be restored, but her devotion to the Virgin Mary could at long last find a voice. Ironically, Catholicism provided Mary the sexual liberation she had sought since her first night in Hiram's bedroom.

In *Marriage,* Mary quoted from a letter she had written to a single woman who was living with a married man. To this troubled "mistress," Mary wrote: "You are to cultivate in yourself constantly the feeling of

fidelity, not to man, but to God; or in other words, to the highest in yourself. . . . [Your lover] must be worthy of your love . . . else you have no divine right to be his. . . . 'He that would save his life shall lose it, but he that
would lose his life for Christ's sake, shall find it.' People are nothing to me
now, only as they are worthy."[17] Mary had begun to live for Christ long
before the fateful séances. And Thomas had long lived for Mary.

The purifying experience of baptism also appealed psychologically to
the Nicholses, who either had never been baptized as infants or did not
know if they had. The ceremony of using water to cleanse one's life of *all
prior sin* symbolically honored and preserved the hydropathic aspects of
their work while purging that which the church condemned. In 1853
Mary had written, "I believe in daily baptism in pure water. . . . It corresponds to the baptism of Truth in the Spirit." But at that time, she had
added, "If my neighbor . . . believes in the ordinance of baptism in a more
restricted mode, being confined to one immersion . . . in a life time, I have
no fault to find with his faith, though I feel sure that I am more religious
than he."[18] The Catholic Church had reason to wonder at the Nicholses'
newfound faith.

Yet even earlier Mary had written a letter to the editor of the Fourierist *Phalanx* in which she attributed American doubts about passional
freedom to a generalized "want of Faith." There she confessed that she
too had first "looked upon the actualization of this great Idea as something in the far distance, something if I must confess it, like the planning
of journeys to the moon." Though Mary was referring to the promise of
associationism and free love, her words foreshadow a more religious quest:

> The fact was, I lacked Faith in God and Man. And this I opine is the
> condition of the majority of our race. They do not believe that the Des-
> tiny of man is holiness or *wholeness*, and consequently happiness. . . .
> This want of that Faith, which is the *substance* of things hoped for, the
> Divine energy or substance out of which and by which one whole or
> holy Ideal is created, leaves men sunk in inaction, or weak and puerile
> action. We want more Faith.[19]

Ever since her sudden adoption of Quakerism as a teenager, Mary had
sought "faith." The religious language that suffused her writing reflected
more than a rhetorical fashion of the era. She genuinely equated personal

wholeness with holiness. Thus it was in Catholicism, not the phalanx, that Mary ultimately found a satisfyingly rich measure of Harmony. Spiritualism had tended to disrupt faithful communities. It could not answer Mary's hunger for close, living bonds. For years, she and Thomas had weathered displacements, rejection, slander, and financial loss. Catholicism offered the glimmering promise of acceptance, influence, and immortality.

Less than a week after her conversion, Mary wrote to her old friend in Lynn, Alonzo Lewis, to share her news. "On Sunday last my husband and myself our daughter Mary Wilhelmina and Franstina Hopkins were all baptised into the Holy Roman Catholic Church," she wrote. "This may seem strange to you; indeed it does to us, but we are now humble believers. . . . We are unspeakably happy in the faith, and ask only to be allowed to live and die humble Catholic Christians." She added that Elma, who was living in Cincinnati and "doing *well,*" was "High Church Episcopal and has to hold on to keep from 'going over to Rome.'" In this cheerful letter, Mary acknowledged that "of course all our 'Reform' are charged to us now. We move only with the approbation of the Church."[20]

Archbishop Purcell had not casually welcomed the Nicholses' request for conversion. In a letter to Bishop Peter Paul Lefevre of Detroit, written a month before the nationally newsworthy baptisms, Purcell had sought his colleague's guidance: "What do you think, Monseigneur, of my receiving into the Church the Mother Abbess of the Free Lovers?" He went on to explain that another family from Memnonia had adopted Catholicism. From them, presumably, he had gained a sense of the Nicholses' teachings. "You know," he wrote, "they hold that, under the old dispensation, a woman had not the possession of herself, her individuality. And that one of her sacred rights is that of choosing the father of her child. Surely God can have, or make, his elect everywhere. And His holy grace is never more triumphant than when he subdues such souls."[21]

Purcell wrote similar letters of concern to the archbishops of Baltimore and St. Louis. One of them, Peter R. Kenrick, expressed apprehension. While in principle he saw "no difficulty in receiving converted Spiritists and Free Lovers into the Church," Kenrick did not find the Nicholses' story of spirit guides particularly reassuring. "I believe that the whole affair is pure Deviltry, and should hesitate before receiving into the Church those who would have no other motive than that which might be derived from such a source," he wrote.[22] But by then Archbishop Purcell had sanctioned the conversion, with the requirement that the Nicholses publicly recant their former teachings. Mary and Thomas received their first Holy Communion in July 1857.[23]

Late in life, when Thomas once again recounted the strange story of their conversion, he attempted to reconcile their previous spiritualism with what had followed. While "no religious organization is more strenuous [than Catholicism] in requiring the assent of all its members to what is defined as 'of faith,'" he wrote, "no one can give more freedom as to the right of private judgment in [other matters]. As Spiritualism deals almost entirely with phenomena which are matters of fact, of course no religious teacher could condemn what belongs not to faith, but to science."[24]

SYNTHESIS

After converting, the Nicholses left Yellow Springs and spent several months at a large Ursuline convent in Brown County, Ohio. A train carried the family deep into the woods and deposited them six miles from their destination along a rutted and difficult wagon road. Finally, a clearing in the forest revealed the large brick convent, several cottages, and a small log chapel. The nuns of St. Ursula wore black robes and veils, with leather belts at their waists and wooden crosses around their necks. Novices wore white veils. The Mother Superior of the Brown County Convent was herself a convert from Protestantism who had scandalized her British relatives by converting while at school in France. Two French priests supervised life at the convent. One, in his seventies, served as spiritual adviser. The other, thirty-five years old, oversaw the farming and conducted services. The nuns also ran a school for girls, many of whom were Protestant. Mary shared her knowledge of hygiene and hydropathy with the nuns and their students. She and Thomas also spent much of their time observing the rituals of convent life and studying Catholic texts.[25]

But what of their views on marriage? In the letter he sent to Archbishop Purcell in 1857, Thomas wrote with reverence of "the Sacrament of Holy Matrimony . . . from which souls may be born for life and happiness instead of death and misery." Three years earlier, the *Nichols' Journal* had asserted that "marriage enslaves men and women, annihilating their individuality, and converting their very virtues into sources of misery." Mary and Thomas had argued that marriage "produces disease." Regarding the inequities of marriage, Thomas had bluntly asserted, "The canons of the Church and the civil law alike prove the truth of our allegations."[26] There was no easy way to reconcile the Nicholses' earlier writings on free love and individual sovereignty with Catholic doctrine. The church viewed premarital and extramarital sex as sin. It forbade divorce. Its Bible declared that "what God therefore has joined together, let no man put asunder." Yet the *Nichols' Journal* had implored its readers: "Remember that the same Bible appoints and enforces both marriage and slavery. Its authority is as good for one as the other; but no authority can justify any wrong. 'Thus saith the Lord,' cannot make anything true or right."[27] Mary and Thomas had much to disown.

In 1864 Thomas broached this difficulty in his broad-ranging and entertaining two-volume *Forty Years of American Life*, published in England. With a journalist's detachment, he described American institutions and customs, ranging from apple-peeling, skating, and quilting to slavery, religion, and the periodical press. His cool and ironic tone belied Thomas's deep involvement with many of the subjects described, including Fourierism, hydropathy, spiritualism, and opposition to traditional marriage. "It is scarcely known, I believe, in England, to what extent anti-marriage theory has been maintained in the Northern States of America," he wrote, without mentioning his own role in that cause. Speaking in the past tense of a movement he and Mary had helped to spearhead, Thomas portrayed his earlier antimarriage philosophy in terms that were fundamentally compatible with Catholicism; he recast what had been the disparagement of *all* indissoluble marriage as a very specific disparagement of *civil* marriage: "[By the antimarriage movement, I mean] the very prevalent doctrine that the relations of the sexes were matters with which the State, the Government, and the laws had no proper business. Every one, it was said, should be free to enter upon such relations without the interference of the civil magistrate. If marriage was held to be a sacrament, as among Roman Catholics, then it was an affair of religion, with which American governments had nothing to do."[28] This summary did not exactly misrepresent the antimarriage crusade. Mary and Thomas had written as much in regard to Mormon polygamy ten years earlier when the House of Representatives had spent two days debating the subject.

The Nicholses' defense of free love implicitly included acceptance of the choice to seek permanent and exclusive Catholic union, but given the prevalence of indissoluble wedlock and its then repulsive quality to Mary and Thomas, they had never written in its theoretical defense. In fact, Mary had been more inclined to challenge the faith. In *Marriage* she wrote, "I was recently conversing with a popular clergyman on the subject of evil marriages and their indissolubility. He was giving some instances to show how fiend-like people can be to each other when bound remedilessly in a bundle of antipathies. I said, 'Do you believe in such marriage?' 'No,' said he, 'but I tell people I do, for fear they will fall into something worse.' Something worse!" Mary and Thomas could not foresee the day when they would come to view the laws of nature as synchronous with the teachings of the Catholic Church. Only three years before their conversion, Thomas wrote: "The Church assumes that men *ought* to believe, in a certain way, and *ought* to love in a certain way; as if belief and love were voluntary actions. Both are out of the domain of volition. . . . How can a man say, 'Now, I will believe in this religious doctrine, and I will love that woman?' He may promise both, pretend both, and in both be a hypocrite."[29]

There is no evidence that Thomas and Mary ever renewed or revised their original wedding vows before a Catholic priest. The sacramental records of St. Xavier's Church in Cincinnati make no reference to the Nicholses, whose Swedenborgian wedding would not have satisfied the Catholic Church as fulfilling the sacrament of marriage. Most likely, Mary and Thomas renewed their vows after conversion and had their marriage blessed by a Catholic priest. This would have required the annulment of Mary's first marriage to Hiram, which probably would have been granted on the grounds that Mary agreed to that marriage in the context of undue external pressure and had not freely desired to marry Hiram Gove. However, the possibility that Mary and Thomas did not renew their vows suggests other theories, one of which is that her marriage to Hiram could not be voided for some reason and therefore Mary would never be allowed to remarry. Another possibility (assuming the successful annulment of the Gove marriage) is that Mary and Thomas preferred that their marriage not be recognized by the church, in which case neither would be bound by Catholicism's sanction against divorce; they could, presumably, seek a civil divorce and remarry, creating what the church would view as their first marriages, if within the faith. Of course, given that they did not separate, this possibility would also imply that Mary and Thomas viewed each one of their sexual unions as a sin demanding confession and penance, or that they remained chaste for the rest of their lives. Given their chastity-oriented teachings prior to conversion and the extreme unlikelihood of their seeking additional children (Mary was forty-seven), this last scenario seems possible.

In 1872 Thomas produced a new book, *Human Physiology: The Basis of Sanitary and Social Science,* a 479-page tome addressing some of the questions raised by the couple's conversion. Regarding divorce, Thomas wrote:

> There are those who believe that love alone can justify the most intimate relation of the sexes. Without mutual love, they say, marriage is but legalised prostitution. They would justify a husband in denying conjugal rights to his wife, or a wife in refusing herself to her husband, if either ceased to love the other. If mutual love be the sole justification of sexual union—if it be false, unnatural, abhorrent, where such love does not exist, then the cessation of love on the part of either would be the end of marriage—a divorce, or at least a separation.

Thus far, Thomas had explained the Nicholses' earlier position on the subject. Yet he continued,

> But the interests of children, families, and society, as it is now constituted, do not permit of divorce for sentimental grievances. The intimate relations of two married partners must be regulated by themselves, and in this, and in all that pertains to marriage, they must follow the law of charity, do as they would be done by, and what, all things considered, seems to them best for all concerned. Where there is no positive sin, no violation of conscience, we must seek the greatest good, even in a choice of evils; and we are not to seek our own good merely, but to make sacrifices, if need be, for the good of others. [30]

This may well be one of Thomas's most opaque paragraphs. Clearly, he was striving to condemn a frivolous attitude toward divorce and to endorse the greatest good "for all concerned," even to the point of personal "sacrifices." Yet he has left an implicit loophole for those cases in which there *is* "positive sin" and where there *is* "violation of conscience." Thomas artfully obscured this opinion in rather muddled, highly qualified prose. He did not suggest who should be the arbiter of such gray areas—but what could be more personal than a "violation of conscience"?

Earlier in the text, Thomas had quite clearly explained and dismissed the "theory of social morals [known as] Free Love," a theory he now considered "abhorrent . . . yet consistent." He described the doctrine as "one of unrestrained, universal, promiscuous intercourse, extending to every person of both sexes" and derived from a scientific error that held that "the generative organs . . . are subject, like all other organs, to the law of exercise." In fact, Thomas explained, "the generative organs differ from all others in being adapted to long periods of perfect repose. We have seen that in vegetables and many insects they are used but once in a life time; and that in all the higher animals they come into use only at long intervals, in many, intervals of years, and for one specific purpose." In this way, Thomas had used scientific observation to revise his own earlier beliefs about the proper expression of sexual passion: "The law of nature is intercourse for reproduction. Throughout the vegetable and animal world there is no other. Pleasure is a secondary consideration." Despite his unequivocal censure of free love, however, he could not help but soften the blow: "Based upon a fallacy, [free love] is yet more reputable than the partial and absurd conventional morality of society, which has one law for men and another for women, and sacrifices thousands of women to provide for the vices of one sex and protect the virtue of the other."[31]

Thomas and Mary accepted Catholicism's vision; on the fine points, however, it seems some tension persisted. Who does not question certain aspects of their chosen religion? Even zealous faith in water cure had led the Nicholses into controversy with fellow practitioners. In print, Mary took issue with others' hydropathic approaches. Likewise, when it came to Catholicism, Thomas preserved in later editions of *Esoteric Anthropology* the very doctrine that Archbishop Purcell had found most disturbing: "If a woman has any right in this world, it is the right to herself; and if there is anything in this world she has a right to decide, it is who shall be the father of her children. She has an equal right to decide whether she will have children, and to choose the time for having them."[32] Though Thomas had generally purified the text—limiting, for example, his tolerance for abortion to cases that threaten the mother's life—he had refused to eliminate or remotely dilute his conviction of woman's "right to herself." His discussion of the subject lost no force over the years. Later, addressing the matter in *Human Physiology*, he wrote: "But what can be done when lustful men . . . compel their wives to submit to their embraces, when they are utterly unfit to bear children, [and] . . . during pregnancy, at the risk of producing abortion, and during nursing, to the great injury of mother and child?" His answer challenged the church: "First of all, there should be no such unnatural husbands. But it is hard to say how wives can protect themselves from them, where they exist, any more than they can from being abused or outraged in any way. In such cases, it would seem that the wife ought to have a right to protect herself and her offspring. No man has a right to force a child upon a woman against her wishes: and for every wrong there should be a remedy."[33]

Twenty-four years after her conversion, seventy-one years old and still a practicing Catholic, Mary briefly referred to her first marriage in language suggesting the tenacity of her commitment to married women's rights: "I was first married when too young to know the fearful responsibilities of married life, and knowledge would have been of no use to me, for law and custom require submission of the wife."[34] Her wording implies that arbitrary law and custom— rather than infallible divine law— demand a wife's submission to her husband. This passage suggests that Mary never accepted St. Peter's command that wives "be in subjection to your own husbands" or St. Paul's teaching that "The wife hath not power over her own body, but the husband."[35] When fighting to abolish the institution of marriage, Mary had written, "The Church said the Scripture saith, 'obey your husband.' The Church did not add 'in the Lord,' [as directed by the Lord] who had said, 'call no man master.'"[36] Clearly, Mary read Scripture with a close and critical eye, just as she had always approached her medical texts. In many ways, the Nicholses' conversion to Roman Catholicism consolidated rather than contradicted their past.

ON THE ROAD

In September 1857, two months after his first Communion, Thomas offered the church his services as a lecturer. Writing to the *Catholic Telegraph and Advocate* (a paper that had endorsed him to Catholic literary societies), Thomas proposed to speak on the "Doctrines, Sacraments, and Influences of the Catholic Church, as well as the Principles and Ultimations of Protestantism." The obsequiousness of this letter bears no resemblance to the arrogant tone of Thomas's early newspaper columns or to his prior flippancy regarding religion. In *Esoteric Anthropology* he had sarcastically classed religion with the "passional diseases": "In its mild form it is enthusiasm; in its severe, fanaticism; in its repulsive, it is bigotry. This disease is often acute, and commonly epidemic. It is also clearly contagious. It spreads like small-pox or measles, through a community; disappears for a long time, and then comes back again. It is probably kept alive by chronic cases." Now Thomas adopted a different tack: "I wish to be guided . . . by the principle of entire submission to the will of God, and consequent obedience to my spiritual superiors; recognizing that in whatever relates to the welfare of the Church, I have no more right to act without their express approbation, than a soldier would to engage in military operations without the sanction and direction of his commanding officer." He had no intention of making trouble. "With humility, with submission, I ask that I may be permitted in this way to make some amends for past errors."[37]

In November Thomas delivered five lectures in the basement of Cincinnati's cathedral. Despite his history as an outspoken infidel and his novice's understanding of Catholic dogma, Thomas received favorable reviews for these introductory presentations—historical sketches, doctrines, and critiques of Catholicism and Protestantism. "Notwithstanding the length of some of the lectures," commented the *Catholic Telegraph and Advocate*, "the pure style of language in which they were composed and the pleasing manner of their delivery secured the attention of the audience to their close." These talks initiated two years of lecturing throughout the Midwest and South and subsequently resulted in a book, *Lectures on Catholicity and Protestantism.*[38]

After leaving the Ursuline convent, Mary and Thomas had first moved to Cleveland, where Thomas lectured at a local seminary while Mary taught at a convent school.[39] Not long after their move, however, Mary was entreated by the bishop of Cleveland to assist at a Catholic orphanage stricken by an epidemic of scarlet fever. Mary applied the water cure to nearly a hundred children and to more than one priest; she also taught the nuns how to manage the crisis. Only one child died under her watch. As a consequence, Cleveland's bishop strongly recommended Mary to the bishops of Detroit, Chicago, and Natchez, Mississippi, as well as to the archbishops of St. Louis and New Orleans. Throughout 1858 and 1859, Mary and Thomas visited dozens of Catholic institutions from Michigan to Mississippi. She lectured on hygiene, while he lectured on religion. Willie, who was eight years old when the family left Ohio, would experience the United States almost exclusively in the context of circumscribed communities founded on distinctive political or religious ideology.

At a convent near the University of Notre Dame, Thomas remembered Mary relieving the sprained ankle of the mother superior with her "'gift of healing' or magnetic, or mesmeric power." He recalled that Mary "laid her hand upon the . . . tortured limb, and in a few moments the pain had ceased." "It was a beautiful cure," Thomas wrote, "and was of course considered miraculous." Perhaps it was flirtation such as this with superhuman forces that inclined Archbishop Purcell to warn Archbishop Blanc of New Orleans: "I am told Mrs. Nichols needs watching."[40] Years after the Nicholses' conversion, the clergy thus continued to monitor the couple. They would have been encouraged by the letter Mary sent from Jersey City, New Jersey, to Alonzo Lewis in September of 1859:

I was *glad* to get your letter this morning—but somewhat surprised that *you* should not understand me better. Somehow I expect you to know all I mean. With regard to the Church it is to me no myth, or supposition, but an Entity established by Christ with an order infallible, whilst it is not departed from, to do men the most good they are capable of receiving. And we have Christ's promise that He will always abide with His Church, and therefore it shall not fail. Individuals may do wrong—Popes and Priests may be bad—but the Church of our Lord remains for She is His body among men and her order and Her consolations and her saving power remain always to the end of time, to bless all honest souls, whether they know of its existence, or not. If we fear to do wrong, and humbly desire to do right, we are as well off in the present, and the *sure* future, as the highest arch angel. . . .

It is well for you to forget your kindness and fidelity to me, when I was poor and maligned. I can *never* forget. . . . If you were Catholic you would be perfectly happy. Your soul was made for order, for harmony, and for generous deeds. If I could give you my Faith in our Lord of His Church I would gladly suffer much. . . .[41]

Her newfound religion enabled Mary to feel *guaranteed* future harmony. She understood the failure of the church to be impossible. After so many of her own community-building initiatives—Port Chester, Desarrollo, the Progressive Union, Memnonia—had come up short, Mary found peace in a faith whose growth and achievements seemed to withstand any setback.

During her travels to Catholic institutions, the opportunity to lecture before teachers especially excited Mary. This contact seemed to promise future influence—something Mary had always craved. "I have impartially laboured for Protestants, Infidels, and Catholics," wrote Mary. "The latter," she continued,

> have the advantage of combined orders which live through centuries, and conserve and carry forward the knowledge of laws and principles, and apply them with unflagging devotion. For this reason it is a greater good to instruct the superior of a religious order than the head of a Protestant seminary. The Protestant may live and labour successfully for half-a-century, but a religious order may last a thousand years and the wisdom of one superior embodied in the rule and life and teachings of an order may be spread over continents and carried out by a long line of his successors. When I instruct one, in such a case, it is a comfort to think I may be teaching thousands, and doing a good work for future generations. My failing life will live on in others."[42]

This perceived immortality, an idea that had long attracted the couple, fortified the Nicholses' dedication to the Faith.

Mary and Thomas saw no contradiction between personal freedom and full religious compliance. To show his understanding of others' confusion, Thomas paraphrased the objection in unmistakable capitals: "CATHOLICISM IS A SYSTEM OF DESPOTISM. THE CHURCH CLAIMS TO BE INFALLIBLE, AND DEMANDS OBEDIENCE. I COULD NEVER SUBMIT TO SUCH TYRANNY." In response, Thomas reminded his readers of a fundamental freedom: "If any man's freedom of opinion, exercise of self-government, and individual sovereignty lead him to believe that God has constituted a Church on the earth; one, visible, united body, upheld by His Omnipotent Power, and guided by His Holy Spirit, and consequently infallible . . . it is his right to believe in this Church [and] to submit to its requirements."[43] He and Mary had followed precisely this trajectory.

The Nicholses had always defined "right" as that sanctioned by God's laws and evidenced by health. Thomas had written, "When we say a thing is right, we wish to be understood as meaning that it is in harmony, or accordance with the laws of nature, or, what is the same thing, the laws of God."[44] Roman Catholicism, with its canon law and sacraments, provided Mary and Thomas a specific codification of their philosophy. Unlike Fourierism or Equitable Commerce—philosophies that lacked both history and successful implementation—Catholicism had, since its inception, continued to spread throughout the world. As to the notion that Catholicism tyrannically demanded submission of its flock, Thomas explained that "to obey the Church is to obey God himself; and that is never inconsistent with the highest freedom of any creature."[45]

In fact, Thomas considered Catholics exceptionally broad-minded and diverse in their opinions. The more Catholics obey their clergy "in spiritual matters," wrote Thomas, "the more they repel interference in temporal affairs. I knew an instance in which a popular priest, having a large congregation, tried to induce his flock to vote *one* way, with the result that all but two of them voted the *other*." In contrast, Thomas depicted Protestant clergymen as consistently overstepping their rightful bounds of influence.[46] Repeatedly, Thomas described the Catholic love of independent thought: "They have cultivated mathematics, astronomy, geology, natural history, mental and moral philosophy, and the whole range of human learning with zeal and devotion. . . . Catholicity founded and built up almost every University in Europe."[47] Beyond his reverence for Catholic scholarship, Thomas admired the relative "order" of the Catholic Church, in contrast to what he considered the chaotic fragmentation of Protestantism. Without suppressing the life of the mind, Thomas argued, the structured, infallible faith of Catholicism looked toward the promise of a harmonic future. Mary and Thomas understood Catholicism to encompass all they had rightly worked for; the warmth with which they were received during their travels must have seemed a soothing balm after the iciness of Yellow Springs.

In New Orleans, Mary was invited to visit a large girls' school, proud of its resilience to fatal epidemics of cholera and yellow fever. When Mary met the lady superior of the school, she learned that her own book, *Experience in Water-Cure,* had been the institution's guiding text through these frightening outbreaks of disease. They had not lost a single pupil. This must have gratified Mary, another sign that her medical teachings reflected God's laws. As Mary continued to tour and lecture at various convents in New Orleans, Thomas lectured throughout the region, traveling to Mobile, Alabama, and Galveston, Texas. While visiting with the bishop of Galveston, Thomas remembered, the two shared a lively dinner with M. Victor Considerant, a French disciple of Fourier who had recently failed in an attempt to establish a phalanstery in Texas. The dinner must have underlined for Thomas the relative success of Catholics in building lasting harmonic communities, and it surely reaffirmed his new life direction.[48]

Writing years later of their extended lecture tour, Thomas stressed the sacrificing generosity, good cheer, broad vision, steady competence, and noble ambition of the many Catholics he and Mary had come to know. He also respected the self-possession and leadership of Catholic women, whose enterprising and autonomous work belied any notion of female inferiority. Describing the superior of New York City's Ladies of the Sacred Heart, he wrote that Madame Hardy was "equal . . . to the duties of any department of State; and one who would be the right woman in the right place, as the governor of an important colony."[49] Thomas's description of his visit to Indiana's Notre Dame evokes the idyllic quality of a Fourierist phalanx. Nestled in a spectacular forest clearing, glittering with lakes, orchards, and vineyards, the college buildings included workshops, classrooms, a laundry, a dining hall, dormitories, and a chapel. All members of the community seemed bound in sympathetic devotion, studying, relaxing, and praying in turns. Though the sexes did not intermingle, and though the air chimed with hymns, a closer approximation of Desarrollo Thomas had probably never seen.[50]

At the start of their travels, Mary and Thomas had imagined lecturing at all the English-speaking convents in the world. By the end of their tour of the South, they realized the overambition of this dream and instead returned to the North to reestablish their own home.[51] Winding through Memphis and then Cincinnati, they finally arrived back in New York. In April of 1860, Mary and Thomas released a one-page circular promoting their new home, "EMMET MANSION, corner of Fifty-ninth Street and Second Avenue, New York, for the treatment of a limited number of invalids." The house, advertised in the *Water-Cure Journal* as a "Hygienic and Hydropathic Establishment," was surrounded by greenery and sat between Central Park and the East River.[52] (It is not clear why Trall accepted an advertisement for the Nicholses' establishment after seeking to dis-

credit them in the same journal seven years earlier. Possibly this seeming reconciliation was an editorial oversight, as no copies of the advertisement appear in immediately previous or subsequent issues.) The
Nicholses described their therapeutic philosophy as "Hydropathic, combined with such Medicinal (Homœopathic), Dietetic, Gymnastic, and
Electric treatment as each case may require."

Mary, as has been noted, had long doubted the efficacy of homeopathy,
considering it harmless at best. However, she seemed by 1860 to have
gained faith in its methods. In his 1887 memoir, *Nichols' Health Manual*,
Thomas described an experience remarkably similar to the Jesuit spirit
visitations that can help pinpoint in time (if not satisfactorily explain)
Mary's heightened interest in homeopathy:

> One day, at our residence, near Cincinnati, Ohio, we were talking of
> homœopathy, in which she had more confidence than I had. Suddenly
> her whole appearance changed. Her face looked like that of an old
> man; her voice and mode of speaking corresponded to her appearance.
> She seized my hands, and went on for ten minutes, with great energy
> explaining a theory of the action of homœopathic medicines in the
> cure of disease. I have no reason to believe that she had ever held such
> a theory, or read, or heard of it. It was her belief that she was possessed
> for the time by the spirit of Hahnemann, who wished to convert her
> to his system. She was suffering at the time from disease of her lungs;
> and he told her what medicine to get for her relief. She had never
> heard of such a medicine; but on visiting a homœopathic physician
> whom we knew in Cincinnati, she got the one prescribed. . . . I have no
> doubt as to the facts. The only question is as to whether her knowledge
> was the exercise of her own clairvoyance, or that of some friendly spirit
> who gave her the information. . . . Of the verity of the facts there is
> no room for doubt.[53]

According to Thomas, Mary had later prescribed "homœopathic prophylactic belladona" to the Catholic orphans afflicted with scarlet fever.
In 1881 Mary wrote, "Before I was convinced of the efficacy of homœopathic remedies, I believed that all curable diseases could be cured by
water; and now, whatever confidence I may have in other means of cure,
water is to me more nearly an universal remedy, or panacea, than any

other curative agent, except the life of love that we give one another in harmonious relations, and in a divine charity."[54]

Because their new house would accommodate only twenty patients, Mary and Thomas felt it "their duty to give a preference to invalid Clergymen, Religious Teachers, and Young Ladies, or Children, who, from failing health or delicacy of constitution, are unable to attend to their studies." For these last, tutors would be provided. Patients would be expected to supply their own blankets, sheets, and towels, and to pay a weekly fee of from ten to fifteen dollars, depending on the size of their room and the intensity of their treatment.[55]

It is not clear why this grand plan did not succeed. Perhaps hostile competition from Russell Trall's successful Hygeio-Therapeutic Cure prevented Emmett Mansion from acquiring a sufficient clientele; perhaps the Nicholses' reputation had been irreparably tainted in New York City by 1855 reviews of *Mary Lyndon*, by the Nicholses' association with free love, or by reports of their strangely inspired conversion to Catholicism. Perhaps more mundane obstacles—lack of money—interfered with their plans. Before long, however, Mary and Thomas moved into a cottage on Staten Island, with a grand view of New York Harbor and Brooklyn.[56]

In April of 1861, Thomas inaugurated a new weekly newspaper, the *New York Age*, philosophically devoted to social and sanitary science but overtly political in its first number. Pleading for peace in the face of imminent violence, Thomas managed to publish only one issue of his paper before the Civil War erupted. With thousands of other somber onlookers, he watched as the naval armada steamed out of New York Bay, ostensibly to resupply the garrison at Fort Sumter, but clearly, in Thomas's mind, a provocation to attack. Having advance notice from Lincoln of the fleet's arrival, Jefferson Davis ordered his Southern troops to open fire in a preemptive strike at 4:30 in the morning on April 12, 1861. The Northern ships, waylaid by heavy seas, never even launched their supply boats.[57]

The Confederate firing on Fort Sumter horrified Thomas, who had "not believed in the possibility of a civil war." Even worse to him seemed the Northern response to this bloodshed: total galvanization in defense of the Union. Where only the day before New York City had rumbled with division over appropriate government policy, it seemed after Sumter that every window billowed forth an American flag. A quarter of a million people gathered to rally for the Union. Blazing patriotism allowed for no dissent. Prominent leaders who had advocated peace either reversed their opinions or kept silent. Thomas, opposed to violence and sympathetic to the Confederacy, perceived the gravity of his situation. In Lincoln's determination to retain federal control over the port of Charleston, Thomas saw a once-free republic demanding its citizens' allegiance by force. He did not issue a second number of the *New York Age*. He felt unable even to remain in the "United" States of America.[58]

LEAVING AMERICA

"It was not heroic to run away," Thomas wrote from London in 1864. "I admit it and feel it, sometimes more deeply than I care to express."[59] Unlike Mary, whose political views of the war must largely be surmised, Thomas left an extensive record of his thoughts and feelings regarding the conflict. He wrote *Forty Years of American Life* soon after arriving in England. Of this two-volume work, Thomas devoted eleven chapters to the Civil War and its causes—naturally topics of timely interest. Later editions of *Forty Years* eliminated all but five of these chapters.

In July of 1861, President Lincoln had given Secretary of State William H. Seward command of the nation's internal security. Seward had approached this new responsibility with zeal, imprisoning anyone suspected of "treason." By February of 1862, when Lincoln relieved Seward of this much-abused power, two hundred political prisoners had been herded into jails. Seward had also forbidden any citizen to leave the country without a passport, the acquisition of which required an oath of loyalty to the Union. The Nicholses had no passports. The *New York Age*—where Thomas suggested that only a "military despotism" could hold the South against its will—had been suppressed. Shaken by reports that an outspoken Democrat had been shot dead during an argument in a coffeehouse and that another New Yorker had scarcely survived a lynching for having compared the Union cause to fighting for the rights of kings, the Nicholses decided to sell their furniture and seek asylum abroad. Thomas could not have forgotten his own frightening experiences in Buffalo more than twenty years earlier: the street attack suffered at the hands of local militiamen; the destruction of his printing offices; and months of imprisonment for libel. These events had occurred in peacetime. In the midst of war fever, with a deeply loved wife and child, Thomas lost all appetite for making personal enemies.[60]

Noting that the London-bound ships carried fewer passengers than packets headed elsewhere, Thomas calculated that the former would be less carefully surveyed by the police. He also chose to engage a small cabin on a merchant's sailing ship rather than risk involvement with the passenger steamers.[61] The family was fortunate. Without interference from government authorities, Thomas, Mary, and Willie made their escape in the spring of 1861. Smooth weather eased their month-long crossing. On board, they had compatible shipmates. A secessionist editor from Missouri and his family had also fled New York in fear. Other company included Northern Irishmen who had been fired from their jobs so as to be compelled to volunteer for the Union. Thomas wrote of a ship of exiles, with only two Unionists on board, and recalled the "joy when our feet pressed the soil of the old fatherland." Two steam-tugs guided the Nicholses' ship up the Thames and to the docks of East London. In St. John's Wood, an area rich in gardens, Mary, Thomas, and Willie found an inexpensive unfurnished house. Though the Nicholses had little money and only a few letters of introduction with which to renew their lives, they did not despair. For Thomas, the sense of relief subsumed all misfortune.[62]

How could Thomas—so outraged by the bondage of indissoluble marriage that he compared it to chattel slavery—deeply sympathize with the South? How could he and Mary have kept such distance from the abolitionist movement? How could they defend the slave owner? In her autobiography, Mary admits that she once directly confronted leading abolitionist William Lloyd Garrison with the assertion that "the Northern wife is worse off than the Southern slave, for her mental cultivation gives her a keenness of anguish that the want of spiritual culture saves her Southern sister from." However, she reflected, "This was hard saying to the man of one idea, and I now think it is not true. Chattel bondage is the lowest of all—but those who are oppressed by marriage, and find no escape but by the loss of name and fame, food and children, may well be excused from seeing a parallel to the institution of marriage in that of slavery."[63] Though brief, this passage provides some limited insight regarding Mary's relationship to the abolitionist movement. It is the clearest surviving statement of her views on the subject. Unlike Thomas, who wrote at length on the institution of slavery, Mary maintained a relative silence. Perhaps she and Thomas disagreed as to whether "chattel bondage is the lowest of all." Whatever her opinion on the subject, however, it is obvious that Mary did not devote a great deal of energy to the cause of Southern emancipation.

Thomas, we know, considered the war "unconstitutional": "I could see no right that one portion of the country had to subject the other—no reason why twenty States should compel the rest to remain united with them, or failing that, should invade, conquer, subjugate, or exterminate them." Thomas fundamentally rejected the notion of coerced Union, and he blamed the "intermeddling fanaticism" of abolitionists for the war and its resultant "inhumanity, barbarism, and extermination."[64] Governments, he felt, had no place mandating indissoluble ties—not between spouses and not between states. Though Mary and Thomas had long argued against "slaveries," it was the bondage of the Southern states' legislatures, not the bondage of the black slave, that most alienated them from their country. "I became a 'traitor,'" wrote Thomas.

> It was "treason" to assert the sovereignty of the States; "treason" to quote the Declaration of Independence; "treason" to talk of the rights of peoples.... Lincoln had upheld the sacred right of revolution; Seward had denounced the folly of a war to restore the Union, comparing it to the conduct of a husband who should beat his wife to compel her to live with him as his loving companion; Greeley had declared that six millions of people in the South had as clear a right to separate from the Union as three millions of colonists had to rebel against Great Britain.... They changed their principles, and became patriots. I adhered to mine, and was a "traitor."[65]

For Thomas, comparisons to marriage cast the Confederate government as subjected wife and Lincoln's administration as abusive husband. The actual plight of black slaves seemed less troubling to him.

"I was educated in the horror of slavery," Thomas explained, writing for a British and predominantly abolitionist readership. "My opinions were modified by much observation of the condition of free negroes in the North, and of slaves in the South." Thomas's portrayal of American race relations conveys his deep condescension toward the Negro population. Whereas his deprecation of Negro capabilities reflected an entirely

conventional viewpoint for the era, his admiration for the peaceful inter-
mingling of races (where it existed) was relatively progressive. He even
sought to call the bluff of Northern abolitionists, not more than a dozen
of whom, he imagined, "could contemplate the idea of having a son-in-
law with Negro blood in his veins, without an emotion of horror." In contrast, Thomas wrote, "The master has been born and brought up among
his slaves. Slaves nursed him in his infancy, slaves were the playmates of
his childhood. He knows them thoroughly, and they know him. He has
none of that colour-phobia, that horror of a black man because he is black,
which prevails in the Northern States." At the same time, Thomas
speculated that a "natural instinct" against miscegenation might have
been "implanted by nature for some wise purpose." His tentative support
for this theory derived from his perception of the relative health and
longevity of "pure blooded" American Negroes as compared with
"mulattoes."[66]

Thomas's understanding of the Negroes' ability for self-government informed his political views of slavery. While he and Mary had long argued
for the human right to individual sovereignty, they had always qualified
this demand by excluding those unprepared for freedom. Recall Mary's
argument that "the man who cannot govern himself, without bringing
evil upon himself and others, must be governed, as whoso has broken legs
must have crutches—and yet all men have the natural right of unbroken,
useful legs." Writing metaphorically of marriage, Mary had conceded that
"slavery is no preparation for freedom." In Thomas's view, it would be as
cruel to emancipate the Southern slave population as it would be to deprive a crippled man of his crutches. It would be the same as turning "a
shop-full of canaries loose in Regent's Park."[67] The South, he believed,
was effectively educating, civilizing, and Christianizing its slaves.

Thomas's opposition to emancipation seemed to originate most strongly
from perceptions of what life was like for free blacks in the North. He
quoted at length the replies sent from governors and legislators of Northern states to General Cobb of Georgia, who, according to Thomas, had
sent queries regarding the moral, physical, and intellectual conditions of
the free black population. "Their condition is debased," wrote New Jersey, "with few exceptions very poor; generally indolent, generally ignorant, far below the whites in intelligence. Immoral; vicious animal propensities; drunkenness, theft, and promiscuous sexual intercourse quite

common." Pennsylvania, Indiana, and Illinois echoed these observations. Thomas considered these assessments "mainly candid and true," though he also granted that many exceptions existed. His acceptance of slavery found legitimation in Thomas's utter inability to conceive of a workable social alternative. "I have no wish to maintain that the four millions of negroes in the Southern States of America are in the best possible condition," he wrote. "But I seriously doubt whether any change yet proposed for them might not be for the worse." Thomas not only believed that all but the extremely exceptional slave owner protected and cared for his slaves, providing a guarantee of housing, medical care, clothing, and food, but also that Southern slaves were, "on an average, better off in these respects than the agricultural labourers of Great Britain."[68] He simply did not believe the stories of Northern abolitionists. His own encounters with Southern slavery did not corroborate their horrors.

But Thomas well knew that only the "softest and most amiable aspects" of slavery would be presented to visitors. In 1854, recall, he had observed with outrage that "thousands of women suffer [from spousal abuse] where one complains." And yet, ten years later he would write of slavery that "the regular increase of the slave population proves that they have not been very hardly treated." Thomas went so far as to suggest the possibility of slavery's "redeeming features," as indicated by "the fact that English, Irish, and the Northern American emigrants to the South, whatever their former opinions, generally follow the customs of the country, and become the owners of slaves." Given the era's deep racism and sexism, what is more surprising than Thomas's attitude toward other races is his ability to conceive of women as worthy of political equity. That he could devote his life to the liberation of women and yet remain aloof to the condition of Southern slaves seems to current sensibilities a glaringly obvious contradiction—and one that Thomas never adequately addressed. The strain in his views is perhaps most succinctly conveyed by Thomas's statement: "I love liberty, but I see the necessity of authority and obedience."[69]

MARY AND THOMAS spent the second half of the nineteenth century in England. Neither ever returned to the United States. Nearly broke, they had arrived in London with a letter of introduction to Cardinal Wiseman. Their earliest and most helpful friends in England included writers William and Mary Howitt and their daughter Anna Mary Howitt-Watts; Dr. Garth Wilkinson; William White (biographer of Swedenborg); and Charles Dickens, whom Thomas later described as "one of our best friends, and a frequent visitor." These literary associates quickly helped the Nicholses find work. Mary wrote for the *Athenaeum, Frazer's Magazine,* and *Household Words;* Thomas published articles for *Temple Bar* and *Once a Week* that would soon become *Forty Years of American Life.* He also wrote an entertaining and descriptive account of two American mediums, entitled *Biography of the Brothers Davenport*—a work that revealed his sustained belief in spiritual manifestations. William Howitt introduced Thomas to Robert Chambers, from whom he accepted work writing for *Chambers' Encyclopedia*—beginning, he recalled, with "Fourier." Thomas also acted for eight years as London correspondent to the *New York Times,* traveling occasionally to Paris, Metz, and other cities on the Continent. The family summered at Brighton, Eastbourne, and Hastings.[1]

Excerpts from *Forty Years of American Life* indicate the intellectual distance Thomas had traveled from his most earnest devotion to Josiah Warren and Charles Fourier: "How men are to be prevented from injuring others in the exercise of their own freedom, I do not think Mr. Warren has very clearly explained," he wrote in 1864. Furthermore, he admitted that "very few understood the doctrines or the system of Fourier or what it required, and those who comprehended it were not prepared for so thorough a revolution in morals and social organization. It is a form of life that may exist on some other planet, but can scarcely be expected to take root on ours; yet no one can read Fourier without being fascinated with its beauty, splendour, and apparent practicability." In 1863 Mary published her "Reminiscences of Edgar Allan Poe" in *Sixpenny Magazine* and in 1864 finished a novel, *Uncle Angus*. Years after her death, Thomas described Mary's novels as "sanitary" and attributed their lack of broader success to Mary's being "too much in earnest as an advocate of physical and moral reformation." But for all their literary productivity, 1864 would prove to be the worst year of their lives. In 1864, Mary Wilhelmina, only fourteen years old, died of bronchitis.[2]

"I know that the question will arise,—How is it that with all your knowledge of the laws of health, and your sanitary habits, your own child, in spite of your care, should die at the age of fourteen?" wrote Thomas, sitting in the same house where his only child had died. "It is a fair question, and requires an answer." The burden of responsibility and grief could not have been heavier. Thomas later came to doubt whether "persons with strong tendencies to consumption" should even get married at all. "You have seen that the beloved mother of this beloved child struggled through her life with hereditary tendencies to disease," Thomas labored to explain. "Mary Wilhelmina was born when both her parents were engaged in very earnest, active mental work. [A child's] intellectual precocity is often unfavourable to longevity, because the brain robs the body, and especially the stomach and the nutritive system. Health requires an equitable distribution of the forces of life. Cerebral activity may favour the development of dyspepsia or consumption." Thomas had deeply admired Willie's intellectual talent, which flourished either despite, or thanks to, the Nicholses' decision not to send her to school. "Until almost the end, I did not give up the hope of her recovery," Thomas continued.

She knew that she was going, and was content to go, only pitying us. She had no fear of death, but dreaded the pain of dying. A few days before she died, she said, "Papa, please lie down beside me; I want you to tell me something. Tell me just how it will be when I go. What will be the process of dying?"

"As you grow weaker," I said, "you will not be able to clear your lungs; your blood cannot get oxygen, your brain will lose consciousness; you will fall asleep, and then stop breathing."

. . . A few days after, sitting near her as she slept in the early morning of January 2, 1864, I felt *silence*. She had simply stopped breathing, while holding a glass of water in her hand, without spilling a drop.

Mary could not bear the loss of her daughter. Though she tried to seek comfort in work, frequent uncontrollable tears weakened and, Thomas believed, finally extinguished her vision. From the beginning of 1864 through 1868, Mary was completely blind from cataracts and from grief. Visits from Willie's spirit helped Mary and Thomas regain equilibrium after her loss. Thomas recalled that years after Willie's death, "we not only saw her, but heard her speak to us in her own voice and her peculiarly distinct articulation, felt her delicate fingers—saw, heard, and felt her, when quite alone by ourselves, on one occasion, in our own bed-room, at one o'clock in the morning."[3]

In 1867 the Nicholses moved from London to the hills of Malvern, where they rented a large house, Aldwyn Tower, and established it as a residential water-cure. "We went to Malvern for a month and stayed eight years," wrote Thomas. Mary had hoped to found a new "School of Life" at Malvern, but her blindness made such work impossible. To the patients under their care, the Nicholses did provide daily lectures and instruction. Mary felt that her treatment of individual patients was most useful as legitimizing proof of her medical beliefs, which she hoped would help a much greater number. "I have cured the sick to illustrate my teaching," she wrote. Upon arrival in England, Mary chose not to discuss her medical background, cautiously adopting the more acceptable identity of a magazine writer until she and Thomas established themselves. But by 1868, despite physical incapacity and mourning, she had resumed her role as a water-cure physician and decided to republish *A Woman's Work in Water-Cure*. After five years of blindness, the dependence of which left Mary desperately frustrated, she finally consented to undergo two surgeries at the Nottingham Eye Infirmary. Dr. Charles Bell Taylor successfully removed Mary's cataracts and fully restored her vision.[4]

The Nicholses never stopped working. In 1873 they issued the first number of the *Nichols' Journal of Sanitary and Social Science,* soon replaced by the penny monthly *Herald of Health* and an additional weekly newspaper called *Our Living Age*, both of which Thomas edited, and neither of which proved adequately profitable. Soon Thomas sought stockholders and founded "Nichols and Company," which enabled him to open a shop at 23 Oxford Street in London called the Health Depot, where he sold "sanitary and philanthropic inventions" as well as health food. He was spending three days each week in London while Mary, full of energy and once again independently mobile, traveled frequently on medical consultations. These were very busy years for the two. They republished more of their writings and began composing new texts on health, sanitary science, women's rights, and dress reform.[5]

In the *Herald of Health*, Thomas promoted a variety of items available at the Health Depot, most notably his "Food of Health," eaten as "Porridge, Blancmange, Puddings, etc." and intended for invalids and children. Advertisements described the food as a substance "on which one may entirely live," even at one meal per day. Nichols and Company also sold baking powder; Count Rumford's Vegetable Soup (a powder packet); fragrant and antiseptic soap made from olive oil; and "milk solvent"—"a chemical compound, which, when added to the milk of the cow, gives it the properties of mother's milk." Thomas also invented and advertised a life preserver to be worn around the neck when swimming and a hot-air vapor bath. His shop sold sponges, brushes, bottle injection instruments, siphon enemas, and two therapeutic substances that Mary had personally invented and magnetized with healing powers: "Sapolino," and "Alma Tonic." Mary described Sapolino as "a creamy fluid, oleaginous, or rather saponacious *[sic]*, which destroys both vegetable and animal germs and parasites, and at the same time softens, soothes, and gives the physical conditions of cure." Mary claimed to have developed Sapolino in 1855 when treating a patient with severe facial burns. Alma Tonic, derived from concentrated grape juice, was recommended in small doses for a variety of general disorders. Nichols and Company also helped establish the Alpha Food Reform Vegetarian Restaurant at 429 Oxford Street, and promoted the Food of Health Restaurant on Farrington Road and the Food of Health Cafe at 170 Fleet Street, a cafe which, despite its noble health mission, advertised the "Best tea and coffee in London."[6]

Two evenings each month Thomas participated in open debates on the subject of food in relation to health, disease, drunkenness, and foreign competition. Mary filled her extra hours working for charities on behalf of invalids and the poor; she also began developing plans for an organization that would help to place orphans in loving families, devoted to hygienic living. Yet despite the couple's hard work and social activism, Nichols and Company was in financial trouble. In retrospect, they flatly called the company "a mistake," but they comforted themselves with the knowledge that no shareholder had lost money in the venture.[7] This seems to have required tremendous sacrifice. Thomas simply *gave* the struggling business to James Salsbury (the manager and presumably a shareholder in the Health Depot) and continued writing and editing the *Herald of Health* without pay. Mary assured readers of the *Herald*, "We have no personal interest in, or control of, or pecuniary benefit from the business of Nichols & Co., and the Sanitary Depot, and Vegetarian Restaurant, at 429 Oxford Street. Dr. Nichols, some years ago, handed it over unreservedly to . . . Mr. James Salsbury, and has never since interfered with it in any way, except to help as he could by writing and editing the HERALD OF HEALTH, which he engaged to do without compensation." Living largely on publishing royalties, Mary and Thomas moved in 1877 to a spacious house in South Kensington that was large enough to accommodate inpatients. Thus, the Nicholses continued to practice water cure, preserving a medical system that in the United States had already begun to acquire historical interest.[8]

Back home, the Civil War had brutalized American dreams of universal health and happiness. Never had the country seemed less perfectible or harmony more elusive. The optimistic water cure had failed to redeem society. It had promised too much. Though many of its preventive health tenets survived, the water-cure movement steadily lost ground in America after the 1850s. Meanwhile, the advance of germ theory led to an appreciation of hygiene among regular physicians, who began to adopt and endorse the lifestyle recommendations of hydrotherapists that were previously considered radical. Technological advances such as indoor plumbing and better universal sanitation diminished the frequency of contagious disease and made personal hygiene more convenient. Water-cure advocates likewise grew more sympathetic to the value of diverse medical treatments; in the late 1850s many water-cure retreats began to change their names. They became "resorts" or "sanitariums" or "medical institutes," reflecting the awareness that water had not proven to be a panacea.

Germ theory presented a new site of faith. Opportunities for women were also expanding; thus, the empowering aspects of the water-cure became part of a larger selection of socially relevant and personally validating activities that included the suffragist movement, labor activism, and higher education. By the end of the century, hydrotherapy had lost its original cohesion. It ceased to offer a complete "system" by which to live.[9]

At the water-cure retreats that did survive the Civil War, baths were warmed. Treatments grew gentler. By the end of the century, what had begun as a rather harsh regimen of cold-water bathing and abstemious diet had given way to luxurious spas. But all was not failure. That Americans generally bathe regularly; aspire to regular exercise; praise a low-fat, high-fiber diet; and wear nonconstricting clothing all reflect the water cure's early influence. Yet with the exception of concern over the cost of health insurance, the virtue recognized in these personal choices today stems less from their relationship to the social good than it did in antebellum America; though "health" is still weighted with moral overtones, little current rhetoric seeks to save "humanity."

Until 1886, Thomas continued to edit the *Herald of Health* and to maintain the annual publication of the *Almanac of Health*, which first appeared in 1877.[10] Meanwhile, Elma, who had followed Mary and Thomas to England before departing to study art in Paris, Dresden, and Italy, had returned to Malvern in 1869 and there had met her husband, Thomas Letchworth, Esq., a Quaker from Bedfordshire. He was visiting Malvern for health and had brought a letter of introduction from Anna Howitt-Watts, the Nicholses' friend from London. Elma and Thomas Letchworth married in Malvern; established a home in Bournemouth; and had two children, Mabel and Thomas, for whom Mary wrote stories. The Nicholses visited them frequently. To the American health lecturer and suffragist Paulina Wright Davis, with whom she had established a warm correspondence, Mary wrote of her son-in-law, "The husband and father is as good as ever—one of the best of good men." She added, "Elma is *stout* and ruddy—looks better than in many years and has taken to dressing herself prettily—of which I am very glad." A month later she wrote to Paulina again: "[Elma] is loving and elegant, the best wife, and mother of the *old school*—Her little girl is a delight. Her boy strong and fine. . . . One can hardly see where her husband got his Catholic tastes, and charming manners, unless from his genius—He could not be better to me, if he had been born to me." Mary characterized the 1870s as "perhaps, the most useful [years] in our lives."[11]

In 1881, Mary fell on the front steps of her home, breaking her left thigh bone in its lower third and injuring it above. The fracture healed, but the bony callus formed above pressed on the sciatic nerve, causing chronic pain and limiting her mobility. However, her treatment of patients had come to rely heavily on her magnetic powers, which fortunately did not require the great physical exertion of wet sheet packs. By passing her hand over injuries or providing magnetized materials, Mary claimed to cure without physical contact or medication. As Thomas explained, "A piece of blank paper, held and breathed upon, retains the vital force which has been given to it, and makes upon a sensitive spirit the impression it was intended to make. Mrs. Nichols sends leaves of very delicate paper which are laid upon diseased portions of the body—lungs, heart, stomach, uterus, etc.—and works a rapid cure."[12] Mary would soon apply such treatment to herself, for the following year she developed breast cancer.

Every morning and every evening she magnetized her body for ten minutes. She ate two simple meals per day, bathed often, and sought homeopathic remedies. Still, the cancer advanced. Through all this, Mary maintained her correspondence, and she treated patients as best she could until twelve days before her death. "Then, all at once, she broke down utterly. Her stomach rejected food—her brain failed. She sank into a state of unconsciousness—a kind of trance—and unable to take any food, in twelve days she simply ceased to breathe." She had expressed her wishes to be buried at Kensal Green, without great ceremony. "I gave no invitations," wrote Thomas, "but friends gathered in the chapel, clustered around the open grave, and covered the coffin with sweet and beautiful flowers, the roses and lilies that she loved." Mary died on May 30, 1884; she was seventy-four years old.[13]

Three months after Mary's death, Thomas wrote in the *Herald of Health*, "I beg to express my grateful appreciation of all the kind letters which have been written to me during the past month—the greater portion of which I have been unable to answer. I have felt more than ever the value of human sympathy. Though I *know* that separation and loss are only in the outward, they still are painful, and we need the consolations that come to us. Time itself is a softener of sorrow—and it requires a little time to arrange ourselves in a new position." For their public condolences, Thomas specifically thanked the *Dietetic Reformer,* the *Light,* the *Boston Independent,* and the *Banner of Light* of Boston.[14]

A friend who had been one of Mary's last patients described her six-week stay in the Nicholses' home during the two months just before Mary's death: "Well do I remember day after day . . . the hall table covered with letters," she wrote, "sometimes *twice* a day, all addressed with violet ink in the familiar hand; . . . many of these had been written in the night, when . . . she would . . . try, in the alleviation of others' pain, to forget her own. . . . Her last care in this world was for a poor woman, in whose behalf the last words she ever penned were written, begging my help for her, and for whom she further sought to enlist my sympathy when I bade her farewell!"[15]

Several years before her death, Mary had begun to express interest in compiling her most useful medical writings. She had hoped to include in this work a full description of obstetrics, and "the principles that . . . will secure painless birth and healthy children." She regretted not having written such a work sooner: "If I had given [my many correspondents] a book clearly and exhaustively teaching principles and methods, they could have kept it, and studied it, and lived in accordance with it. Then where I reach ten persons a book may reach a thousand. I feel the need of this work on health, disease, and cure, which shall comprehend midwifery and nursing to the smallest details. . . . But for me to continue the kind of practice that I have long been for years engaged in, is to destroy the possibility of completing my book."[16] Yet despite the dream of writing such a book, Mary continued to work.

Her leg injury and spreading cancer impeded her further, and when she knew herself to be dying, she asked Thomas to finish her imagined project, which he did. "I promised to devote what remained of my life to doing what she wished me to do—" recalled Thomas, "and what, had she been able to stay with us longer, she would have done."[17] Mourning her loss, Thomas spent three years in Mary's archive, listening to her voice preserved on paper. Considering the pages, Thomas wrote, "My difficulty is not so much as to what I wish to give in this permanent form, but what I am compelled to omit." When complete, his *Nichols' Health Manual: Being Also a Memorial of the Life and Work of Mrs. Mary S. Gove Nichols* came to 452 pages. Filled with love and respect for Mary, the work offers excerpts from nearly all of her writings on health and social reform as well as from her diaries. Thomas could scarcely bear to edit his wife's prose.[18]

"Woman is strong only in love, and until man is redeemed her love is her bane, her destruction," Mary had written in 1869. She continued:

> Woman would live chastely, lovingly, in holiness and health, if she could have the blessed strength of a spiritual love to sustain her. What is wanted now for the world's redemption is wisdom and self-restraint in man. Only as he comes to a loving and living and chaste unity with woman, can either be saved for this world. Marital union, only for wise and healthy birth, is the law of health and holiness for those who are to inaugurate physical and spiritual redemption. . . . Only the highest and holiest love can aspire to a life of marital chastity—of continence except for pure birth.

To this quotation, Thomas appended the simple remark, "I give the above 'for what it is worth'. . . . I do not expect that it will find a large acceptance, but thoughtful and earnest men and women may read and consider."[19] In the end, Mary Gove Nichols found only one way to reconcile herself to sexual intercourse—an act so profoundly tainted in her early personal experience that decades of anatomical study, idealistic prose, radical social philosophy, and loving matrimony could not redeem it. Mary's ambivalent relationship to the body found its comfort in the spiritual. Sexual love remained her "bane." Thomas had also revised his views on the physiologic need for sexual expression. Ironically, it was only in the extremes of free love and chastity that Mary and Thomas found adequately strong protection of "a woman's right to herself."

"When people are able to rise above the bondage of the sensual life, then their mistakes will not curse thousands of their descendants," wrote Mary. "The sublimation of the sensual force; its use in giving health and material power . . . ; its use in producing harmonies of music, architecture, and painting, in the prophecy and teaching of inspired poets, in the living words of a divine philosophy—all, and the myriad multiplication of all, are contained potentially in the sensual life of man. This sensual force is the fertile soil which produces the highest beauty he can conceive and create." Three years later, in his own book, Thomas wrote, "Chastity is the conservation of life and the consecration of its forces to the highest use. Sensuality is the waste of life and the degradation of its forces to pleasure divorced from use. Chastity is life—sensuality is death."[20]

Mary and Thomas had come to realize that liberated sexuality would not result in social equality for women. Free love alone would not grant women lives of intellectual rigor, spiritual fulfillment, physical safety, or political power. A century later, the sexual revolution of the 1960s has yielded similar lessons. Neither effective birth control nor accessible abortion have fully answered the Nicholses' wish for women's freedom. Despite progress, we have yet to create a society in which sexual happiness and gender equality coexist harmoniously. Tireless reformers, the Nicholses opened discussions of the relationship between power and sex that propel us still.

Mary and Thomas had fully anticipated the centrality of marriage reform in the fight for women's rights. Yet by the time America's most famous feminists had come to advance the Nicholses' earlier perspective, Mary's definition of sexual freedom had evolved into the realm of chaste spirituality. On July 20, 1857, four months after Mary's conversion to Catholicism, Elizabeth Cady Stanton echoed the Nicholses in a letter to Susan B. Anthony: "So long as our present false marriage relation continues, which in most cases is nothing more nor less than legalized prostitution, woman can have no self-respect, and of course man will have none for her; for the world estimates us according to the value we put upon ourselves. Personal freedom is the first right to be proclaimed, and that does not and cannot now belong to the relation of wife, to the mistress of the isolated home, to the financial dependent."[21] Three years later Stanton wrote:

Woman's degradation is in man's idea of his sexual rights. Our religion, laws, customs, are all founded on the belief that woman was made for man. Come what will, my whole soul rejoices in the truth that I have uttered. . . . How this marriage question grows on me. It lies at the foundation of all progress. I never read a thing on the subject until I had arrived at my present opinion. My own life, observation, thought, feeling, reason, brought me to the conclusion. . . . I feel a growing indifference to the praise and blame of my race, and an increasing interest in their weal and woe.[22]

Stephen Pearl Andrews, with the Nicholses, had both predicted and worked for this ultimate attention to marriage (if not for the denial of their influence). "The whole body of reformers . . . bring up sooner or later against the legal or prevalent theological idea of marriage," Andrews had written in 1852.[23] It took time. Nearly a decade later, Elizabeth Cady Stanton was still explicitly hoping to avoid letting "free lovers get the platform" at the very convention in which she had condemned restrictive divorce laws. Yet after another ten years she admitted: "We are all free lovers at heart, although we may not have thought so."[24] Ultimately, Stanton encouraged women's resilience to public scorn—courage that Mary Gove Nichols had long demonstrated. In a reflective letter to Lucretia Mott, Stanton wrote:

> Most women, who, like some tender flower, perish in the first rude blast, think there must be some subtle poison in the hardy plant. . . . We have already women enough sacrificed to this sentimental, hypocritical prating about purity, without going out of our way to increase the number. Women have crucified the Mary Wollstonecrafts, the Fanny Wrights and the George Sands of all ages. Men mock us with the fact and say we are ever cruel to each other. Let us end this ignoble record. . . . If . . . woman must be crucified, let men drive the spikes.[25]

The idea that God intended women for "hardy plants" had found two of its strongest and most prolific advocates in Mary Gove and Thomas Low Nichols.

Though their religious conversion effectively distanced the Nicholses from other social reformers, Catholicism undermined none of Mary's devotion to women's rights. In 1870 she wrote to Paulina Wright Davis:

> I cannot come [to your planned women's rights convention], but my interest in the freedom of woman has not in the least abated during thirty years of labour and prayers for her emancipation. I claim one right for Woman which includes all human rights. It is that she be free to obey the Divine law of her own life—that she be not subjected to the lustful despotism of one man, or to the selfish or unwise legislation of many.

As a Roman Catholic I claim for woman that she be free to become the pure daughter of the Mother of Our Lord, either as virgin or wife. . . . [and that children] be not forced upon her in fear or hate.

. . . In the Church the name of St. Scholastica is more than the shadow of that of her glorious brother, St. Benedict. St. Clara was not the mere echo of St. Francis. St. Catherine of Sienna, St. Bridget of Sweden, St. Theresa, St. Gertrude were in effect Doctors of the Church. St. Catherine of Genoa wrote a treatise on Purgatory which is the most highly esteemed book on the subject. Rose of Castile (the mother of St. Louis), St. Jane Frances de Chantal, Helena Cornaro, Mrs. Seton, Mother Margaret, and hosts of other women in every incident of their lives give us ample proof that the Church never desired to silence woman or diminish her usefulness, when she has spoken wisely or done well.[26]

Combing Catholic history, Mary had found validation of women's intellectual worth and many precedents of respect for women's teachings. She discovered this veneration in a religion that worshipped a virgin mother and that established cloistered, chaste homes for its holiest women. Free of sexuality's complications, nuns had achieved "rooms of their own" in which to think and work.

Devoted to the quest for women's happiness and fulfillment, Mary had never found a satisfying way to integrate women's sexual cravings with their political and intellectual longings. Yet she dared to open this can of worms—one that we have yet to close or conquer. And she risked this pursuit without the cultural support of gender studies programs, libraries full of women's scholarship, or an accessible pantheon of female mentors. Today the topic of sexuality is incorporated into school curricula and framed as a normal part of physiology and psychology. Medical students are taught to include the "sexual history" as part of a patient's full health history and to ask screening questions about domestic violence. There is no longer a "deep hush" about these most intimate and consequential topics.

The last work Thomas published was *Social Life: Its Principles, Relations, and Obligations,* which appeared in 1895, when he was eighty years old. Thomas had written nearly thirty books. He had helped to create and had contributed to dozens of periodicals; published many controversial pamphlets; and delivered hundreds, if not thousands, of lectures. In July of 1902, the London *Herald of Health* included the notice: "From a reliable source we learn that in the summer of last year Thomas Low Nichols, the pioneer of food reform, passed away at the age of eighty-five at Chaumont-en-Vezin, France."[27] Further details have been lost.

THE REACH OF RADICALS

By the end of the nineteenth century, the turmoil and pressure to create a perfect society had subsided. Religious passion no longer seemed the best guide to social reform. A more practical vision came with the rise of scientific objectivity, symbolized by the Nicholses' interest in inventing life preservers, treating patients, and selling soap rather than devising single solutions to multiple miseries. Even Mary called the 1870s the most "useful" years of her life—a decade of relatively ordinary work, reflection, writing, and family visits when compared to the Nicholses' earlier undertakings. Their personal story tells a much larger one.

Perhaps the couple's most important contribution was to clarify the fact that the "personal" is indeed "political." Mary and Thomas advanced the belief that the individual body and the social body more than mirror one another—that the two are inextricably bound. Physiology informed all of their reform efforts and supplied their most resilient metaphors: "The miseries of mankind are but the symptoms of its errors, of thought and life. There is no disease without a cause, and the cause is closely related to the remedy," wrote Thomas.[28] Consistently, the Nicholses advocated both self-help and social restructuring. As reformers, they were unusual in their ability to integrate physiology, anatomy, sociology, and religion. When they spoke of "natural laws" or "God's laws," or even of "spiritual manifestations," they brought to the discussion a respect for scientific empiricism. Their clinical work kept them grounded in earthly reality, even as their séances took them to the spirit world.

Mary and Thomas explored widely before finding stability in Catholicism. The misunderstood and radical peers of their youth had sought to remove whatever social corsets drove thousands into lives of boredom, poverty, disease, and sadness. Repression of instinct had seemed the curse. "Curb the erratic action of human nature ever so craftily in one direction, it darts off into some opposite evil," noted Mary. "Only by giving legitimate direction and occupation to all man's faculties and powers is the whole evil that rests on Humanity to be removed." This was a grand aim. Fourierism had intellectually answered their longing for communal spirit, but it offered no practical home. Optimistically though, Thomas believed that it "requires exertion, oppression, and repression to keep men in error. The tendency of the mind is to truth."[29] In fact, Thomas attributed much of his own stamina as a reformer to the voices of conservatism, asserting that "next in usefulness to the apostles and leading spirits of a true reform, are its most violent opponents and persecutors. They bring out the truths, they stimulate zeal, and invigorate exertion. . . . [C]onservatives . . . will preserve to us all the good of the past, while their efforts to perpetuate its evils, though strenuous, will be unavailing."[30] Both as radicals and as Catholics, Mary and Thomas believed that with patience, the future harmony for which they worked and prayed would someday find its realization.

Intellectual collaborators for thirty-six years, Mary S. Gove and Thomas Low Nichols lived by their belief that despite innate differences in body, soul, and mind, women and men should not be relegated to separate spheres of experience or influence. As Thomas once put it, "If woman, for the past century, had not been shut out from her rightful share of the advantages of education and opportunities for culture, the world would have made more rapid advances. The great mistake of men has been, to leave her behind, and to endeavor to get along without her."[31]

Even as Mary's language of spiritual love and harmonic progression lost its resonance in a culture turning toward technological promise and away from the soul, she and Thomas clung to their idealism. They left the United States when national ironies and disappointments grew overly fierce, departing for England saddened by the failures of the society they were leaving behind and aware that universal happiness would not come in their lifetimes. As Mary and Thomas believed, "The end of all being is the enjoyment of being; and man fulfils his destiny when he . . . fills his capacity for happiness. The work of the reformer, the educator, the philanthropist, is to aid in bringing about such conditions in individuals and in society." And so they did good work. Witness to her own slow fading, Mary bravely wished that "the books we have written, and those we hope to write will still be left, and, we hope widely circulated, so that 'being dead, we may yet speak' to the coming generations."[32]

NOTES

ABBREVIATIONS

AAS American Antiquarian Society

BMSJ *Boston Medical and Surgical Journal*

GJ *Graham Journal of Health and Longevity*

Godey's *Godey's Magazine and Lady's Book*

MG Mary Gove

MGN Mary Gove Nichols

NJ *Nichols' Journal of Health, Water-Cure, and Human Progress*

NM *Nichols' Monthly: A Magazine of Social Science and Progressive Literature*

TLN Thomas Low Nichols

UNDA University of Notre Dame Archives

UVA University of Virginia Archives

VC Vassar College Library

WCJ *Water-Cure Journal, and Herald of Reforms*

INTRODUCTION

1. *New York Morning Herald*, 10 April 1839, 2.

2. Jackson, *Hints on the Reproductive Organs* (1852), 30.

3. MGN and TLN, *Marriage* (1854), 265.

4. TLN, *Nichols' Monthly Extra* (ca. 1856), 3.

5. Alexis de Tocqueville, *Democracy in America*, ed. J. P. Mayer; trans. George Lawrence (13th ed., 1850; Garden City, N.Y.: Doubleday, 1969): 592–94, 502, as quoted in Hartog, *Man and Wife in America*, 102.

6. Quoted in TLN, *Nichols' Health Manual* (1886) (hereafter, *Health Manual*), 392–93.

7. Quoted in ibid., 217. For overviews of the antebellum medical turf wars, see Starr, *Social Transformation*, 30–59; Cassedy, *Medicine in America*, 33–39; and Green, *Fit for America*, 3–29.

8. See especially Cayleff, *Wash and Be Healed*; and Donegan, *"Hydropathic Highway to Health."*

9. For discussion of the social construction of the body and its subsequent power to reify culture as "natural," see Rosenberg and Smith-Rosenberg, "The Female Animal"; M. Douglas, *Natural Symbols*; and Smith-Rosenberg, *Disorderly Conduct*, 11–52.

10. Russell T. Trall, "March Matters," *WCJ* 15, no. 3 (March 1853): 61.

11. TLN, *Woman, in All Ages* (1849), 229.

12. "Women's Rights," *Nichols' Weekly* 2, no. 1 (7 January 1854): n.p., third sheet.

13. Isenberg, *Sex and Citizenship*. As Isenberg writes, "Separate spheres has resulted in separate histories, with women dominating the moral domain, men the political, and feminists have been forced to fall within either the feminine sphere of moral reform or the masculine realm of partisan politics" (10). The near-loss of Mary Gove Nichols from collective memory illustrates the dangers of such an approach.

14. "The World's Conventions," *NJ* 1, no. 7 (1 October 1853): 55.

15. Noever, "Passionate Rebel," 3–8.

16. John Neal, "Literary," *Brother Jonathan* 5, no. 1 (6 May 1843): n.p.; MGN, "A Letter to Women," *NJ* 1, no. 1 (April 1853): 6.

CHAPTER 1. THE FORMATIVE YEARS

1. Hadley, *Goffstown*, 2–28, 171, 232.

2. TLN, *Health Manual*, 18–19.

3. Ibid., 12, 8.

4. Ibid., 12–13, 18.

5. Quoted in ibid., 17.

6. MGN, *Mary Lyndon*, 17–18.

7. Ibid., 17; and TLN, *Health Manual*, 7.

8. On the perceived influence of novels, see Davidson, *Revolution and the Word*, 40–41: "Timothy Dwight took time out from presiding over Yale, Jonathan Edwards from fomenting a religious revival, Benjamin Rush from attending to his medical and philosophical investigations, Noah Webster from writing dictionaries, and Thomas Jefferson and John Adams from presiding over a nation—and all to condemn the novel." For the Neals' attitudes toward writing, see TLN, *Health Manual*, 13–14.

9. Quoted in TLN, *Health Manual*, 13; Noever, "Passionate Rebel," 30, n.10.

10. MGN, *A Woman's Work*, 10.

11. MGN, *Mary Lyndon*, 32. I do not know the real name of Mary's sister.

12. Ibid., 34.

13. Ibid., 36.

14. Ibid., 36, 38.

15. Ibid., 40.

16. TLN, *Health Manual*, 8, 20; MGN, *Mary Lyndon*, 54–58.

17. MGN, *Mary Lyndon*, 67–69.

18. Ibid., 70–73, 77.

19. Ibid., 74.

20. Ibid., 91–103.

21. Ibid., 20.

22. Ibid., 99–102, 106.

23. Ibid., 107.

24. Ibid., 110; MG to John Neal, 3 July 1841, quoted in Richards, "Mary Gove Nichols and John Neal," 350.

25. MGN, *Mary Lyndon*, 62.

26. *Anatomy*, by John Bell and Sir Charles Bell, was originally published in Edinburgh in 1793 and saw many editions, first in Scotland, then in England and the United States. Mary was likely to have encountered the third American edition, based on the fourth English edition and titled *The Anatomy and Physiology of the Human Body. Containing the Anatomy of the Bones, Muscles, and Joints, and the Heart and Arteries* (New York: Collins & Co., 1817). This work also included descriptions of the lungs, the brain and nerves, the viscera of the abdomen, the organs of the senses, and the male and female generative organs. The first American edition of this widely read textbook appeared in 1809 under the shorter title, *The Anatomy of the Human Body*. Two other influential works she read not long after were Robley Dunglison's *Human Physiology* (Philadelphia: Carey, 1832) and Anthelme M. B. Richerand's *Elements of Physiology* (Philadelphia: Moore, 1823 [orig. 1803]). "[These texts] were in my first and last waking thoughts. I got almost crazed with this mental feast" (TLN, *Health Manual*, 21). Her later medical reading broadened considerably and included the works of pathologist François Joseph Broussais and anatomist Xavier Bichat.

27. MGN, *Experience in Water-Cure* (1850), 21–22. Though Mary studied Latin independently, she received tutoring in French from no less eminent a neighbor than Governor Crafts of Vermont. See TLN, *Health Manual*, 20.

28. MGN, *Mary Lyndon*, 111–12.

29. Ibid., 114.

30. Ibid., 119.

31. MGN and TLN, *Marriage,* 194.

32. MGN, *Mary Lyndon,* 121.

33. Ibid., 121–23.

34. MGN and TLN, *Marriage* (1854), 192. In the 1830s the concept of "mental health" or "psychology" as a distinct branch of human experience did not exist. Everything from inherited predisposition, to environment, to behavior could explain one's afflictions. Body and mind were necessarily linked and interactive. Germ theory would not be accepted for another half-century. Thus, insomnia might be addressed by a change in diet or by a change in scenery. Physicians today tend to subdivide health into "physical health" and "mental health," granting with more lip service than substance the notion that the two always influence one another.

35. Little, *History of Weare* (1888), 878; Gove, *Gove Book* (1922), 204–5.

36. MG to John Neal, 1 February 1842, quoted in Richards, "Mary Gove Nichols and John Neal," 354.

37. *International Genealogical Index,* The Church of Jesus Christ of Latter-day Saints, 1994; MGN, *Mary Lyndon,* 127. By studying anatomy, Mary must also have been seeking explanation for her many failed pregnancies, for which there is no evidence—other than her misery with Hiram—to suspect intentional abortion.

38. MGN, *Mary Lyndon,* 128, 119, 129, 135.

39. MGN and TLN, *Marriage,* 198.

40. Ibid., 194.

41. MGN, *NJ* 1, no. 5 (August 1853): 37.

42. Lewis, *History of Lynn* (1829), 235–56. Also see Faler, *Mechanics and Manufacturers.*

43. "Notices of New Books," *Democratic Review* 26 (March 1850): 286. With rare and brief exceptions, Alonzo Lewis spent his entire life in Lynn. This and subsequent personal descriptions of Lewis come from a memorial written by James R. Newhall; see 544–66 of Lewis and Newhall, *History of Lynn, Essex County.*

44. MGN to Alonzo Lewis, 2 January 1850. Given Mary's friendship with an outspoken abolitionist like Alonzo Lewis, it is even more difficult to explain her subsequent distance from the antislavery movement. Many Quakers were involved in abolitionism, and it is a possibility that Mary had simply grown averse to the company of a sect that must have reminded her of Hiram. She did, however, attend antislavery meetings while in Lynn and continued, for a time, to speak and write in the manner of the Society of Friends. (See MG to John Neal, 29 February 1840, quoted in Richards, "Mary Gove Nichols and John Neal," 344.)

45. MG, *Lectures to Ladies* (1842), 98.

46. Before the end of September 1837, Sarah and Angelina had addressed more

than 13,000 people in twenty-three towns. "Men came in their shirtsleeves directly from fields and workshops . . . and women flocked to the talks, many carrying small children in their arms." See Mayer, *All On Fire*, 233–34. Also see Bartlett, *Liberty, Equality, Sorority*, 59.

47. Sylvester Graham would not recognize our modern graham crackers, the sugar-coated legacy, ironically, of a man devoted to plain food. For extended analysis of Graham's teachings, see Nissenbaum, *Sex, Diet, and Debility*.

48. MG, "Statement by the Editor," *Health Journal and Advocate of Physiological Reform*, 4 November 1840, 102.

49. "Boarding School," *Lynn Record*, 28 March 1838; "Graham Boarding School," *GJ* 2, no. 8 (14 April 1838): 128.

50. MGN, *Mary Lyndon*, 136–37.

51. MGN, "To the Friends of Truth," *NJ* 1, no. 6 (September 1853): 45.

52. Hunt, *Glances and Glimpses* (1856), 139. Also see Bartlett, *Liberty, Equality, Sorority*, 27–28. Bartlett quotes the response of the *Louisville Focus* to Wright's lectures, as reported in the *Free Enquirer*, 12 August 1829, 329: "Miss Wright . . . has with ruthless violence broken loose from the restraints of decorum, which draw a circle around the life of a woman, and with a contemptuous disregard for the rules of society, she has . . . laid hold on the avocations of man, claiming a participation in them for herself and her sex. . . . Miss Wright stands condemned of a violation of the unalterable laws of nature, which have erected a barrier between man and woman, over which neither can pass, without unhinging the beneficent adjustments of society, and doing wanton injury to the happiness of each other."

53. Quoted in Morantz, "Making Women Modern" in Leavitt, ed., *Women and Health*, 347–48; and Verbrugge, *Able-Bodied Womanhood*, 51.

54. Hudspeth, ed. *Letters of Margaret Fuller*, 1:86–89.

55. Ibid. In 1848 Elizabeth Cady Stanton would found the Seneca Falls Conversation Club, based on Fuller's model (see Conrad, *Perish the Thought*, 137). Other women's organizations had been established much earlier. The Female Moral Reform Society (FMRS) had been founded in New York City in 1834; by 1837 its weekly journal, *Advocate of Moral Reform*, was reaching 16,500 subscribers. By 1839 the organization had 445 auxiliaries. In New York the FMRS established a house of refuge for reformed prostitutes, and throughout the country its members advocated temperance and female solidarity in the fight against America's seeming moral degradation. See Smith-Rosenberg, *Disorderly Conduct*, 109–28.

For a description of the literary activities among Lowell factory workers, see Robinson, *Loom and Spindle* (1898). For a rich treatment of women's diverse health-reform initiatives in Boston during the nineteenth century, see Verbrugge, *Able-Bodied Womanhood*. College students, too, were forming clubs devoted to physiological living. At Wesleyan University, a club of six men "commenced boarding upon a pretty thoroughly reformed mode, determined to give 'Grahamism' a fair trial," wrote a member to the *Graham Journal.* "They agree . . . that pure water shall be their only drink; that neither butter, sugar, molasses, or any condiment whatever, excepting salt, shall be used; that no animal food shall be used, excepting an occasional meal of milk, and that but one kind of food shall come upon the table at a meal" (*GJ* 3, no. 6 [13 April 1839]: 95).

56. This Gag Rule—which had been initiated by Southerners and passed only with the aid of Northern Democrats—was rescinded on December 3, 1844, as a consequence of the withdrawal of Northern support. Abolitionists roundly condemned this federal denial of the right of petition. See Chase et al., eds., *Dictionary of American History.*

57. *GJ* 2, no. 18 (1 September 1838): 288. Women were beginning to form social networks that broadened their public influence. These organizations also enhanced the legal status of married women. As historian Nancy Isenberg explains, "By incorporating, benevolent societies . . . expanded women's ability to exercise certain legal rights, allowing them to own and manage property, to make legally binding contracts, and to control their finances. . . . Such societies permitted married women to meet the requirement of the bourgeois public sphere as property owners" (*Sex and Citizenship,* 59).

58. *GJ* 2, no. 18 (1 September 1838): 288. Thomas Low Nichols described William Alcott as a neighbor and friend to Mary as well as a friend to Ralph Waldo Emerson and a teacher of Sylvester Graham (*Health Manual,* 28).

59. *GJ* 2, no. 18 (1 September 1838): 2. Marlboro' Chapel served as the site for many lectures sponsored by the American Physiological Society (APS). On February 12, 1839, the president of the Oberlin Collegiate Institute, Asa Mahan, delivered a talk before the APS on the "Intimate Relation Between Moral, Mental and Physical Law" in which he argued: "Esteemed [woman] cannot be till she exhibits a respect for herself, by the exhibition of a sacred regard for the laws of her constitution" (*GJ* 3, no. 10 [11 May 1839]: 158).

60. Alcott, *Library of Health and Teacher of the Human Constitution* (November 1838): 357. Despite his support for female health reformers, Alcott did not argue for a broad expansion of women's roles. As Carroll Smith-Rosenberg has noted, *The Young Wife; or Duties of Woman in the Marriage Relation* (1837) emphasized the virtues of "domesticity," "obedience," "submission," and "cheerfulness." See Smith-Rosenberg, *Disorderly Conduct,* 25. Also see TLN, *Health Manual,* 28.

61. Anna Breed to Abby Kelley, 11 November 1838, AAS; TLN, *Health Manual,* 22.

62. It seems probable, given Fuller's move to the Boston area in the late winter of 1839, that she had just missed her opportunity to attend Mary's lecture series in that city, since Mary initiated her New York lectures in the spring of 1839. See Hudspeth, *Letters of Margaret Fuller,* 1:36–37.

63. *New York Morning Herald,* 10 April 1839, 2–3. Some of the *Herald*'s purported quotations seem more like sheer invention than exaggeration or mild distortion. For example, while the following may have soothed more than shocked contemporary sensibilities, it seems unlikely that Mary ever told her audience: "A wife must persuade by gentleness . . . and not bring her will to bear in opposition to her husband. Man is the head of the family, and where there are two heads to one subject, it must be a monster" (*New York Morning Herald,* 26 April 1839, 2).

64. Combe, *Phrenological Visit,* 2:32, 216. Combe's 18-month tour greatly enhanced the popularity and credibility of phrenology, a science of human psychology that relied on a mapping of skull contours to identify character traits. The theory, based on cerebral anatomy, had been founded by a German physician, Franz Joseph Gall, who began promoting his theories in Europe in 1802. His pupil, Johann Spurzheim, coined the term *phrenology* and helped popularize the science. Mary respected phrenology and recommended the works of George Combe to her audiences. See *Lectures to Ladies,* 206.

65. *GJ* 3, no. 11 (25 May 1839): 181.

66. Ibid., 19 January 1839, 37; *GJ* 3, no. 19 (14 September 1839): 309.

67. MGN, "Human Culture—No. II," *NJ* 1, no. 2 (May 1853): 15; *GJ* 3, no. 2 (19 January 1839), 37; TLN, *Health Manual,* 23.

68. MGN, *Experience in Water-Cure,* 20–21.

69. *GJ* 3, no. 4 (16 February 1839): 69. Mary also lectured to smaller groups. On Tuesday, August 13, 1839, for example, she met with the Ladies Physiological Society at 23 Brattle Street in Boston, a Graham boarding house that provided free shower baths to all boarders at all hours. See *GJ* 3, no. 16 (3 August 1839); the prior issue of the *Graham Journal* contained an advertisement for "Portable Shower Baths" manufactured by Messrs. Cushing and Robie, who described their apparatus as an "article [that] occupies but a small space in a sleeping room, and makes a very neat part of the furniture" (20 July 1839, 248).

70. Quoted in TLN, *Health Manual,* 25. In 1845, Paulina Kellogg Wright Davis would follow Mary's example and begin offering her own public lectures to women on anatomy, physiology, and health reform. For four years she lectured throughout the East and Midwest. Davis, an abolitionist and advocate of women's rights, did not publish her medical lectures, but went on to found the *Una,* a women's rights journal established in the early 1850s. The *Una* included articles condemning excessive sensuality in marriage and the legal dominance of husbands

over their wives. Davis also founded the Providence Physiological Society in 1850. See Brodie, *Contraception and Abortion*, 128–29; and Battenfeld, "'She hath done what she could.'"

71. MG to John Neal, 4 April 1841, quoted in Richards, "Mary Gove Nichols and John Neal," 347. Mary hoped for Neal's approval in this action and also asked him whether he had read Mary Wollstonecraft's *Rights of Woman* (ibid., 346).

72. Quoted in TLN, *Health Manual*, 24 (italics in original). In this diary entry, Mary also wrote that she had "called on L.M. [most likely Lucretia Mott]. She is, take her for all in all, one of the most remarkable women I ever met" (ibid., 23).

73. MG to John Neal, 3 July 1841, quoted in Richards, "Mary Gove Nichols and John Neal," 350.

74. For these observations on the brain, see *GJ* 2, no. 21 (13 October 1838): 328; and on the stomach, see *GJ* 2, no. 22 (27 October 1838): 340.

75. *GJ* 2, no. 23 (10 November 1838): 357. Mary knew what it meant to be a "slave" to bad habits. She admitted that at around the age of twenty-one, "[I] mostly left the use of snuff and tea. I had all along thought it impossible to give up snuff. I most sincerely pity any one who uses tobacco in any form. It requires great moral courage to break the spell. . . . After leaving the use of tea, I became enslaved by coffee, and almost lived upon it. This injured me greatly and I finally abandoned it because I found I could not perform my duties as a teacher if I continued its use. I had great weakness, trembling, and palpitations of the heart, in consequence of taking coffee." See MG, "Statement by the Editor," *Health Journal and Advocate of Physiological Reform* 1, no. 25 (21 October 1840): 98.

76. MG, *Lectures to Ladies*, 217–18.

77. MG to John Neal, 1839, 5th day, night, 11 o'clock, quoted in Richards, "Mary Gove Nichols and John Neal," 341.

CHAPTER 2. A PROFESSIONAL ESCAPE

1. *BMSJ* (11 November 1840): 228; MG, *Solitary Vice*, 5. The first childcare manual to appear in the United States was written anonymously by "an American matron" in 1811 and published by Isaac Riley in New York. Entitled *The Maternal Physician: A Treatise on the Nurture and Management of Infants, from the Birth until Two Years Old. Being the result of sixteen years' experience in the nursery*, the text did not treat the subject of masturbation, but it did suggest treatments for a wide range of physical disorders as well as guidance regarding the training of habits such as obedience and regular sleeping patterns. For a concise overview of this work, see Charles E. Rosenberg's Introduction to the 1972 Arno Press edition of *The Maternal Physician*.

2. Nissenbaum, *Sex, Diet, and Debility*, 26; MG, *Solitary Vice* (1839), 6, 18.

3. Ibid., 6. The antebellum cultural response to masturbation resembles today's concern over teen smoking. Writers argued that innocent children were initiating a dangerous practice too addictive to abandon with ease. The only effective treatment was abstinence. As for the question of explicit sexual education for children, the debate over whether or not to "risk the silent course" remains unresolved.

4. In an undated letter to her friend John Neal, Mary claimed that Graham's *Lecture to Young Men on Chastity* had saved her own brother from ruin. See Richards, "Mary Gove Nichols and John Neal," 342.

5. Tissot, *Onanism* (1832), v; Graham, *Lecture to Young Men on Chastity*, 42. Health writer William Alcott described Graham as "far-famed, and very far-hated," and believed that "while the public odium was ostensibly directed against his anti-fine flour and anti-flesh eating doctrines, it was his anti-sexual indulgence doctrines, in reality, which excited the public hatred and rendered his name a by-word and a reproach" (*Physiology of Marriage*). Speculatively, one can easily detect personal reasons for Graham's leadership of the sexual temperance crusade. From a Freudian perspective, he seems to have devoted his life to condemning the sexual drive that could produce enough children to drive a mother mad. It may have seemed logical to Graham that if his father had been less sexually active, then his mother might have preserved her sanity and peace. "Health does not absolutely require that there should be an emission of semen from puberty to death, though the individual live an hundred years," he wrote (ibid., 75). The self-punishing and extreme qualities of Graham's teachings suggest that he was not simply a representative of his times. Graham was motivated by personal trauma as well as by larger cultural and economic forces.

6. In antebellum America, youth constituted nearly 30 percent of the population. Many of these young, unattached people migrated in and out of cities, entirely free of the close supervision so integral to rural communities. Heightened concern over masturbation correlated in time with anxiety over the moral management of so many independent, unaccountable young people. See Cohen, *Murder of Helen Jewett*. Masturbatory "waste" of sperm was akin to fiscal irresponsibility in a newly commercial era that valued sound investment and delayed gratification. See Cominos, "Late-Victorian Sexual Respectability," 18–48, 216–50; and Barker-Benfield, "The Spermatic Economy," 45–74.

7. MGN, "To the Friends of Truth," *NJ* 1, no. 6 (September 1853): 45. In March 1839 the *Graham Journal* quoted the Boston *Morning Post*'s notice that "in Europe, a knowledge of physiology is considered essential in the education of females. . . . In Paris . . . they have models of diseased portions of the human frame, and real skeletons of infants, hung up in some of the shop windows, like any other articles of merchandise. Mrs. Gove's lectures would be considered as nothing strange in that part of the world, while here they are quite a sensation." See "A

Knowledge of Anatomy and Physiology Should Be Accessible to All," *GJ* 3, no. 5 (2 March 1839): 84.

8. MGN, "To the Friends of Truth," *NJ* 1, no. 6 (September 1853): 45.

9. A Friend, "Case of Mary S. Gove," *Reformer* 1, no. 2 (November 1839): 24.

10. Bacon, *Valiant Friend,* 43–45; Joseph Wall, "Society of Friends in Great Britain Versus Society of Friends in America," *Reformer* 1, no. 3 (December 1839): 1. For more on the Hicksite schism, see Bonner, *"The Other Branch"*; and Ingle, *Quakers in Conflict.*

11. "From The Golden Rule," *Reformer* (15 February 1840): 32; B.J. Tefft, "Testimony in Favor of Mary S. Gove," *Reformer* (18 January 1840): 27.

12. MG to John Neal, 29 February 1840. See Richards, "Mary Gove Nichols and John Neal," 345. The *Health Journal and Advocate of Physiological Reform* was sent to all subscribers of the defunct *Graham Journal,* "As ours is designed to take the place of that paper." See *Health Journal and Advocate of Physiological Reform* (3 June 1840). The editors simply asked that readers either return the unrequested issues or pay the subscription fee.

13. She elaborated further: "What *shall* I do? I know Smith. He is a good fellow. . . . But I dread being known to him as A.B. I fear I shall lose my ground in the paper and I do want to occupy it exceedingly. . . . Smith urges me to see him. . . . He told a medical friend of mine a short time since, that he 'would trap that fellow yet, for he had written some of the best articles he had ever had—and he was determined to find him out'" (MG to John Neal, quoted in Richards, "Mary Gove Nichols and John Neal," 344–45). I do not know why Mary chose the initials A.B.

14. "Critical Observations on Dr. Durkee's 'Remarks on Scrofula,'" *BMSJ* 21, no. 19 (18 December 1839): 297. The term *scrofula* referred to what in today's medical lexicon is known as cervical tuberculous lymphadenitis, a swelling of the lymph glands in the neck.

15. Ibid., 298.

16. "Respiratory Apparatus—Mr. Bronson, &c.," *BMSJ* (26 August 1840): 49–51. For reference to her lessons with Bronson, see MG, "Statement by the Editor," *Health Journal and Advocate of Physiological Reform* (4 November 1840): 102. On Bronson, see Verbrugge, *Able-Bodied Womanhood,* 51–52. Bronson was the author of several popular works on elocution and music, including *Abstract of Elocution and Music* (1842) and *Elocution; or Mental and Vocal Philosophy* (1845).

17. "Quotations and Remarks on the Blood—No. 1," *BMSJ* (19 February 1840): 24–27, "Quotations and Remarks on the Blood—No. 2," *BMSJ* (26 February 1840): 43–45. François Magendie (1783–1855) was a French physiologist most famous for his advocacy of an empirical approach to scientific investigation and for his many physiology experiments using animals. He was also a pioneer in experi-

mental pharmacology. His works include *An Elementary Summary of Physiology* (1816); *An Elementary Treatise on Human Physiology, on the Basis of the Précis Élémentaire de Physiologie* (1844); and the *Journal de Physiologie Experimentale et Pathologique*, published in Paris. John Eberle (1787–1838) was an American physician who taught at the Medical College of Ohio and who was a founding editor of the *American Medical Recorder*, a quarterly journal first published in 1818, and the *Western Medical Gazette*, founded in 1832. Eberle's 1823 *Treatise of the Materia Medica and Therapeutics* became a standard textbook in medical curricula and saw five editions.

18. Bacon, *Valiant Friend*, 73–74; MGN, *Mary Lyndon*, 164. The first lyceum organization in Lynn had been founded in 1828 and lasted until 1834. In 1841 the new Lyceum of the Town of Lynn was built on Market Street. This meeting hall seated one thousand people and accommodated many antislavery lecturers; a bank and a post office occupied its first floor. John Quincy Adams would have been the lyceum's inaugural speaker, had he not been sick on opening day. See *Records of the Lynn Lyceum*, Lynn Historical Society.

19. MGN, *Mary Lyndon*, 166–67.

20. MG to John Neal, 1 February 1842, quoted in Richards, "Mary Gove Nichols and John Neal," 353; Johnson, ed., "John Neal," *Dictionary of American Biography*, 398–99. David S. Reynolds credits Neal with writing "our earliest full examples of the American Subversive Style . . . [which] tried to be deliberately outrageous, inflammatory, disquieting. It spit in the face of conventional literature. . . . It represented a form of autocriticism within American society, a turning inward of the rebelliousness that had once been directed at foreign tyrants" (*Beneath the American Renaissance*, 200). Whether or not Mary Sargeant Neal Gove Nichols was related to John Neal has been a matter of historiographic dispute. In a letter dated February 3, 1875, to John Ingram (who was seeking information for a biography of Edgar Allan Poe), Mary refers to Neal as being "of my blood." And Thomas Nichols called John Neal Mary's "cousin" in his *Health Manual* (28). But historian Irving Richards could find no genealogical evidence to connect them as first cousins. He suggests the possibility that the two were related through Mary's mother, whose maiden name began with an "R." If that "R" stood for "Roberts," Richard suggests the relationship might have been through Neal's grandmother, Elizabeth Roberts. See Richards, "Mary Gove Nichols and John Neal," 335–55.

21. MGN, *Mary Lyndon*, 130; MG to John Neal, 1 February 1842, quoted in Richards, "Mary Gove Nichols and John Neal," 353.

22. MGN, *Mary Lyndon*, 158–59.

23. Hiram Gove eventually became a practicing homeopathic physician. Few

details of his medical career exist, though it is tempting to wonder if he had been influenced by his famous wife's devotion to sectarian medicine. He is listed as a graduate of 1842 "from NY" [?] in Abrahams, *Extinct Medical Schools*.

24. MG to John Neal, February 1, 1842, quoted in Richards, "Mary Gove Nichols and John Neal," 353–55.

25. Ibid. One of Neal's letters to Mary (30 November 1846) has been preserved in the Boston Public Library. It discusses Neal's feelings about the reception of his own creative writing, especially regarding a cold review written by Edgar Allan Poe, one of Mary's friends at the time.

26. MGN, *Mary Lyndon*, 169, 131.

27. *BMSJ* 26, no. 6 (16 March 1842): 97–98; *New York Herald*, 18 March 1842.

28. MG, *Lectures to Ladies*, 264.

29. Ibid., 284, 97.

30. Ibid., 98 (italics in original), 97, 95.

31. Ibid., 106.

32. Ibid., 99, 103 (italics in original).

33. "Lectures to Ladies on Anatomy and Physiology," *BMSJ* 26, no. 6 (16 March 1842): 97–98; and MG, *Lectures to Ladies*, 216.

34. MG, *Lectures to Ladies*, 273, 272; and MGN, *A Woman's Work*, 149.

35. MG, *Lectures to Ladies*, 272.

36. Ibid., 32.

37. MG to John Neal, 10 August 1841, quoted in Richards, "Mary Gove Nichols and John Neal," 351–52 (italics in original).

38. Bedell, *Alcotts*, 121, 17–18, 102–3, 129.

39. Ibid., 167–68; advertisement for Alcott House reproduced in ibid., n.p.

40. For a description of Wright, see MGN, *Mary Lyndon*, 179; and Bedell, *Alcotts*, 179. The quality of Wright's relationship to his wife, Elizabeth, is not entirely clear. Elizabeth Hardwick had been a follower of Greaves. She and Wright claimed to have been secretly married late in 1841; she gave birth to their child in July 1842. It was likely a concocted shotgun wedding to avoid scandal at Alcott House. Elizabeth and Henry's relationship infuriated Greaves, a lifelong bachelor and celibate, as well as Lane, who had separated from his wife and had spent three years in court, successfully fighting for custody of their son. According to one Alcott biographer, Greaves and Lane were "certainly woman haters" and possibly also homosexuals. Lane became a staunch defender of celibacy and eventually joined the Shakers. See Bedell, *Alcotts*, 183–84.

41. On their attitudes toward clothing and vegetables, see Richardson, *Emerson, Mind on Fire*, 381–82. For further discussion of Emerson's relationship to popular reform, see Reynolds, *Beneath the American Renaissance*, 92–98.

42. Letter from Charles Lane to William Oldham, 31 December 1842, Harland typescript, cited in Bedell, *Alcotts,* 197–98.

43. Noever, "Passionate Rebel," 94–95. Joseph Wall had died of tuberculosis in October of 1842 at age twenty-five.

44. *Health Journal and Independent Magazine* (April 1843): 58–60.

45. Cayleff, *Wash and Be Healed,* 21–24; TLN, "Vincent Preissnitz [*sic*]," *NJ* 2, no. 1 (7 January 1854): 4.

46. Letter from Andrew J. Colvin to Joel Shew, M.D., quoted in Shew, *Water-Cure Manual,* 268–69; Horsell, *Hydropathy for the People,* 102.

47. MGN, *Mary Lyndon,* 221. On water's therapeutic uses through history, see Green, *Fit for America,* 54–67; Cayleff, *Wash and Be Healed,* 18–24; and, though undocumented, Russell Trall's 1853 *Hydropathic Encyclopedia,* "Medical Testimony in Favor of the Remedial Use of Water" (1:36–52), wherein Trall cites more than eighty medical authorities, from Hippocrates to the American physician John Bell, who advocated water treatment. The American physician Benjamin Rush, famous for his "heroic" therapeutics, recommended applications of cold water for the treatment of "tonic madness." These included placing bladders of cold water or ice on the head while submerging the feet in warm water, immersing the whole body in cold water for several hours, and daily shower baths. See Rush, *Medical Inquiries* (1827), 196–201.

48. Bedell, *Alcotts,* 198–99; MGN, *Mary Lyndon,* 225; Noever, "Passionate Rebel," 96–97. Plans for a future association discussed in a letter from MG to James Russell Lowell, 30 June 1843, Houghton Library, Harvard University, cited in Noever, "Passionate Rebel," 97.

49. Quoted in Bedell, *Alcotts,* 231. For an extended discussion of Fruitlands, see ibid., 177–231; and Francis, *Transcendental Utopias.*

50. Richards, "Mary Gove Nichols and John Neal," 336; Noever, "Passionate Rebel," 99; MGN, *NJ* 1, no. 6 (September 1853): 45. In *Mary Lyndon,* Mary describes Elma as ten years old when Hiram took her away, which would make the year 1842. This appears not to have been the case, and perhaps Mary chose to portray her daughter as a younger and therefore more helpless victim. In her autobiography, Mary claims to have learned of Elma's abduction from a clairvoyant, a "magnetized boy." This version of events strains a skeptic's patience. Mary tells the story of a visit to a twelve-year-old boy, who had been sent into a deep sleep by an aged mesmerist; in his trance, this boy had the power to describe the unknown. The elderly man laid Mary's hand on the boy's and made passes between them. Then, as Mary imagined herself in different cities, the boy accurately narrated her mental journey, even down to the slightest and most quirky detail. What began as a pleasant and highly entertaining experience turned grim when the boy

described an "ugly man" carrying away a crying girl in a wagon, with his hand covering her mouth. The hypnotized boy reassured Mary that she and the girl would ultimately be reunited and happy but that it would take time. The prophecy turned out to be true (*Mary Lyndon*, 249–50). Mary wrote this version of events in the mid-1850s, a period during which she was heavily involved with spiritualism and called herself a medium. The belief in mesmeric power to communicate with the spirit world or to exhibit clairvoyance had great popular appeal in antebellum America; thus, her story may have seemed more plausible to its original readers.

51. The reader should bear in mind that the subsequent narrative of Mary's quest to recover Elma is drawn entirely and without other corroboration from *Mary Lyndon*.

52. MGN, *Mary Lyndon*, 254, 256, 258.

53. Fuller, *Woman in the Nineteenth Century*, 31–32.

54. MGN, *Mary Lyndon*, 252–65, 314; Mintz and Kellogg, *Domestic Revolutions*, 62. For an excellent analysis of marital law during this period, see Hartog, *Man and Wife in America*.

55. Fuller, *Woman in the Nineteenth Century*, 163–64. "Orvietan" was a composition thought to be an antidote to poison.

56. *Boston Moral Reformer* 1 (1835): 184, quoted in Shryock, "Sylvester Graham," 174.

57. *A Description of the Brattleboro Hydropathic Establishment, with a report of 563 cases treated there during the years 1845, 1846 and 1847, and the rules and regulations of the establishment* (Brattleboro, Vermont, 1848), 8. For description of the region, see ibid., 5–8.

58. Ibid., 8; R. T. Trall, F. D. Pierson, and G. T. Dexter, "Crisis," *American Journal of Hydropathy* 1, no. 1 (1 June 1847): 2–3. Publications advocating the water cure were not above using graphic and revolting images to encourage readers' compliance with hydropathic regimen. Consider the warning posed in the *New Grafenberg Water-Cure Reporter*: "If you are too irresolute to bathe all over frequently, and too careless in changing your soiled for clean clothes, and thus become covered with the excrementitious matters of dried perspiration; then even the kind brutes will take pity on you, and the flies, lice, and fleas will become useful to you, by generously rooting up and tearing off this unwholesome coating that smothers the life of your skin" (2, no. 1 [January 1850]: 16).

59. MGN, *A Woman's Work*, 23; *A Description of the Brattleboro Hydropathic Establishment*, 8–9. For a typical list of supplies patients were asked to provide, see advertisement for "Dr. Wesselhœft's Water-Cure Establishment at Brattleboro, Vermont," *WCJ* 11, no. 6 (June 1851): 158; and the advertisement on the back cover of the *New Grafenberg Water-Cure Reporter* 2, no. 1 (January 1850).

60. Beecher, *Letters to the People*, 117–18.

61. MGN, *A Woman's Work*, 20, 26.

62. Donegan, *"Hydropathic Highway to Health,"* 21, 29.

63. Russell T. Trall, "Death of Dr. Shew," *WCJ* 20, no. 5 (November 1855): 104–5; Donegan, *"Hydropathic Highway to Health,"* 19–24.

64. MGN, *Mary Lyndon*, 280–84. Later, in her autobiography, Mary made a special point to defend Marie Shew's reputation. She seemed to think Marie's popularity with the attractive young men in her house had caused others to make unfair assumptions about her friend's character. Fear for the preservation of reputation often limited women's range of activities in this era—a fact that Mary found extremely frustrating. It is not surprising that she was immediately drawn to a woman who refused to let such concerns dictate her lifestyle.

65. Ibid., 287–89.

CHAPTER 3. PASSION UNLEASHED

1. MGN, *Mary Lyndon*, 311–24.

2. Ibid., 311–12.

3. Ibid., 319–20.

4. MGN, *Experience in Water-Cure*, 30. There is some discrepancy as to dates. In this text, she claims to have arrived in New York in the fall of 1844, not 1845, and to have opened her own water-cure house in May of 1845. Other sources, however, suggest that these are typographical errors. According to its own annual reports, for example, the Brattleboro Hydropathic Establishment began receiving patients on May 29, 1845.

5. Manuel and Manuel, *Utopian Thought*, 582–83. Greeley's *Tribune* advanced many controversial positions, including women's rights (if not women's suffrage), the free-soil movement, abolition, temperance, high tariffs on imports, and the legitimacy of spiritualism. An ambitious politician, Greeley (1811–72) had launched his career by editing Whig campaign weeklies, first the *Jeffersonian* starting in 1838, then the widely circulated *Log Cabin,* starting in 1840. He founded the New York *Tribune* on August 10, 1841. Unlike Bennet's *New York Herald,* which thrived on sensational stories, the *Tribune* sought a higher moral tone and placed greater emphasis on the intellectual life of the city. Greeley served in Congress for three months in 1848–49 and unsuccessfully ran for reelection in 1850. He subsequently failed to rewin a seat in Congress in 1861, 1863, 1868, and 1870. See Johnson, ed. *Dictionary of American Biography,* 528–34. Horace Greeley and Mary Gove Nichols became close friends in the late 1840s. TLN, *Health Manual,* 89.

6. MG, "Letter to The Editor," *Phalanx, or Journal of Social Science* 1, no. 5 (5

February 1844); MG, *Lectures to Ladies*, 214–15; Fourier, Archives Nationales, 10 AS 8(4), quoted in Manuel and Manuel, *Utopian Thought*, 666. Mary's name had appeared on a list of thirteen regular contributors in the *Phalanx's* first issue, 5 October 1843. There, she intended to finish articles begun in the ill-fated *Health Journal and Independent Magazine*. See Noever, "Passionate Rebel," 97–98.

7. Guarneri, *Utopian Alternative*, 15–20, 292–320; Manuel and Manuel, *Utopian Thought*, 643–58. Fourier did preserve private property in the phalanx, however, and rewarded shareholders in proportion to their investments. He considered economic communalism unnatural, but this did not imply acceptance of differential happiness among members of the phalanx. To Fourier, the psychological payoff of living in an emotionally fulfilling environment where all passions enjoyed free and full expression would make disparities in wealth irrelevant. See Manuel and Manuel, *Utopian Thought*, 666–67.

8. Fourier, Archives Nationales, 10 AS 8(4), quoted in Manuel and Manuel, *Utopian Thought*, 660.

9. Fourier, *Design for Utopia: Selected Writings of Charles Fourier* (New York: Schocken Books, 1971), 80, quoted in Noever, "Passionate Rebel," 83; Guarneri, *Utopian Alternative*, 130–31.

10. Rexroth, *Communalism*, 251. Associationists familiar with Earth's thirty-two stages believed that the creation of phalanxes would enable humanity to skip the sixth and seventh stages and establish Harmony forthwith. See Guarneri, *Utopian Alternative*, 17–18.

11. Lazarus, *Passional Hygiene*, 255–56; 121. An excellent assessment of the Fourierist movement by one who lived through it can be found in Noyes, *History of American Socialisms* (1870).

12. MGN, *Mary Lyndon*, 343; Albert Brisbane, *Social Destiny of Man, or Association and Reorganization of Industry* (New York: Greeley and McElrath, 1843), 5, quoted in Noever, "Passionate Rebel," 88. The literati and social reformers who gathered at 261 Tenth Street varied their meeting places. One of New York's most popular hostesses was Anne Charlotte Lynch, a teacher and poet who established an elite intellectual salon in her home, frequented by the city's most prominent thinkers and writers—among them Margaret Fuller, Horace Greeley, Elizabeth Oakes Smith, Lydia Maria Child, Edgar Allan Poe, Catharine Sedgwick, Mary Hewitt, Ann Stephens, William Cullen Bryant, Richard Henry Stoddard, Rufus Griswold, Elizabeth Ellet, Frances Osgood, Albert Brisbane, Charles A. Dana, and, when in New York, Ralph Waldo Emerson, Bronson Alcott, and John Neal. Mary Gove was a regular guest as well. As historian Janet Noever has noted, with the exception of Elizabeth Oakes Smith, all of the women typically found at Anne Lynch's gatherings remained distant from the organized women's rights

movement that emerged in the 1850s ("Passionate Rebel," 145–46). For more information on Anne Lynch and her peers, see Madeline B. Stern, "The House of The Expanding Doors: Anne Lynch's Soirees, 1846," *New York History* 23, no. 1 (January 1942): 42–51; and Conrad, *Perish the Thought.*

Margaret Fuller left for Europe in August of 1846, approximately eight months after Mary had arrived in New York City. Though I have found no surviving correspondence between Mary Gove and Margaret Fuller, it is likely that the two women had met as early as 1842, when Fuller was living in Jamaica Plain, a suburb of Boston, and Mary was living in Lynn. Fuller was then editing the transcendentalist *Dial* and working closely with Ralph Waldo Emerson and Bronson Alcott, close associates of Henry Gardiner Wright. In December of 1842 (within a month of Henry Gardiner Wright's decision to move into Mary's house), Fuller wrote to Emerson that she was on her way to hear a "conversation by A. B. Alcott in which Messrs. Lane and Wright will participate." Even if they had not met in 1842–43, Margaret Fuller and Mary Gove surely knew of one another's work and reputation. See Hudspeth, *Letters of Margaret Fuller,* 1:36–45, 104.

13. MGN and TLN, *Marriage,* 217; quotes from MGN, *Mary Lyndon,* 312–13; MGN, "To the Friends of Truth," *NJ* 1, no. 6 (September 1853): 46.

14. TLN, *Health Manual,* 88; MGN, *Experience in Water-Cure,* 30; "Literary Notices," *Boston Quarterly Review* 5 (April 1842): 255; Walt Whitman, *Brooklyn Daily Eagle,* 26 September 1846, quoted in Reynolds, *Whitman's America,* 209; MGN, *Mary Lyndon,* 318.

15. MGN, "Human Culture—No. 11," *NJ* 1, no. 2 (May 1853): 15; MGN, *Experience in Water-Cure,* 27. Homeopathic medicine, founded in 1810 by Samuel Hahnemann, based its methods on the principle of "infinitesimals" and the belief that "like cures like." While allopathic medicine employed heavy doses of drugs to counteract the symptoms of disease, homeopathic treatment prescribed minute quantities of substances that, if given in large amounts, were believed to induce the same symptoms as the disease. See Gevitz, ed., *Other Healers.* For more information about homeopathy, see Kaufman, *Homeopathy in America* and Coulter, *Homeopathic Science.*

16. MGN, *Experience in Water-Cure,* 25–28. Mary cites Billings, Boerhaave, Cullen, Bruno, and Darwin as advocates of nervous pathology.

17. Ibid., 8–9, 33.

18. Ibid., 45; Cayleff, *Wash and Be Healed,* 25, 29–30.

19. Bartlett, *Liberty, Equality, Sorority,* 52; MGN, *Experience in Water-Cure,* 18.

20. Eliza W. Farrar, *The Young Lady's Friend,* quoted in *GJ* 3, no. 10 (11 May 1839): 164. The editors of the *Graham Journal* followed this excerpt with a qualifier that the *Journal* did not approve all manner of "intercourse" that physicians

sought to practice: "We allude to . . . obstetrics and accoucheur." They argued that these specialties emerged in response to preventable disorders and that women, if "properly instructed by teachers of their own sex, [would] manage their own affairs." Mrs. Farrar, also a strong advocate of physiologic self-knowledge for women, spurred her readers to greater study: "Would you not like to hear how your lively feelings depend on your circulations. . . . Will you not be willing to learn how the stomach operates on the food . . . and why the pound-cake gives you the headache?" (*Young Lady's Friend*, 144–45).

21. MGN, *Experience in Water-Cure*, 17. One of Mary's strongest allies in this cause was Samuel Gregory, the man who had quoted *Solitary Vice* in his own work on the dangers of masturbation. In 1848 Gregory wrote a pamphlet entitled *Man-Midwifery Exposed and Corrected*, and in 1850 (the copyright year of Mary's *Experience in Water-Cure*) he published another pamphlet, entitled *Letter to Ladies, in Favor of Female Physicians for Their Own Sex*. For several years he had been lecturing on the value of female medical education, and he had helped to found the first women's medical school in the United States: the Boston Female Medical School, which opened on November 1, 1848, to an incoming class of twelve pupils. Despite their shared interests, there is no evidence that he and Mary ever met.

22. MGN, *Experience in Water-Cure*, 18. On the life of Elizabeth Blackwell, see Sahli, "Elizabeth Blackwell"; Kline, *Elizabeth Blackwell;* and Burby, *Elizabeth Blackwell.*

23. For a lively (if undocumented) portrait of Sarah Josepha Hale as covert feminist, see Woodward, *Bold Women*, 181–200. Though a strong advocate of women's education and the creator of *Woman's Record, or, Sketches of All Distinguished Women from the Creation* (1855), Hale also encouraged women to pursue intellectually lifeless, nonpolitical interests such as needlework and did not support the suffrage or dress-reform movements. As Woodward puts it, "For the acres of doilies and knickknacks produced by American housewives in their spare time during the past century, *Godey's* bears a Judgment Day responsibility" (ibid., 194). Even women whose work had a dramatic effect on the political culture evidenced the power of this limited feminine ideal. Harriet Beecher Stowe, for example, declined to submit biographical material or a personal daguerreotype for Hale's *Woman's Record*, as she "had no pretensions" to status. See Kelley, *Private Woman*, 185.

24. Many historians have concluded that nineteenth-century women embraced the "cult of domesticity" as a desperate and ultimately futile strategy for retaining some measure of social control in a political and economic climate that increasingly denied their relevance. As Kelley has written (*Private Woman*, 309): "The impulse to envision themselves as morally superior and as beings of a higher and separate sphere was a response of those who felt excluded from and denied a place in the world." Even highly productive professional writers like Lydia Sigour-

ney, Sarah Josepha Hale, and Harriet Beecher Stowe idealized the religious, domestic wife. To suggest that woman's moral influence must guide men and children in the regeneration of a corrupted world was to speak the language of
power—but it did not equip women with its reality. Middle-class women seem to
have been anxiously aware of their relative uselessness—complaining of nervous
disorders while they read stories portraying women as little more than decorative
symbols of purity and virtue. Jane Tompkins argues in *Sensational Designs* (176–77)
that sentimental fiction taught women how merely to survive political invisibil-
ity and repression through prayer, self-sacrifice, and suppression of personal will.

The prominent exception to this sorority of sentimental female writers was
Margaret Fuller, who lamented the female ideal offered by women's magazines.
"Will there never be a being to combine a man's mind and woman's heart, and
who yet finds life too rich to weep over?" she asked, "Never?" (Quoted in A. Douglas, *Feminization*, 269). Fuller, one of the most thoroughly educated American
women of her generation, edited the transcendentalist *Dial*; wrote for the *New
York Tribune*, and in 1845 published *Woman in the Nineteenth Century*, a feminist
critique of gender inequity.

Nancy Isenberg has recently challenged historians' tendency to view women's
civic role as a "contribution that only adds feminine influence or domestic concerns to the public sphere." She argues that the religious and political domains
overlapped greatly, and that women "have been neglected in traditional studies
that focus on elections, the party system, and presidents—and that discount fem-
inized politics—or women have been distorted to fit secular and masculine models of political engagement" (*Sex and Citizenship*, 10).

On the cultural role of sentimental fiction and the creation of "woman's
sphere," see Blair, *Clubwoman*; Cott, *Bonds of Womanhood*; Epstein, *Politics of Do-
mesticity*; A. Douglas, *Feminization*; Freedman, "Separatism as Strategy"; Kelley,
Private Woman; Kerber, *Women of the Republic*; Melder, *Beginnings of Sisterhood*;
Sklar, *Catharine Beecher*; Smith-Rosenberg, "Beauty, the Beast, and the Militant
Woman"; and Tompkins, *Sensational Designs*.

25. Mary Orme [MG], "Marrying A Genius," *Godey's* (September 1844): 104–7;
and MGN, *Mary Lyndon*, 125.

26. Mary Orme [MG], "The Artist," *Godey's* (April 1845): 156. Mary Gove's
medical reading also reinforced the idea that parents' dispositions and behavior
influenced their children's health. Hence the early death of Sophia's idiot child.
The notion that "PARENTAGE is EVERYTHING" found one of its strongest if not
earliest expressions in Orson Fowler's 1851 work, *Love and Parentage*—a text that
eventually sold over 40,000 copies. Fowler elaborated that "[parentage] exerts an
influence on character almost infinitely more powerful than all other conditions
put together" (quoted in Reynolds, *Whitman's America*, 21).

27. "The Artist," 154–55. As Kelley has noted, "The woman of fashion . . . symbolized the materialism of an age, but she also provided unholy evidence that regardless of social status, women were narcissistic and pampered and led lives that were idle, unproductive, and without redeeming value. The awful thought was that they were the playthings of men" (*Private Woman*, 314).

28. Stowe, *Pink and White Tyranny*, quoted in Kelley, *Private Woman*, 269.

29. Mary Orme [MG], "The Evil and the Good," *Godey's* (July 1845): 36–38. When she was seventy-one, Mary still held to the belief that "the highest condition of health is love. . . . And water is the next." See MGN, "A Retrospect—VI," *Herald of Health*, no. 44 (August 1881): cover. Sociologist Steven Seidman describes a progressive "sexualization of love" that evolved over the nineteenth century in America: "The Victorian language of love as a spiritual communion was either marginalized or fused with the language of sensual desire and joy" (*Romantic Longings*, 4). However, Mary's own discussions of love and sex took a different trajectory. Well ahead of her peers, Mary promoted the physical aspects of sexual love; yet by the time most people accepted this sexualization of love, Mary had returned to an earlier emphasis on love's spirituality.

30. Mary Orme [MG], "Mary Pierson," *Godey's* (January 1846): 39–41.

31. Mary Orme [MG], "Providence," *United States Magazine and Democratic Review* 18, no. 92 (February 1846): 141.

32. Poe, "Literati," 16.

33. J. G. Varner, "Osgood, Frances Sargent Locke," in Johnson, ed., *Dictionary of American Biography*, 653–55. With the exceptions of Marie Louise Shew and Frances Osgood—both of whom Mary came to know in the context of the mixed-sex hydropathic and literary circles of New York—Mary describes no close friendships with individual women. This apparent lack of interest in bonding with other women was not typical. See Smith-Rosenberg, "Female World."

34. MGN, *Reminiscences of Edgar Allan Poe* (New York: Union Square Book Shop, 1931 [orig. *Sixpenny Magazine*, February 1863]). The brief introduction to this 1931 reprint incidentally refers to Mary's seven-page portrait of Poe as "the one thing worthy of her epitaph."

35. MGN, *Mary Lyndon*, 343.

36. The poet Richard R. Stoddard remembered Frances Osgood as "a paragon. For loved of all men who knew her, she was hated by no woman who ever felt the charm of her presence" (quoted in Griswold, *Passages from the Correspondence*, 214).

37. MGN, *Mary Lyndon*, 333. Note that the following description of the Christmas party is drawn entirely from *Mary Lyndon*.

38. Ibid., 337–44.

39. Because no letters have survived, it is impossible to know whether these letters were actually "faithfully transcribed," as Mary and Thomas both claimed,

or whether they are fiction. Their respective voices are convincing, however, and I am inclined to believe that they are not far from the truth. But even if they reflect nothing more than Mary's own midlife fantasy of her early romance with Thomas, they still reveal a great deal about her character. The following account of their exchanged notes is drawn entirely and without other corroboration from *Mary Lyndon*, 345–82.

40. In his 1887 *Health Manual* (89), Thomas claimed to have been a water-cure patient of Mary's during their courtship: "Somewhat overworked, and needing the purifying action of packs and douches, I became a patient—a friend—a warm admirer, and after some months of this acquaintance our lives and our work were united." The intimacy of hydropathy's methods—baths and rubbing—seemingly enabled Thomas and Mary to "play doctor" figuratively as well as literally. During that time, some of Mary's critics were apparently living in or near Lynn, Massachusetts. In February of 1848, Mary wrote a letter to Alonzo Lewis, reassuring him of her indifference to the slander he must have reported to her in a prior letter: "Do not be troubled about me, my very good friend. If they have stolen your letters from me, it is no great loss and I am sure I am very willing they should read them or print them. I do not live in the world of those who malign me. I live in a world of great happiness and usefulness. I have no need to be careful and I have asked my husband to come and spend some time here that he may know my life and Elma's. . . . *All is well* with your friend, Mary." In the margin, she added, "Write me something besides warnings please—Many thanks for your good will however." This letter indicates that someone had stolen Mary's earlier letters to Lewis, hoping to find evidence of Mary's immorality. It is also interesting that Mary claims to have invited Hiram to New York City during the peak of her romantic infatuation with Thomas; perhaps she knew Hiram would not come, or perhaps she truly sought recognition for the restraint she was exercising.

It is clear, however, that Mary's reputation was under siege by Hiram. A letter dated 17 October 1847 from Oliver Porter to his wife Aurora (quoted in Bowers, *Waterford Water Cure*, 93) describes Mary's request for their legal testimony in defense of her character. The Porters were followers of the water cure who lived in Lynn.

41. Mary Orme [MG], "Minna Harmon, or, The Ideal and the Practical," *Godey's* (December 1848): 335–38.

CHAPTER 4. THE NEEDFUL MATURATION OF
THOMAS LOW NICHOLS

1. TLN, *Forty Years*, 1:14; TLN, *Journal in Jail*, 129.
2. TLN, *Forty Years*, 1:98.

3. *Catalogue of the Officers and Students of Dartmouth College* (Newport, N.H.: Simon Brown, 1834); TLN, "Personal Experience of a Vegetarian Diet," *Herald of Health* 25 (January 1880): 293. In Thomas's *Ellen Ramsay,* a novel whose plot largely paralleled his own life, the protagonist's mother encourages her resisting son to become a minister, a physician, or a lawyer.

4. TLN, "Letter From Dr. T. L. Nichols," *American Vegetarian and Health Journal* 1, no. 2 (February 1851): 41–42.

5. TLN, *Forty Years,* 1:109.

6. TLN, "Suppression of Jesuits in Spain," *Standard* 1, no. 2 (6 October 1835): 3. Seven issues of the *Standard* survive in the collections of the American Antiquarian Society in Worcester, Massachusetts. Thomas did later assert that "at twenty I edited a weekly newspaper." See *Nichols' Monthly: Extra* (Cincinnati, 1856): 1.

7. TLN, "Americans, Read!" *Standard* 1, no. 1 (29 September 1835): 1, 4; and no. 2 (6 October 1835): 2. Thomas claimed to have published two thousand copies of the first issue.

8. TLN, *Standard* 1, no. 15 (6 January 1836): 1.

9. TLN, *Lecture on Immigration,* 3. Virulent anti-Catholicism had a long history in the New England colonies. As one historian writes, "Expressions of anti-popery could be found in the churches, schools, taverns, streets, and newspapers of colonial New England. . . . Eighteenth-century New Englanders were Protestants in the most fundamental sense. They were opposed to the Roman Catholic Church. Whatever their other theological, intellectual, political, or social differences, almost all New Englanders agreed on this point" (Cogliano, *No King, No Popery,* 2). Cogliano argues that because the success of the American Revolution depended on the help of French Catholics, a greater toleration of Catholics followed the war. However, in 1835, Thomas Nichols was still unlikely to offend most potential readers by promoting anti-Catholic sentiment.

10. For a detailed account of Rathbun's role in Buffalo history, see Whitman, *Rise and Fall.*

11. Ibid., 100; TLN, the *Buffalonian* 1, no. 1 (25 December 1837): 1.

12. TLN, "The Wonder Increases," *Buffalonian* 1, no. 3 (8 January 1838): 2; and no. 2 (1 January 1838): 3.

13. TLN, *Forty Years,* 1:135–36.

14. According to Rathbun's biographer, Thomas's attacks so confused the public that many began to see "the erstwhile rascal Rathbun as a martyred hero" (Whitman, *Rise and Fall,* 188).

15. Ibid., 189; TLN, *Buffalonian* 1, no. 3 (8 January 1838): 2; TLN, *Buffalonian* 1, no. 15 (16 March 1838): 1; TLN, *Journal in Jail,* 11.

16. TLN, *Journal in Jail,* 17–18, 20, 28; Whitman, *Rise and Fall,* 191. On May 27,

1840, Governor William H. Seward rejected a clemency appeal on behalf of Rathbun, who was imprisoned at the state penitentiary. Seward explained his refusal by reiterating the prosecution's version of events: "The amount of forged paper remaining unpaid when the prisoner was arrested exceeded one and one-half millions of dollars. Including what was issued for the various purposes of renewal, postponement and payment, the whole amount forged must have been more than twice that sum. It is believed that these forgeries surpassed in boldness and perseverance all similar offenses in this and every other country" (quoted in Whitman, 202). The Buffalo and Erie County Public Library today occupies the former site of the Erie County Jail. (It is fun to imagine that my reading of the *Buffalonian* took place in the space of Thomas's former cell.)

17. TLN, *Forty Years*, 1:142; TLN, *Journal in Jail*, 71.

18. TLN, *Journal in Jail*, 32–33, 38, 159–61.

19. TLN, *Buffalonian* 1, no. 5 (29 January 1838): 1; TLN, *Journal in Jail*, 81, 35, 151.

20. This rare pamphlet can be found at the American Antiquarian Society in Worcester, Massachusetts.

21. TLN, *Journal in Jail*, 75.

22. TLN, *My Notions*, 20.

23. Ibid., 25–26.

24. Ibid., 18. Walt Whitman succeeded Thomas as editor of the *Aurora*. Apparently Thomas had printed a libelous article just before his departure from the paper. See Reynolds, *Whitman's America*, 98.

25. TLN, *Ellen Ramsay*, 59. Information regarding Thomas's connection to the brothels comes from personal communication with scholar Patricia Cline Cohen, who has encountered a number of admittedly suspect and teasing references to Thomas's friendships with known prostitutes in New York's "flash" penny newspapers of the early 1840s. These papers, however, were known for their sensationalism and questionable veracity; Thomas also socialized with their editors, who, Cohen believes, may have been ribbing him in print.

26. TLN, *Forty Years*, 1:160 ff.

27. MGN, *Mary Lyndon*, 354.

28. TLN, *Health Manual*, 90; MGN, *Mary Lyndon*, 385. In the colonial period divorce was exceedingly rare and often attainable only through an act of legislature. Often divorcees were not permitted to remarry. Over the nineteenth century, however, states gradually began to liberalize divorce laws, transferring the responsibility of judging petitions from the legislature to the courts and recognizing as legitimate a wider range of grounds for divorce, such as adultery, abandonment, physical abuse, prolonged absence, failure to fulfill proper role, and nonsupport. Laws differed significantly from state to state. See Mintz and Kellogg,

Domestic Revolutions, 61. However, it was not unusual during this period for couples to separate and remarry without legal sanction, becoming what Hendrik Hartog calls "functional bigamists." As Hartog writes, "The United States was an unimaginably large country, and many could disappear permanently from discarded pasts" (*Man and Wife*, 87). Given Mary's public presence, however, this would have been relatively difficult.

29. MGN, *Mary Lyndon*, 385; TLN, *Illustrated Manners Book*, 239. Hiram Gove went on to marry Mary Ann Thurbur of Farmington, New Hampshire, on September 3, 1848. See Gove, *Gove Book*, 204–5.

30. MGN and TLN, *Marriage*, 121.

31. Swedenborg, *Heaven and Its Wonders*, 201–2.

32. *Report of the Woman's Rights Convention*, 8–9. Mary described the details of her wedding in an undated letter to Alonzo Lewis, UVA.

CHAPTER 5. SEMINAL INFLUENCE

1. MGN to Alonzo Lewis, 13 March [1850], and 20 November 1849, UVA.

2. MGN, *Mary Lyndon*, 382; "Society of Public Health," *WCJ* 10, no. 1 (July 1850): 27; Cayleff, *Wash and Be Healed*, 170–71. For a history of the AMA and of disputes among medical systems vying for status in the mid-nineteenth century, see Starr, *Social Transformation;* Cassedy, *Medicine in America;* and Gevitz, ed., *Other Healers.*

3. TLN, "The Curse Removed. A Statement of Facts Respecting the Efficacy of Water-Cure, in the Treatment of Uterine Diseases, and the Removal of the Pains and Perils of Pregnancy and Childbirth," *WCJ* 10, no. 5 (November 1850): 167–73. For quotes, see 167, 171.

4. Advertisement at back of TLN, *Introduction to Water-Cure;* TLN, *Health Manual*, 90; MGN to Alonzo Lewis, 2 January 1851, UVA.

5. Noever, "Passionate Rebel," 174; MGN, *Mary Lyndon*, 387; MGN, "Water-Cure in Childbirth—Again," *WCJ* 9, no. 4 (April 1850): 117.

6. MGN, "Human Culture—No. II," *NJ* 1, no. 2 (May 1853): 15.

7. The review praised Mary's "enthusiasm," asserting: "That she has been brave and resolute, her life . . . bears witness; [and reflects] . . . that lofty and religious feeling . . . which has made her regard her professional work as a sacred duty, to which Providence called her, and in the prosecution of which, for the benefit of science, and the good of her sex, she has shown something of the devotion of a Joan of Arc . . . ; and sure we are that whatever of good may be contained in the Water Cure system, will be fully developed by so able a practitioner as Mrs. Nichols, with or without a diploma" (*Democratic Review* 26, no. 141 [March 1850]: 284–86).

8. Donegan, *"Hydropathic Highway,"* 70–73; TLN, "The Diseases of Women," *WCJ* 11, no. 5 (May 1851): 123–24. Differences between hydropathic and allopathic management of pregnancy and parturition were stark; Donegan treats these distinctions at length. Regarding the debate over localized versus constitutional etiology of disease, Thomas suggested that more doctors read John Abernethy (1764–1831), a British surgeon and anatomy professor who in 1809 had published a work entitled *Constitutional Origin and Treatment of Local Diseases.*

9. TLN, *Woman, in All Ages,* vi, 158.

10. Donegan, *"Hydropathic Highway,"* 169–70, quoting TLN, *WCJ* 10, no. 6 (December 1850): 235.

11. For more on the history of women's medical education, see Peitzman, *New and Untried Course.*

12. Donegan, *"Hydropathic Highway,"* 33; MGN, "Woman the Physician," *WCJ* 12, no. 4 (October 1851): 74, quoted in Cayleff, *Wash and Be Healed,* 70.

13. TLN, "The Diseases of Women," *WCJ* 11, no. 5 (May 1851): 122, 124. For a history of medicine's relationship to female sexual responses, see Maines, *Technology of Orgasm.*

14. "Letter from Dr. Thomas Low Nichols," *American Vegetarian and Health Journal* 1, no. 2 (February 1851): 42; "American Hydropathic Convention," *WCJ* 10, no. 1 (July 1850): 14–15; "American Vegetarian Society," *WCJ* 10, no. 1 (July 1850): 6, cited in Cayleff, *Wash and Be Healed,* 100–101, 112. Established in June of 1850, the American Hygienic and Hydropathic Association of Physicians and Surgeons—apparently dissatisfied with its predecessor, the American Hydropathic Society, founded only a year earlier—was the second organization of its kind in the United States. The Association did not thrive, and by 1851 fewer than twenty attended its annual meeting.

15. "American Hydropathic Institute," *WCJ* 11, no. 4 (April 1851): 91.

16. Ibid., 171; TLN, "Letter from Dr. Nichols," *American Vegetarian and Health Journal* 2, no. 3 (March 1852): 39.

17. J. H. H., "The Class of the American Hydropathic Institute," *WCJ* 12, no. 5 (November 1851): 115; *WCJ* 13, no. 2 (February 1852): 41; *WCJ* 12, no. 2 (August 1851): 30, cited in Donegan, *"Hydropathic Highway,"* 171. Those graduates who headed their own cures included William F. Reh (in Newport, Rhode Island); W. H. Stevens and Isabel Pennell Stevens (in Forest City, New York); Hiram Frease (in Sugar Creek Falls, Ohio); Mary Ann Torbet (in Auburn, Alabama); and Hester A. Horn (in New York City, New York). Graduates Thomas Fearnside (Galesburg, Illinois), T. T. Williams (Monongahela City, Pennsylvania), and Esther C. Wileman (Marlborough, Ohio) practiced water cure as private practitioners. Thomas and Mary proudly advertised their graduates as skillful and trustworthy. See *NJ* 1, no. 1 (April 1853): 4. Among the first class of graduates was Harriet N.

Austin (1825–91), who went on to become a leading hydrotherapist at James Caleb Jackson's highly successful Glen Haven Water Cure, located on the western shore of New York's Skaneateles Lake.

18. Donegan, "*Hydropathic Highway,*" 24. For a detailed summary of this journal's history, see Cayleff, *Wash and Be Healed,* 24–27.

19. *American Vegetarian and Health Journal* 2, no. 10 (October 1852): 152–53; TLN, "Letter From Dr. T. L. Nichols," ibid. 2, no. 5 (May 1852): 73; William A. Alcott, "American Hydropathic Institute," ibid. 2, no. 5 (May 1852): 73.

20. MGN, "Esoteric Anthropology," *NJ* 1, no. 1 (April 1853): 8.

21. TLN, "Esoteric Anthropology," *NJ* 1, no. 1 (April 1853): 8, quoting original notice of the work published in the *WCJ* 14, no. 5 (November 1852).

22. *NJ* 1, no. 1 (April 1853): 8. These letters have not been preserved; therefore, the reader must choose whether or not to trust the Nicholses' published descriptions of their mail. An endorsement from Stephen Pearl Andrews follows the excerpts, in which he writes, "Having examined the original letters, from which these extracts are made, I certify their genuineness." The fourteenth edition of *Esoteric Anthropology* was published in London in 1916.

23. TLN, *Esoteric Anthropology,* 51, 56.

24. Ibid., 152–53.

25. Ibid., 153, 197–98.

26. Ibid., 200.

27. Pulte, *Woman's Medical Guide,* 142–43, 28, 200–204. Pulte's treatment of childbirth (152–53) even manages to avoid any reference to the vagina: "The appearance of the . . . labor-pains, soon terminates the state of gestation, expels the child, together with the after-birth, and allows the womb to contract." Antebellum anatomy and physiology texts aimed at younger readers evidenced draconian modesty. As Charles E. Rosenberg writes, "The reproductive system was simply ignored. The body in the prebellum classroom was one that began with the head and ended at the waist. It was also not a gendered body" ("Catechisms of Health," 187). Thomas Nichols did later acknowledge that "objection has been made to a few of [*Esoteric Anthropology*'s] engravings; but those to which some fastidious persons object, are of the greatest practical necessity, and every one is copied from standard works of Anatomy, Physiology, and Obstetrics" (*Nichols' Monthly Extra,* 4).

28. TLN, *Esoteric Anthropology,* 222–23, 172–73, 218.

29. Ibid., 151, 172–73, 197. The three most popular books describing contraception that preceded *Esoteric Anthropology* were Robert Dale Owen's *Moral Physiology* (1831); Charles Knowlton's *Fruits of Philosophy; or, the Private Companion of Young Married People* (1832); and Hollick's *The Marriage Guide* (1850). The first remained in print for forty years; the second underwent ten editions; and the third saw three hundred editions in twenty-five years. Owen recommended with-

drawal (though he also described condoms and the vaginal sponge); Knowlton advised the use of postcoital vaginal douches; and Hollick discussed condoms, douches, and the rhythm method. The candor regarding sexual physiology evident in the 1840s and 50s did not last; the Comstock Act of 1873 squelched free discussion and made the distribution of contraceptive advice a crime. See Smith-Rosenberg, *Disorderly Conduct*, 222, 236; D'Emilio and Freedman, *Intimate Matters*, 59–60; and Brodie, *Contraception and Abortion*. Alcott's *Physiology of Marriage* also briefly discussed abstinence, male withdrawal, and the rhythm method (190–92).

30. Noyes, *Male Continence*, 10–11; Noyes, *Bible Argument* (1848), quoted in *Male Continence*, 12, 14.

31. Noyes, *Male Continence*, 8.

32. Noyes, *Bible Argument*, 1848, quoted in *Male Continence*, 13; *Male Continence*, 17–18.

33. Historian Steven Nissenbaum has noted the ironic similarity between the attitudes of Sylvester Graham and John Humphrey Noyes in regard to sexual orgasm. Both Noyes (who practiced and advised frequent sexual intercourse) and Graham (who recommended near chastity) mistrusted male orgasm as potentially dangerous to health. Noyes sought to make sexual intercourse "a quiet affair, like conversation," and one that would avoid "the sensual crisis." See Noyes, *Male Continence*, 14; and Nissenbaum, *Sex, Diet, and Debility*, 166.

For an intriguing study of Noyes and the Oneida Community, see Klaw, *Without Sin*. Also see Fogarty, ed., *Special Love*. The original Oneida Community Mansion House has been preserved as a historic museum and is open for guided tours.

34. Noyes, *Male Continence*, 15; TLN, *Esoteric Anthropology*, 190. In 1860 James Ashton published an even more radical defense of abortion in a 64-page tract entitled *The Book of Nature*. In addition to outlining the era's five most reliable methods of contraception (withdrawal, condoms, the vaginal sponge, douching, and the rhythm method), Ashton's work also explained, without apology, the most effective means and timing for inducing miscarriage. See Brodie, *Contraception and Abortion*, 128, 185–87. *The Book of Nature* was republished in 1861, 1865, 1870, and most recently in 1974. See Rosenberg, ed., *Birth Control*.

35. TLN, *Esoteric Anthropology*, 435, 442–43, 449, 205. This is not to suggest that Thomas was a staunch suffragist. He and Mary both considered the reform of marriage laws far more crucial to justice than the right to vote.

36. Alcott, *Physiology of Marriage*, 117, 119.

37. TLN, *Esoteric Anthropology*, 223, 212, 85. A more typical excerpt of the era can be found in Horsell's *Hydropathy for the People* (1850), 209: "Let us not complain that Providence has made self-denial necessary . . . it is for our interest. Organic and moral law here hold one language, and our own souls bear witness to

the teaching of Christ, that while it is eminently calculated to promote our health of body, it is also the 'narrower way which leadeth unto life.'" Horsell's discussion of self-denial extends for over twenty consecutive pages.

38. TLN, *Esoteric Anthropology*, 477–78.

39. "Esoteric Anthropology," *NJ* 1, no. 3 (June 1853): 21; Nichols, "American Hydropathic Institute," *New York Daily Tribune*, 22 July 1853, 7. In 1856, Thomas claimed to have sold more than 26,000 copies (TLN, *Nichols' Monthly Extra*, 4).

40. TLN, "The Reason Why," *NJ* 1, no. 1 (April 1853): 5.

41. Trall, *Hydropathic Encyclopedia*, 381–83; TLN, *Esoteric Anthropology*, 333. To treat jealousy, for example, Thomas looked first to society: "Enlarge the spheres of both sexes, and we should have the soul flowing out into other channels. . . . The cure . . . is [to] . . . give rest and equilibrium, by bringing other passions into play" (ibid., 335).

42. TLN, *Esoteric Anthropology*, 220–21. Recall that this may have been an informed opinion, as Thomas had become friends with a number of prostitutes during his freelance journalism days in New York City. The social world of New York's early brothels has been beautifully documented by Patricia Cline Cohen, who alerted me to Thomas's one-time participation in it. See *The Murder of Helen Jewett.*

43. Ibid., 201, 219, 208–10, 217.

44. Trall, *Hydropathic Encyclopedia*, 2: 445, 493, 494 (italics in original).

45. TLN, "The Reason Why," *NJ* 1, no. 1 (April 1853): 5. The Nicholses claimed on the first page of this issue to have gratuitously distributed 100,000 copies of the journal's first number by way of introduction. Though Thomas thoroughly granted that Trall had acted within his rights as editor, he still felt that "in a certain sense, those who had read our articles for two or three years were our readers. It would seem as if our wishes and theirs might have been consulted" (*NJ* 1, no. 1 [April 1853]: 5).

46. TLN, *Ellen Ramsay*, 52–53; TLN, "Port Chester, New York," *NJ* 1, no. 1 (April 1853): 7.

47. TLN, *Human Physiology*, 315; MGN, "Letter from Mrs. Gove Nichols," *WCJ* 14, no. 3 (September 1852): 68; *NJ* 1, no. 1 (April 1853): 6.

48. *NJ* 1, no. 1 (April 1853): 6; MGN and TLN, "Our School of Life," *NJ* 1, no. 3 (June 1853): 22.

49. TLN, "Port Chester, New York," *NJ* 1, no. 1 (April 1853): 7; *NJ* 1, no. 3 (June 1853): 21.

50. Swisshelm, *Letters to Country Girls*, 89–91.

CHAPTER 6. THE COSTS OF CONVICTION

1. *New York Daily Tribune*, 21 July 1853, 5.

2. Ibid.

3. TLN, "American Hydropathic Institute," *New York Daily Tribune*, 22 July 1853, 7.

4. *NJ* 1, no. 6 (September 1853): 44–45.

5. TLN, "Hydropathic Colleges, *NJ* 1, no. 6 (September 1853): 46.

6. Russell Trall, "Topics of the Month," *WCJ* 21, no. 2 (February 1856): 37.

7. While Trall never developed sympathy for the cause of free love, he did grow more comfortable writing about sex. In 1861 he published *Sexual Physiology: A Scientific and Popular Exposition of the Fundamental Problems in Sociology.* This book echoed many of the more daring passages of *Esoteric Anthropology*, arguing that "it is [woman's] absolute and indefeasible right to determine when she will, and when she will not, be exposed to pregnancy" and that "whether intended as a love embrace merely, or as a generative act—it is clear that [sex] should be as pleasurable as possible to both parties. . . . Surely if sexual intercourse is worth doing at all, it is worth doing well" (*Sexual Physiology*, 245, 248, and 202, cited in Cayleff, *Wash and Be Healed*, 57).

8. Webber, *Spiritual Vampirism*, 28.

9. MGN, "To The Friends of Truth," *NJ* 1, no. 6 (September 1853): 45–46.

10. *NJ* 1, no. 6 (September 1853): 44.

11. Ibid.; ibid. no.7 (October 1853): 49.

12. *NJ* 1, no. 7 (October 1853): 50. On Modern Times, see Wunderlich, *Low Living*, 2–3, 30–31.

13. A lawsuit followed. Cincinnati publisher Valentine Nicholson ultimately paid the Nicholses' debt on the property intended for Desarrollo. Historian Roger Wunderlich speculates that Nicholson may have paid the debt in place of royalties owed to Thomas. Nicholson published *Marriage* (1854), *Esperanza* (1860), and a reprint edition of *Esoteric Anthropology*. The Nicholses' cottage was sold at auction on January 19, 1856. See Wunderlich, *Low Living*, 208, n.58.

14. TLN, "The World's Conventions," *NJ* 1, no. 7 (October 1853): 55. Historian of Fourierism Carl Guarneri has argued that advocates of individual sovereignty were proposing a significant revision of associationism's core tenets: "In redefining socialism as Individual Sovereignty, ex-Fourierists such as Andrews and the Nicholses reversed a decade of Associationist agitation, attempting a Copernican revolution that placed the self rather than the group at the center of renovated social life. Their program of middle-class villages, 'disconnected interests,' and unfettered self-expression rejected not just excessive organization but the com-

munal goals that underlay utopian socialism. Theirs was a new kind of communitarian program, one without community values" (*Utopian Alternative*, 366).

My reading of their work suggests, on the contrary, that despite their brief affiliation with Modern Times, the Nicholses never strayed far from Fourier's group focus, as Guarneri suggests. While they strongly valued individual freedom and described the limitations of existing Fourierist communities, they persistently sought an ultimate Harmonic Society based on human ties. As Thomas put it, "The first thing to be accomplished is the separating of all arbitrary unions. Individual sovereignty is the repulsive force that drives all asunder—the attractions of society, friendship and love, will draw them together, and where there are conditions of health, intelligence, and freedom, they can come together in harmony, and with the result of general happiness" (MGN and TLN, *Marriage*, 384–87). And Mary later wrote: "Self-love claims good for self with no regard for the neighbour, and stops the circulation of life in the social body, as a ligature stops the circulation of the life-current in the individual body. . . . The love of ourself, excluding the love of our neighbour, and isolating us, as by a ligature, from him—this is death by sin" (quoted in TLN, *Health Manual*, 393, 396).

15. MGN, "A Word to the Believers," *NJ* 1, no. 3 (June 1853): 21.

16. For an extended discussion of the ways in which these tenets were conveyed to children in primary-school textbooks, see Rosenberg, "Catechisms of Health."

17. Some historians have viewed Victorian efforts to distance sexual expression from "ideal" love as a means of empowering women within marriage: "To the extent that sex carried significant dangers for women (e.g., unwanted pregnancy, disease, death, and the stigma of impurity or looseness), minimizing sex and giving women control over this activity expanded their autonomy" (Seidman, *Romantic Longings*, 31). Mary, obviously, did not accept the premise that sex contaminated love. She sought, instead, to encourage women's acceptance of their own sexual desires.

18. This assumption took extreme form. In 1853 Russell Trall wrote, "Many a nursing mother has sent her babe to the grave by indulging a furious emotion, which changed the character of her milk from a bland nutriment to a deadly poison" (*Hydropathic Encyclopedia*, 1:383). Thus, even after weathering the constitutional hazards of conception and gestation, a child still absorbed the contaminants of parental character. Also see Golden, *Wet Nursing*.

19. MGN, "A Word to the Believers," *NJ* 1, no. 3 (June 1853): 21.

20. Ibid. Most popular hygiene literature emphasized the role of behavior in preventing chronic illness and offered less about acute and infectious illness, such as cholera, which seemed by contrast unpredictable and relatively unmanageable. (See Rosenberg, "Catechisms," 184, 193.) Mary, on the other hand, theorized about

contagion and aggressively addressed acute as well as chronic disease in her *Experience in Water-Cure.*

21. Ibid.

22. *NJ* 1, no. 1 (April 1853): 8; and *Nichols' Weekly* 2, no. 1 (7 January 1854): 1. Unfortunately, very little of their correspondence seems to have been preserved. *NJ* 1, no. 5 (August 1853): 37. Given the rarity of this journal today, these subscription claims seem to warrant skepticism. The Nicholses published some version of their own periodical from April 1853 through 1856. For a listing of its many incarnations, see the Bibliography of the Nicholses' Works.

23. "Water Cure Instruments," *Nichols' Weekly* 2, no. 1 (7 January 1854): n.p.

24. "Card—To the Public," *New York Tribune,* 4 April 1853, 5, quoted in "Port Chester, New York," *NJ* 1, no. 1 (April 1853): 7. In describing experimental groups devoted to social reorganization, historian Seymour Kesten persuasively argues against the term *community* as overly weighted with confusing connotations. Because Modern Times preserved the right to private property, as did other utopian settlements, he suggests the term *colony. See Utopian Episodes,* 25.

25. TLN, "City of Modern Times," *NJ* 1, no. 5 (August 1853): 39.

26. MGN, "City of Modern Times," *NJ* 1, no. 5 (August 1853): 39.

27. Josiah Warren, "Positions Defined" (Modern Times: Author, August 1853), quoted in "Individuality—Protest of Mr. Warren—Relations of the Sexes," *NJ* 1, no. 7 (October 1853): 52. As a refugee from Robert Owen's failed experimental community, New Harmony (1825–28), Warren had learned from "Owen's mistake of attacking accepted institutions peripheral to the purpose." Owen had condemned private property, marriage, and organized religion. See Wunderlich, *Low Living,* 74, and, for additional discussion of this dispute with Warren, 73–83.

28. "Individuality—Protest of Mr. Warren," *NJ* 1, no. 7 (October 1853): 52.

29. MGN, "Josiah Warren," *NJ* 3, no. 1 (26 August 1854): 12.

30. Andrews, *Love, Marriage, and Divorce* (1853), 49, 17. On child care at Modern Times, see MGN, "To Women," *NJ* 1, no. 4 (July 1853): 31.

31. Andrews, "Love, Marriage and the Condition of Woman," published as a distinct manuscript in *Love, Marriage, and Divorce,* 1–2.

32. Wunderlich, *Low Living,* 46–48.

33. Josiah Warren estimated that there were 60 to 70 inhabitants in December 1854. The New York State Census reported 85 residents in 1855. See Wunderlich, *Low Living,* 35, 39.

34. Quoted in Conrad, *Perish the Thought,* 42–43.

35. D. P. W., "Modern Times," *New York Weekly Leader,* 29 July 1854, quoted in Wunderlich, *Low Living,* 87–88.

36. MGN, "Letter from Mrs. Gove Nichols," *WCJ* 15, no. 1 (January 1853): 11.

On the rock-throwing incident, see "Letter from Mrs. Gove Nichols," *WCJ* 14, no. 5 (November 1852): 112. Mary also wrote that she had been "mobbed on account of my dress" and that in New York City "more than one scamp has felt the weight of my husband's cane." See "A Letter to Women," *NJ* 1, no. 1 (April 1853): 6.

37. MGN, "A Letter to Women," *NJ* 1, no. 1 (April 1853): 6.

38. Stanton and Blatch, eds., *Elizabeth Cady Stanton*, 50.

39. MGN, "Individuality in Dress," *NJ* 1, no. 7 (October 1853): 56.

40. *NJ* 2, no. 5 (4 February 1854): 3.

41. MGN, "Human Culture—No. 7," *NJ* 1, no.7 (1 October 1853): 51; and MGN, "Human Culture—No. 4," *NJ* 1, no. 4 (July 1853): 29.

42. MGN, *Mary Lyndon*, 387–88, 20, 15.

43. *Nichols' Monthly* (November 1854): 65, 67, cited in Noever, "Passionate Rebel," 221.

44. Lazarus, *Love vs. Marriage*, quoted in MGN and TLN, *Marriage*, 159, 162.

45. Ibid., 162–75.

46. TLN, *Woman, in all Ages*, 211–12.

47. Lazarus, *Love vs. Marriage*, 159, quoted in Charles Shively, "Introduction," in Andrews, *Love, Marriage, and Divorce*, 3.

48. Quoted in Shively, "Introduction," in Andrews, *Love, Marriage, and Divorce*, 3.

49. Andrews, *Love, Marriage, and Divorce*, 24–25.

50. Ibid., 36, 39.

51. Andrews did not include in this collection the contributions of two female writers to the *Tribune* debate: Elizabeth Oakes Smith and an anonymous woman. Smith wrote (15 January 1853) that "it is not possible that entire justice can be done to our sex when all the aspects of our social relation are discussed and adjusted entirely by one half of our humanity, to the exclusion of the opinions of the other half most nearly interested in the question." The anonymous woman criticized society's "double standard" between the sexes and argued for freer access to divorce (27 December 1852). Greeley had disparaged both women, while James and Andrews did not even acknowledge them. See Shively, "Introduction," in Andrews, *Love, Marriage, and Divorce*, 7. Elizabeth Oakes Smith, incidentally, was the first woman to lecture at the Concord Lyceum, the institution at which Henry Thoreau had served as secretary and coordinator of speakers in the fall of 1838 when Mary Gove began lecturing in the Boston area. Smith spoke on "Womanhood" on December 31, 1851. The second woman to speak at the Concord Lyceum was Caroline Dall, who delivered her address nearly a decade later. Personal communication, Robert Gross, William and Mary College. Original source: Concord Lyceum records, Concord Free Public Library. In January 1852, Mary sent a letter to Caroline Healey Dall praising one of Dall's contributions to the

Water-Cure Journal and expressing the desire to meet Dall personally. See MGN
to Caroline Healey Dall (January 24, 1852).

52. Andrews, *Love, Marriage, and Divorce*, 18–19, 46.

53. Two books addressing the subject of divorce laws appeared in the early
1850s: Henry Folsom Page's *A View of the Law Relating to the Subject of Divorce
in Ohio, Indiana and Michigan* (1850) and Joel Prentiss Bishop's *Commentaries on
the Laws of Marriage and Divorce* (1852). In 1849 Connecticut had liberalized its
law by adding as legitimate grounds for divorce "any such misconduct as permanently destroys the marriage relation." This led to 2,065 divorces in Connecticut
over the next ten years, approximately 10 percent of the state's marriages. See
Shively, "Introduction," in Andrews, *Love, Marriage, and Divorce*, 1.

The Married Women's Property Acts of 1848 and 1849 had not impressed the
Nicholses, who advocated the more radical abolition of marriage laws. Thomas
wrote, "To give a married woman rights of property, is an anomaly and an inconsistency. All pretense of such right is a sham. . . . The chief use of such laws is
to enable men to put property into the hands of their wives . . . and out of the reach
of their creditors" (MGN and TLN, *Marriage*, 118). For extended discussion of
married women's property rights, as well as the Property Acts of 1848–62, see
Basch, *Eyes of the Law*. On the history of marital law in the United States, see
Hartog, *Man and Wife*. For a very general overview of the history of family law
in the United States, see Mintz and Kellogg, *Domestic Revolutions*, 60–65. For
more specific examination of eighteenth-century family life, see Cott, "Massachusetts Divorce Records." On divorce history, also see Blake, *Road to Reno*.

54. Andrews, *Love, Marriage, and Divorce*, 51, 67, 59, 79, 82–83.

55. Ibid., 71–72. Also writing in 1852, fellow water-cure physician James Caleb
Jackson noted that matrimony "can exalt a gross licentiousness into Christ-like
purity by putting it through the trouble of a ceremony." Jackson, who was the
chief physician at the long-lived Dansville Water Cure in western New York, also
argued that man's "esteem for woman, and regard for her rights, must be greatly
increased before his notions of what is or what is not her proper sphere, will be
entitled to serious consideration" (*Hints on the Reproductive Organs*, 15, 32). As
previously mentioned, Jackson's close medical associate and adopted daughter,
Harriet Austin, had graduated from the American Hydropathic Institute. The
large Dansville Cure, today a dramatic ruin of crumbling bricks and weeds, welcomed as speakers many of the era's reformers, including Sojourner Truth, Elizabeth Cady Stanton, Susan B. Anthony, Frances E. Willard, Bronson Alcott, Clara
Barton, and Frederick Douglass. See Cayleff, *Wash and Be Healed*, 94–95.

56. Andrews, *Love, Marriage, and Divorce*, 54, 71.

57. Elizabeth Cady Stanton to Susan B. Anthony, 1 March 1853, quoted in Stanton and Blatch, eds., *Elizabeth Cady Stanton*, 2:48. Indeed, the rhetoric of free love

continued to find exponents. "'How long will a true marriage last?' . . . Just so long as love lasts and no longer. . . . If the truly married are not the unfortunate inheritors of crimes and follies, their children will be the world's Saviors," wrote Mrs. H. F. M. Brown. "The evils that call for the hangman and halter are the offspring of outraged souls" (*False and True Marriage* [1859], 18).

58. MGN and TLN, *Marriage*, 81, 180, 89. An anonymous 12-page pamphlet entitled "Slavery and Marriage. A Dialogue" was published in 1850 by the Noyes's Oneida Community in New York. Written as a one-act play, it articulates many of the same objections to marriage that Mary and Thomas voiced at great length four years later. It was reprinted in 1994 by the Oneida Community Mansion House.

59. MGN and TLN, *Marriage*, 100–101, 184, 178, 252.

60. MGN and TLN, *Marriage*, iii, 16. The first edition of *Marriage* was published in New York in 1854 and came to 430 pages; all quotations and page references cited herein are from the revised fourth edition, which was published in Cincinnati the following year and came to 466 pages, included additional chapters and an expanded appendix. Of this fourth edition, Thomas had explicit authorship of 380 pages, while Mary claimed a comparatively succinct 86 pages.

61. MGN and TLN, *Marriage*, 86–87, 123, 292, 119. Intellectual predecessors to this debate include Mary Wollstonecraft, who in 1792 published the formidable and groundbreaking argument for female emancipation, *A Vindication of the Rights of Woman*, and the novelist Charles Brockden Brown, who six years later published a novel called *Alcuin*, in which he wrote, "As soon as the [marriage] union ceases to be spontaneous, it ceases to be just." The British socialist Robert Owen also criticized capitalism's traditional marriage as an institution that encouraged poor women to sacrifice themselves as property in exchange for access to wealth. Owen believed that divorce should be allowed if affection between a couple faded. See Spurlock, *Free Love*, 32–33.

62. MGN and TLN, *Marriage*, 19–24, 199, 250.

63. 1 Timothy 2:12, quoted in ibid., 47, 40.

64. Ibid. 66, 54–55, 71, 48. Thomas acknowledged that his accounts of foreign practice were drawn from works written by "casual visitors to distant countries" who would be liable to error. "Their accounts do not agree with each other; and few of their statements are to be depended upon. We give them for what the reader may think them worth," he wrote (73–74).

65. Ibid., 115–17, 197.

66. Ibid., 85–86, 94.

67. Ibid., 201–2.

68. Alcott, *Physiology of Marriage*, 167.

69. MGN and TLN, *Marriage,* 223, 200, 264–65.

70. Ibid., 221, 214.

71. TLN, "The Question of Marriage," *NJ* 3, no. 2 (2 September 1854): 27; back cover of *NJ* 3, no. 3 (9 September 1854).

72. Hunt, *Glances and Glimpses* (1856), 139. Harriot Hunt further recalled that she had "always quarreled with [Mary's] Grahamism. She told me she had over-tasked—overstimulated—her system; and she urged upon the rational liver the same dietetic abstinence to which she had been compelled. This is frequently the case with the down-right ultras; they ruin their own health, and then prescribe rules for everybody—forgetting that they cannot be judges of cases from their experience, unless they are similar to their own" (ibid.).

73. An advertisement for *Mary Lyndon* published in the *New York Daily Tribune* (4 August 1855, 3) had quoted strong praise for the book from the literary editor of the *New York Daily Times.* This discovery infuriated Raymond, who intended to set the record straight regarding his paper's view. See *Nichols' Monthly* (August/September 1855, 198–99), cited in Noever, "Passionate Rebel," 218. In the *Health Manual,* 428, Thomas speculated that Raymond's acrimony may have derived from Mary's friendship with his professional rival, Horace Greeley, editor of the *Tribune.* Why Mary chose the name "Mary Lyndon" is not clear. In her earlier magazine writing she had used the pen name "Mary Orme," and she had used the name *Mary* for many of her fictional characters (as well as for her second daughter, Mary Wilhelmina).

74. Quoted in Reynolds, *Whitman's America,* 210; see also 213. Whitman, who never officially declared himself a "free-lover," did believe unions should be based in mutual attraction and respect. The Manhattan publishing house of Fowlers and Wells had produced *Leaves of Grass* as well as a wide range of texts devoted to health and social reform; these included TLN's *Woman, in All Ages;* Shew's *Water-Cure Manual;* MGN's *Experience in Water-Cure;* Trall's *Hydropathic Encyclopedia;* Andrews's *Science of Society;* Warren's *Equitable Commerce;* and Lazarus's *Love vs. Marriage.*

While advancing radical social doctrines and the open, scientific discussion of all aspects of physiology, Lorenzo and Orson Fowler and their brother-in-law Samuel R. Wells condemned all lewd or pornographic writing intended merely to stimulate lust. In addition to publishing, the Fowler brothers became famous phrenologists.

Orson Fowler, also an active writer, personally advanced radical views of sex. His 1844 work entitled *Amativeness* (which saw forty editions of more than one thousand copies each) taught that regular sex would help married couples maintain physiological balance. In 1855, after his business partner Samuel Wells suppressed his new work on sex, Orson Fowler left the publishing firm to become a lecturer. The firm changed its name from "Fowlers and Wells" to "Fowler and Wells," and Orson Fowler later published his book as *Sexual Science; Including Manhood, Womanhood, and Their Mutual Interrelations.* One section of this book, titled "Passion Absolutely Necessary in Woman," argued that "the nonparticipant female is a natural abomination." See Reynolds, *Whitman's America,* 21–22, 207–10, and 246–47.

75. "A Bad Book Gibbeted," *New York Daily Times,* 17 August 1855, 2.

76. Ibid.

77. Ibid.

78. Thomas quoted the Norton review in the *Health Manual,* 428–32. See also the *New York Daily Tribune,* 4 August 1855, 3; and 25 July 1855, 1.

CHAPTER 7. SPIRITED ENCOUNTERS

1. *NJ* 3, no. 1 (26 August 1854): 2.

2. *NM* (June 1855): 54–56, 1, quoted in Noever, "Passionate Rebel," 238–39.

3. TLN, *Religions of the World,* 116; TLN, *Forty Years,* 2:55–56; and H. Sears, *Sex Radicals,* 8, 14. In 1880 Margaret and Kate Fox confessed that they had fraudulently produced the mysterious raps by cracking their big toes. Margaret later recanted the confession. See Walters, *American Reformers,* 166.

4. TLN, *Religions of the World,* 112; Cridge, *Spirit-Intercourse* (1854), 50–51.

5. TLN, *Religions of the World,* 112.

6. Moses Hull, quoted in H. Sears, *Sex Radicals,* 16.

7. To underline the relationship between these various influences, historian Hal Sears writes that "when Congress acted on the bill appropriating $30,000 for Samuel F. B. Morse to construct the Washington-Baltimore telegraph, Congressman Cave Johnson attempted to defeat the bill by adding an amendment granting one-half the appropriation to the study of mesmerism. Another suggested that Millerism, a millennialist sect, should also be included. Twenty-two members of Congress then voted to include mesmerism in the bill. That mesmerism should be adduced to ridicule electromagnetism demonstrated the degree of public confusion surrounding both electromagnetism and 'animal' magnetism" (*Sex Radicals,* 14). See also Walters, *American Reformers,* 165–73. On the origins of mesmerism, see Darnton, *Mesmerism.* On spiritualism, see Brandon, *Spiritualists.* On the rise of gothic literature, see Davidson, *Revolution and the Word.*

8. TLN, *Free Love,* 14. After leaving Modern Times, Stephen Pearl Andrews followed a similarly self-promoting path. Like the Nicholses, he began to develop his own vocabulary for social reorganization, calling the harmonic future state a "Pantarchy," of which he intended to be "the Pantarch." He developed a new sci-

ence called "Universology" and a new philosophy, called "Integralism." In 1872, he chartered the Normal University of the Pantarchy, which sought "the Grand Mutual Reconciliation of Humanity" and "the Virtual Inauguration of a Millennial Order on this Planet." See Stern, *Pantarch*, 95, 100, 105, 125.

9. "Social Movements," *NM* (July 1855): 74–75.

10. "The Progressive Union," *NM* (July 1855): 131.

11. Ibid., 130–32.

12. TLN, *Work of Reform*, 15–16; "The Progressive Union," *NM* (July 1855): 125. "Harmonialism" attracted many intellectuals and reformers in the mid-nineteenth century. Derived from a broth of spiritualism, mesmerism, phrenology, associationism, Swedenborgianism, and the writings of health reformers, Harmonialism found one of its most prominent advocates in Andrew Jackson Davis, who described a universal integration of the individual, social, material, and spiritual aspects of the world, united by magnetism and electricity. Davis had written that "all men shall be ultimately joined into one BROTHERHOOD; their interests shall be pure and reciprocal; their actions shall be just and harmonious; they shall be as one Body." Historian David S. Reynolds has written that "the harmonialists thought that electrical magnetism was perfectly in balance in nature and that by plunging into nature people could be physically healed and spiritually refreshed. An almost erotic bonding with nature was seen as a prelude to healing" (*Whitman's America*, 273; see also 270–80). For Davis quotation, see his *Philosophy of Spiritual Intercourse* (New York: Fowlers and Wells, 1851), 176, quoted in Reynolds, 274.

13. *New York Times*, 18 February 1859, 4, quoted in H. Sears, *Sex Radicals*, 10.

14. TLN, *Nichols' Monthly Extra*, 11.

15. This lecture, "phonographically reported," was printed as a 22-page pamphlet, the first number of a tract series. See TLN, *Free Love*. It was apparently not his first lecture at Foster Hall, for he refers to an earlier meeting in which he distributed the prospectus of the Progressive Union. That event most likely corresponds to his tract (not "phonographically recorded") entitled *The Work of Reform: A Tract of the Progressive Union: A Society for Mutual Protection in Right.* It is probable that his lecture relating free love to spiritualism drew unusual attention. For preceding quotes, see TLN, *Free Love*, 3, 13, 5–6.

16. TLN, *Esoteric Anthropology* (1853), 11; TLN, *Work of Reform*, 3; TLN, *Free Love*, 22.

17. TLN, "Oration," *Paine Festival*, 8, 14, 22.

18. Paine quoted in TLN, "Oration," *Paine Festival*, 16–17, 22.

19. TLN, *Work of Reform*, 5.

20. Walters, *American Reformers*, 169–73. See also H. Sears, *Sex Radicals*, which argues in part that spiritualism "filled the needs of those who considered themselves too sophisticated for literal heavens and hells but who still craved eternal

existence and could not face the 'doom of annihilation' of finite life" (7). John C. Spurlock also provides a useful discussion of spiritualism, associating its popularity (like that of associationism and phrenology) with the emergence of the American middle class. See Spurlock, *Free Love*.

21. TLN, *Health Manual*, 94–97. There Thomas emphasized that one should not blindly trust all received communications: "That spirits can appear to us and speak to us is certain—but that what they tell us is true is an entirely different matter. That depends, with spirits out of the body as with those still in it, on two things—intelligence and morality." *NM* (November 1854): 67, quoted in Noever, "Passionate Rebel," 236.

22. *NM* 3 (August 1856): 115–16; TLN, *Health Manual*, 93.

23. TLN, *Forty Years*, 2:48–67.

24. I am inclined to believe that this was a pseudonym for several reasons: first, that Thomas had adopted the name "George Arlington" when he first arrived in Buffalo as a young man, so there is a precedent for his using a false name; second, there are no other anonymous works to which Thomas claimed authorship; third, the "DeValcourt" editions of the book (1865 and 1866) were published in Cincinnati—a notable coincidence of location; fourth, many passages in the work closely echo Thomas's other writings in both style and intent; and lastly, there are no other works by "Robert DeValcourt" listed in the holdings of the Library of Congress. It is also possible that an actual "Robert DeValcourt" simply republished Thomas's book under his own name.

25. TLN, *Illustrated Manners Book*, 300, 302. Thomas was also promoting a free mail-order pamphlet he had written entitled "Letter to a Married Woman, On the Healthy Regulation and Voluntary Control of the Maternal Function": "This letter was never offered for sale, or intended for general circulation, but was sent as professional counsel, with any other the case required, to those who consulted me, as a physician, on this subject, which often affects the health and happiness, and even the life of the patient. . . . I have since incorporated this letter in a little book of sixty-four pages, entitled, 'Maternity,' which, though not sold indiscriminately, can be procured by all who need it, and at a price that must remove from me all suspicion of a mercenary motive" (TLN, *Nichols' Monthly Extra*, 7). I have not been able to find other records of either of these works. For an entertaining and thorough work on the teachings of nineteenth-century etiquette guides (and one that occasionally quotes from *The Illustrated Manners Book*), see Kasson, *Rudeness and Civility*.

26. Dills, *History of Greene County*, 669–79.

27. Tharp, *Until Victory*, 259–61, 278; Dills, *History of Greene County*, 686; Samoff, "Yellow Springs," 49.

28. Dills, *History of Greene County*, 685; *NM* (August 1856): 118–19.

29. Galloway, *History of Glen Helen,* 47–53; Noever, "Passionate Rebel," 239.

30. Gage, "Address to the Friends" (1856); P. Gleason, "Free-Love to Catholicism," 286. Gleason cites *NM* 2 (March 1856): 170, 218–19. The Nicholses did not directly explain the significance of music in the naming of Memnonia, but in her autobiography, describing life in New York City, Mary had written, "A new and most enchanting world was revealed to me in the love of music—a happiness which I had never had suggested to me in any imagining, and one which seems too interior, too sacred to bring into any words which are mine. My life, before this love and appreciation of the harmony of sounds, seems rudely savage compared with my present" (*Mary Lyndon,* 324). Thus, music was harmony, the state that Memnonia sought to achieve for all aspects of human experience.

31. TLN, "The Progressive Union," *NM* (July 1855): 109. In December of 1855, Thomas wrote that "the great truth, which the world is yet to know, is, that Freedom is the Parent of Order, and the condition of Harmony in all relations" (TLN, *Free Love,* 20). Descriptions of individual eccentrics living at Modern Times taken from Wunderlich, *Low Living,* 35–37.

32. Advertising circular, "Memnonia Institute: A School of Health, Progress, and Harmony," Spring 1856. See Archives of Antioch College, Olive Kettering Library.

33. "The Harmonic Home," *NM* (July 1855): 118–19.

34. Galloway, *History of Glen Helen,* 56. Analysis of the water identified many salts and minerals, making it "diuretic, and sometimes laxative" (Walton, *Mineral Springs* [1874], 272). Due to its water management, Yellow Springs had enjoyed a relative immunity from the outbreaks of cholera and typhoid fever that had plagued neighboring towns in the region. In 1849 nearby Clifton lost a greater percentage of its population to cholera than any other Ohio town. Yet less than ten miles away, Yellow Springs did not suffer an outbreak. Geologically speaking, it should have. Both towns sat on thin layers of porous Niagara limestone, below which pooled subterranean drift beds of water that were fed primarily by absorption of surface rain and runoff. The gravelly limestone would have provided an effective natural filter were it not compromised by vertical fractures sometimes a foot wide. By chance rather than medical design, settlers of Yellow Springs preferred the use of cisterns to the cumbersome digging of wells. This habit prevented the mixing of privy water with drinking water and naturally enhanced the town's reputation as a healthful locale. It would be decades before medical scientists could explain the town's epidemiological resilience. In 1848 Yellow Springs simply seemed like an ideal place to establish a hydropathic health resort. See Dills, *History of Greene County,* 675–77.

35. Galloway, *History of Glen Helen,* 58; advertisement in the *Xenia Torchlight,* 22 December 1852, quoted in Samoff, "Yellow Springs," 52.

36. TLN, "Memnonia Institute," 3.

37. "Local and Miscellaneous," *Daily Springfield Nonpareil,* 7 March 1856, 3.

38. Conway, *Autobiography* (1904), 1:263.

39. *Ladies' Repository* 16 (January 1856), 57, cited in Noever, "Passionate Rebel," 259 n. 37. For description of the elaborate and ill-fated financial history of Antioch College, see Dills, *History of Greene County,* chap. 27.

40. Gleason, "Free-Love to Catholicism," 287–88; *NM* (March 1856): 169, quoted in Noever, "Passionate Rebel," 248.

41. *Daily Springfield Nonpareil,* 18 March 1856, 2; Noever, "Passionate Rebel," 249.

42. Gleason, "Free-Love to Catholicism," 288; Mary Mann to Horace Mann, 20 March 1856, Mann Papers, Massachusetts Historical Society. Gleason also cites *Xenia Torchlight,* 2 April 1856, and the *Daily Springfield Nonpareil* 26 March and 9 April 1856.

43. Stearns, "Memnonia," 291 (citing *NM,* May 1856); Horace Mann to Mary Mann, 22 August 1856, Mann Papers, Massachusetts Historical Society.

44. TLN, *Health Manual,* 94; Noever, "Passionate Rebel," 243; Gleason, "Free-Love to Catholicism," 289; Dills, *History of Greene County,* 668.

45. Mann quoted in Tharp, *Until Victory,* 281; *NM* 3 (August 1856): 117–20. Unless otherwise noted, the following account of Jared Gage's experiences are drawn from his own testimonial, "Address to the Friends, Officers, and Students of Antioch College," ca. 1856, pamphlet in Archives of Antioch College Library. See also, according to Gleason, *NM* 3 (September 1856): 180–82, and 3 (September [October] 1856): 233–44. I have unfortunately not been able to access all issues of the rare *Nichols' Monthly.*

46. *NJ* 1, no. 1 (April 1853): 4; Horace Mann to W. N. Hambleton, 4 March 1856, Antiochiana Collection, Antioch College Library; and W.N. Hambleton to the Faculty of Antioch College, 1 March 1856, Antiochiana Collection, Antioch College Library.

47. Minutes of the Adelphian Union Literary Society for 7 November 1856. Antiochiana Collection, Antioch College Library.

48. Cosmelia Hirst, quoted in Galloway, *History of Glen Helen,* 62.

49. MGN, *Mary Lyndon,* 257–58.

50. Quoted in TLN, *Health Manual,* 19.

51. Quoted in Stearns, "Memnonia," 292.

52. *Daily Springfield Nonpareil,* 16 January 1857, 3.

53. Conway, *Autobiography,* 262.

CHAPTER 8. UNSETTLING DEPARTURES

1. Dills, *Greene County,* 672–73; Galloway, *Glen Helen,* 54.

2. *NM* (May 1856): 376, quoted in Noever, "Passionate Rebel," 234.

3. *NM* 3 (November 1856): 283, cited in Gleason, "Free-Love to Catholicism," 297; TLN, *Health Manual*, 106–7.

4. *NM* 2 (April 1856): 306, quoted in Gleason, "Free-Love to Catholicism," 294; "Our Life at Memnonia," *NM* (September 1856), cited in Stearns, "Memnonia," 293, 289.

5. TLN, *Work of Reform*, 16. One strong advocate of free love, James W. Towner, challenged the Nicholses' claim that "material union" was "wasteful and destructive," arguing instead that both love and offspring benefited from frequent sexual intercourse. Mary and Thomas printed his letter to them in the June 1856 issue of the *Nichols' Monthly* (444–47) along with their reply, which emphasized the need of a cleansing, "vestalate" period for civilization. See Noever, "Passionate Rebel," 245–46.

6. TLN, *Health Manual*, 97.

7. Gleason, "Free-Love to Catholicism," 298–300, quote on 299. Gleason based this description of events on the letter Thomas published in the *Catholic Telegraph and Advocate*. In *Religions of the World*, which was published two years before these events, Thomas devoted two pages to Catholicism, four to Swedenborgianism, six to Mormonism, and eight to Spiritualism. In the two pages on Catholicism, Thomas offered a brief history of the faith; its clerical hierarchy; its commandments; its doctrines of Sin, Absolution, and Transubstantiation; its faith in miracles; its requirement of chastity for clerical orders; its worship of the Virgin Mary and the saints; its architecture; its music; and its hope to once again "reign supreme over the whole Christian world." In his *Health Manual*, 97–99, Thomas described Mary's spiritual instruction as follows: "I have no reason to believe that Mrs. Nichols, a Puritan, Quaker, Swedenborgian, Fourierist, had ever read either the Nicene or the Athanasian Creed. . . . She did not know the number or names of the Seven Sacraments. We had no Catholic books—no Catholic acquaintances: yet she gave, day by day, speaking in a kind of trance, so full and clear a statement of Roman Catholic Theology, . . . that a Jesuit Father [endorsed its veracity] 'in every item.' . . . I cannot account in any way [for this experience] except by giving the facts of the case."

8. MGN to Alonzo Lewis, April 2, 1857, UVA; letter from John B. Purcell to Francis Kenrick, 5 February 1857, in the Archives of the Archdiocese of Baltimore, cited in Gleason, "Free-Love To Catholicism," 300. Franstina Hopkins eventually went on to teach English at a Catholic institution in Havana, Cuba. See John B. Purcell to Anthony Blanc, 5 December 1857, Archdiocese of New Orleans Collection (CANO), VI-1-m, UNDA.

9. *New York Daily Tribune*, 7 April 1857, 6. It is not clear why Thomas alone signed this explanatory letter. If Mary recorded her own account of their conversion experience, it has not survived.

10. "Spiritualism and Romanism," *New England Spiritualist*, 25 April 1857; "Letter to Our Friends and Co-Workers," *Catholic Telegraph and Advocate*, 23 May 1857, quoted partially in Gleason, "Free-Love to Catholicism," 305, and in Noever, "Passionate Rebel," 251. One snide response to the Nicholses' conversion came from spiritualist Alfred Cridge, who wrote, "Those who believe in CRUSHING, instead of DIRECTING and admitting of wholesome and spontaneous activity, would confer a benefit to the cause of Reform by leaving its ranks, and going where they belong, as Dr. and Mrs. N have done" (*Social Revolutionist*, 4 July 1857, 6–7, quoted in Spurlock, *Free Love*, 125).

11. "Spiritualism and Romanism," *New England Spiritualist*, 25 April 1857. Other prominent figures who had recently converted to Catholicism and to whom the Nicholses' case was sometimes compared included the famous medium Daniel D. Home, who had converted while on a trip to Italy; transcendentalists Isaac Hecker and Orestes A. Brownson, who had once written that "the religious sentiment is universal, permanent and indestructible; religious institutions depend on transient causes" (*New Views of Christianity, Society, and the Church*, 3, quoted in Richardson, *Mind On Fire*, 225); and Dr. Levi Silliman Ives, the former Episcopalian bishop of North Carolina, who shocked his faith by converting to Catholicism with his wife while on a trip to Rome in 1852.

12. Noyes, *American Socialisms*, 655.

13. "Spiritualism and Romanism," *New England Spiritualist*, 25 April 1857.

14. MGN, *Mary Lyndon*, 36.

15. *Catechism*, 124, 730; letter quoted in Gleason, "Free-Love to Catholicism," 300. On Pope Pius IX and the growth of Mariology, see Noever, "Passionate Rebel," 264, nn.98, 99. I thank Erin Flory for her valuable perspective on the appeal of Catholicism to nineteenth-century women.

16. MGN, *Mary Lyndon*, 129. My own use of the word *rape* is, I grant, anachronistic. As historian Nancy Isenberg has documented, marital rape was not recognized as criminal during this time. In an 1845 Connecticut case, Shaw v. Shaw, the court concluded that the wife's forced sexual submission to her husband constituted "tolerable cruelty" and was not grounds for divorce. "Sexual coercion within marriage was expressly distinguished from rape" (Isenberg, *Sex and Citizenship*, 163).

17. MGN and TLN, *Marriage*, 235.

18. MGN, "Human Culture—No.7," *NJ* 1, no. 7 (1 October 1853): 51. According to the Catholic Church, the sacrament of baptism cannot knowingly be repeated. See *Catechism*, 324.

19. MG, "Letter to the Editor," *Phalanx* 1, no. 5 (5 February 1844).

20. MGN to Alonzo Lewis, 2 April 1857, UVA.

21. Archbishop John B. Purcell to Bishop Peter Paul Lefevre, 22 February 1857, Archdiocese of Detroit Collection (CDET), III-2-i, UNDA.

22. Peter R. Kenrick to John B. Purcell, 15 April 1857, Archdiocese of Cincinnati Collection (CACI), II-4-n, UNDA.

23. John B. Purcell to Anthony Blanc, 6 March 1857, CANO, IV-1-L, UNDA; *Catholic Telegraph and Advocate,* 11 July 1857, cited in Gleason, "Free-Love to Catholicism," 302. The three sacraments required for Christian initiation are: (1) Baptism, which signals the beginning of a new life in Christ; (2) Confirmation, which reflects the strengthening of that new life in the Church; and (3) the Eucharist, which nourishes the transformed recipient with Christ's body and blood. See *Catechism,* 324.

24. TLN, *Health Manual,* 98.

25. TLN, *Forty Years,* 2:102–7. A brief hand-typed notice dated May 16, 1857, is housed in the files of the Ursuline parish in St. Martin, Ohio, which reads in full: "St. Martin Water Cure. Dr. F. L. Nichols and Mrs. Mary F. Grove Nichols [sic] have removed from Yellow Springs and have opened a water cure and Boarding House near the Ursuline Convent in Brown County, Ohio, where they will receive a limited number of patients for treatment. Boarders who wish to be near the Convent School or Day pupils whose health may require special attention [sic]." This notice lacks additional identifying information.

26. "The Question of Marriage," *NJ* 3, no. 1 (26 August 1854): 27; MGN and TLN, *Marriage,* 87.

27. Matthew 19:6. See *Catechism,* 403; and "The Question of Marriage," *NJ* 3, no. 1 (26 August 1854): 27.

28. TLN, *Forty Years,* 2:44.

29. MGN and TLN, *Marriage,* 216, 24, 48, 293; "Polygamy in Utah," *NJ* 2, no. 19 (20 May 1854): 2.

30. TLN, *Human Physiology,* 309–10.

31. Ibid., 300–301, 298, 301.

32. TLN, *Esoteric Anthropology* (Arno Edition, 1972), 100.

33. TLN, *Human Physiology,* 311. The sacramental bond of marriage between two mutually consenting, uncoerced, baptized persons who consummate their marriage is considered indissoluble by the Catholic Church (Codex Iuris Canonici, can.1141). The laws of Moses in the Old Testament had allowed men to divorce their wives, but Christ had eliminated that toleration, which the Catholic Church interprets as Moses' accommodation to man's "hardness of heart" (Matt. 5:31–32; 19:3–9; Mark 10:9; Luke 16:18; 1 Cor. 7:10–11). See *Catechism,* 409, 573.

34. MGN, "A Retrospect—VI," *Herald of Health* 44 (August 1881): 1.

35. 1 Peter 3:1 and 1 Corinthians 7:4.

36. MGN and TLN, *Marriage,* 194.

37. TLN, *Esoteric Anthropology,* 330; TLN, *Catholic Telegraph and Advocate,* 19 September 1857, 1.

38. "Lectures by Dr. Nichols," *Catholic Telegraph and Advocate*, 21 November 1857, n.p. During this time, Thomas also wrote articles for the *Catholic Telegraph and Advocate*. One (11 July 1857) discouraged the impulse to see flirtation as innocent; another (31 July 1858) "compared the failure of socialistic colonies projected by Owen and others with the success of the religious establishment and school founded by the French priest Edward Sorin." Others of his articles appeared on June 6, 13, 20 and August 29, 1857. One of his columns also appeared in the *Catholic Mirror* of Baltimore on June 13, 1857. See Gleason, "Free-Love to Catholicism," 305–6.

39. This transition had likely been facilitated by the French priests at the Brown County convent. Unless otherwise noted, the following account of their travels to Catholic institutions in America comes from MGN, *Woman's Work in Water-Cure*, 140–47; TLN, *Health Manual*, 99–102; and TLN, *Forty Years*, 2:81–118.

40. TLN, *Health Manual*, 100; John B. Purcell to Anthony Blanc, 23 March 1859, CANO, VI-2-a, UNDA. The letter Thomas sent to Archbishop Blanc at the beginning of the following June suggests that Thomas was keenly aware of his own close surveillance as well. "Monsignor," wrote Thomas, "I enclose to you copies of the prospectus of my lectures. I rely upon your kind offices in behalf of this humble effort, and your prayers for its success. Praying for your health, I remain with great respect Your unworthy son in J.C., T. L. Nichols" (3 June 1859, CANO, VI-2-a, UNDA). In his retrospective *Health Manual*, Thomas characterized the Archbishop of New Orleans as "enlightened and friendly" (101).

41. MGN to Alonzo Lewis, 5 September 1859, UVA.

42. MGN, *Woman's Work in Water-Cure*, 147.

43. TLN, *Lectures on Catholicity*, 184–85.

44. MGN and TLN, *Marriage*, 23.

45. TLN, *Lectures on Catholicity*, 186.

46. TLN, *Forty Years*, 2:75–78. Elsewhere he added: "A great number of American preachers, among Presbyterians, Baptists, Methodists, Unitarians, Universalists, have no hesitation in introducing political or social topics into the pulpit. They are often candidates for office, and not infrequently take the stump in presidential electioneering campaigns. . . . The mingling of religion and politics has not been a good to either" (ibid., 1:375).

47. TLN, *Lectures on Catholicity*, 156.

48. TLN, *Health Manual*, 101–2; TLN, *Forty Years*, 1:212–13.

49. TLN, *Forty Years*, 2:100.

50. Ibid., 108–15.

51. MGN, *Woman's Work in Water-Cure*, 147.

52. A copy of this circular is in the Archives of the University of Notre Dame, CANO, VI-2-c. See also "Advertisements," *WCJ* 29, no. 6 (June 1860): 92.

53. TLN, *Health Manual*, 143.

54. Ibid., 99; "A Retrospect," *Herald of Health* 44 (August 1881): 1.

55. MGN and TLN, "Circular," New York City, April 1860, CANO, VI-2-c, UNDA.

56. TLN, *Health Manual*, 102.

57. McPherson, *Battle Cry*, 271–75.

58. TLN, *Health Manual*, 102; TLN, *Forty Years*, 2:348–49; McPherson, *Battle Cry*, 274.

59. TLN, *Forty Years*, 1:10.

60. McPherson, *Battle Cry*, 436; TLN, *Forty Years*, 1:5, 8; TLN, "Peace or War," *New York Age*, 2 April 1861, quoted in *Forty Years*, 2:358–59. Recall that Thomas felt antipathy for William Seward, who as governor of New York in 1840 had refused to pardon Buffalo developer Benjamin Rathbun for forgery of promissory notes.

61. TLN, "A Brief Record of a Well-Spent Life," *Herald of Health* 79 (July 1884): 79.

62. TLN, *Forty Years*, 1:9–10. Thomas seems to have found comfort in the thought that he was returning to the land of his ancestry—a land "which in all beyond this brief century is mine" (ibid.).

63. MGN, *Mary Lyndon*, 269.

64. TLN, *Forty Years*, 1:3, 2:332. The Nicholses' old friend and fellow Fourierist Marx Edgeworth Lazarus had also refused to support the Union cause. According to historian John C. Spurlock, Lazarus went on to practice medicine in the South and maintained his "disgust with all government." Spurlock also notes that the Nicholses' Catholicism may have put them "at odds with the evangelical abolitionists and the anti-Catholic elements of the new Republican party" (*Free Love*, 204).

65. TLN, *Forty Years*, 1:3–4. On the respective positions of Lincoln, Seward, and Greeley, see McPherson, *Battle Cry*, 246–57, 334. Thomas quoted from Seward's speech before the New England Society in New York, December 1860: "When [a family member] gets discontented, begins to quarrel, to complain, does the [good] father quarrel with him, tease him, threaten him, coerce him? No, that is the way to get rid of a family. But . . . if you wish to keep them together you have only one thing to do—to be patient, kind, forbearing, and wait until they come to reflect for themselves. The South is to us what the wife is to the husband" (*Forty Years*, 2:342–44).

66. TLN, *Forty Years*, 2:242, 232, 260, 236–38.

67. MGN, "A Word to the Believers in the Sovereignty of the Individual," *NJ* 1, no. 3 (June 1853): 21; MGN, *Mary Lyndon*, 129; TLN, *Forty Years*, 2:261. For more on the freed-slave population, see Freeman, *Free Negro*; Sterkx, *Free Negro*; Litwack, *North of Slavery*; Brown, *Free Negroes*; and Woolfolk, *Free Negro*.

68. TLN, *Forty Years*, 2: 238–41, 261–63. Thomas could reconcile slavery with the belief that "all men have the right of useful, unbroken legs" because, like the majority of antebellum whites, he believed Negro men to be less than full men. In 1849 he had written, "On this continent, we see the red race gradually fading from existence. A similar change in population seems to be going on in Australia and Polynesia. We may reasonably look forward to the time, when Asia and Africa will be repeopled, by races of a higher order than those by which they are now inhabited. The amalgamated European races, there is reason to believe, will in a few centuries occupy every portion of the habitable globe" (*Woman, in All Ages*, 206). And in *Forty Years*, he had written that the followers of John Brown "are ready . . . to excite four millions of slaves to rapine and murder, to exterminate a white population of eight millions, and make their country a desert of wild beasts and savages" (2: 346).

69. MGN and TLN, *Marriage*, 85–86; TLN, *Forty Years*, 2: 259, 1: 252, 2: 242.

EPILOGUE

1. TLN, "A Brief Record of a Well-Spent Life," *Herald of Health* 79 (July 1884): 79; TLN, *Health Manual*, 428, 444. In 1866 Thomas wrote a letter to Thurlow Weed, asking the favor of having back copies of his *Times* columns sent to him in England for use in a book he claimed to be completing: *Five Years in England.* I have seen no other reference to this work and know no details of Thomas's relationship with Weed. Thomas wrote in this letter that he had in his own possession only five or six of the articles that he had been sending to the *Times* "weekly or oftener." Thomas also wondered whether "Appleton's Cyclopedia's" entry on Weed met with his approval, as Thomas intended to use the published biographical sketch of Weed as a basis for his own profile of Weed in *Chambers' Encyclopedia.* (Thomas also sent his respects to Mr. Raymond, the editor of the *Times* who had savaged *Mary Lyndon* but who in the 1860s was apparently accepting Thomas's correspondence for publication. One is reminded of Thomas's expectation that Mary would stop writing for the *Water-Cure Journal* when Trall refused to advertise *Esoteric Anthropology.* Details of Raymond's possible reconciliation with the Nicholses are unknown.) See Thomas Low Nichols to Thurlow Weed, 21 September 1866, Weed Papers, Archives of the University of Rochester.

2. TLN, *Forty Years*, 2:40, 44; TLN, *Health Manual*, 433.

3. TLN, *Health Manual*, 105–8. On Thomas's doubt about the wisdom of marriage for those with predisposition to disease, see TLN, *Human Physiology*, 310.

4. TLN, "A Brief Record of a Well-Spent Life," 79; TLN, *Health Manual*, 194, 217, 392, 221.

5. MGN to Paulina Wright Davis, 29 June 1875, VC. A chronological bibliography of the Nicholses' writings is appended to this book.

6. TLN, "Methods of Cure," *Herald of Health* 57 (September 1882): cover; advertisements, *Herald of Health* 48 (December 1881); TLN, *Health Manual*, 214. Mary's reference to Sapolino's destruction of "germs and parasites" reveals her assimilation of germ theory, a new notion of disease causation. Yet both Mary and Thomas expressed opposition to legislative proposals for mandatory vaccinations, which they considered dangerous. See *Herald of Health* 15 (February 1879): 161, and 44 (August 1881): cover. Regarding diet, Thomas wrote, "I have never been what may be called a rigid vegetarian, nor am I now a fanatical one." He did eat fish and shellfish. Furthermore, he declared, "In thirty years I have not been disabled by one day of illness—nor ever failed to meet my engagements and to do my work" (*Herald of Health* 25 [January 1880]: 293–94).

7. TLN, *Health Manual*, 394; Nichols, "Our Work," *Herald of Health* 60 (January 1883): 2. The Nicholses also expressed deep gratitude to Sir Walter Trevelyan, who had provided them generous financial assistance during these years.

8. MGN, "To My Friends," *Herald of Health* 48 (December 1881): cover; TLN, "A Brief Record of a Well-Spent Life," 79.

9. For a good discussion of these and other causes of the water cure's fading appeal, see Cayleff, *Wash and Be Healed*, 159–75.

10. Several letters written by Mary during these years have survived. In a letter to Edgar Allan Poe's biographer John Ingram (3 February 1875), Mary referred to the "exceedingly busy life led by my husband and myself, and our two secretaries." Other letters to Ingram indicate the Nicholses' longstanding devotion to Poe and their disgust for the hostile biographical writings of Rufus Griswold. See letters from MGN to John Ingram, UVA.

11. TLN, "A Brief Record of a Well-Spent Life," 78; TLN, *Health Manual*, 445; MGN to Paulina Wright Davis, 29 June 1875 and 28 July 1875, VC; MGN, "To My Friends," cover. Elma Mary Gove became a serious and successful portrait artist, working primarily in crayon and charcoal. Her works were exhibited at the Boston Athenaeum (1859) and the Pennsylvania Academy of the Fine Arts (1855, 1859). She also exhibited at the National Academy of Design (NAD), an organization founded by Samuel F. B. Morse (of Morse code fame) as a non-elite, egalitarian association run by and for artists. Elma was also a member of the Cincinnati Associated Artists, a respected and aspiring organization. The nature of her catalogue listings suggests that she varied her themes and genres with the times. Her oil portrait of Edward W. Nichols, an associate member of the NAD is still held in the association's collections. For a genealogical history of the Letchworth family that extends into the 1940s, see Letchworth, *Letchworth Family*.

12. TLN, *Health Manual*, 211–13. "That persons having the magnetic element can use it to influence the feelings and affections of those they wish to impress, I have no doubt whatever," wrote Thomas. In the 1880s Thomas also endorsed electromagnetic treatments, noting that "sending a strong Faradic current through the body for ten minutes every day or two may strengthen the whole nervous system, and be very useful in many nervous disorders." See "Mesmerism," *Herald of Health* 64 (April 1883): 37; and "The Art of Healing," *Herald of Health* 80 (August 1884): 89. On Mary's injury, see TLN, "A Brief Record of a Well-Spent Life," 79.

13. TLN, *Health Manual*, 219–20; TLN, "A Brief Record of a Well-Spent Life," 79–80.

14. TLN, *Herald of Health* 80 (August 1884): 88–89.

15. Quoted in TLN, *Health Manual*, 443.

16. Quoted in ibid., 218–19.

17. TLN, "A Brief Record of a Well-Spent Life," 79–80.

18. TLN, *Health Manual*, 216. This is now a rare book, with only one known copy in the Library of the British Museum and a photocopy of that text in the National Library of Medicine in Bethesda, Maryland. Its obscurity suggests that the book was not widely printed.

19. Ibid., 288–89.

20. MGN, *Despotism*, quoted in TLN, *Health Manual*, 287; TLN, *Human Physiology*, 297.

21. Letter to Susan B. Anthony, 20 July 1857, quoted in Stanton and Blatch, eds., *Elizabeth Cady Stanton*, 2:69–70.

22. Letter to Susan B. Anthony, 14 June 1860, quoted in Stanton and Blatch, eds., *Elizabeth Cady Stanton*, 2:82.

23. Andrews, *Love, Marriage, and Divorce*, 49.

24. Letter to Martha C. Wright, 2 June 1860, quoted in Stanton and Blatch, eds., *Elizabeth Cady Stanton*, 2:80–81; Leach, *True Love*, 144–45, citing Ellen Dubois, "On Labor and Free Love: Two Unpublished Speeches of Elizabeth Cady Stanton," *Signs* 1 (Autumn 1975): 257–65.

25. Letter to Lucretia Mott, 1 April 1872, quoted in Stanton and Blatch, eds., *Elizabeth Cady Stanton*, 2:136–137.

26. MGN to Paulina Wright Davis, 1870, VC.

27. Quoted in Stearns, "Two Forgotten New England Reformers," 84.

28. TLN, *Esoteric Anthropology*, 9.

29. MG, "Letter to the Editor," *Phalanx, or Journal of Social Science* 1, no. 5 (5 February 1844); TLN, *Work of Reform*, 8.

30. TLN, *Woman, in all Ages*, 219–20.

31. Ibid., 236–37.

32. TLN, *Nichols' Monthly Extra*, ca. 1856; MGN, "To My Friends," 133.

BIBLIOGRAPHY OF
THE NICHOLSES' WORKS

In brackets below each bibliographic entry is the holding library of every primary source located only there or not included in the *National Union Catalog of Pre-1956 Imprints.*

BY MARY SARGEANT NEAL GOVE NICHOLS

by "M.S.G." in the *Graham Journal of Health and Longevity:*
"Reply to a Few Queries Suggested by a Correspondent," *GJHL* 2, no. 21 (13 October 1838): 334–35.
Solitary Vice. Address to Parents and Those Who Have the Care of Children. Portland: Printed at the Journal Office, 1839.
    [United States Library of Congress, hereafter the Library of Congress]
ed., *Health Journal and Advocate of Physiological Reform*, 1840.
    [American Antiquarian Society, Worcester, Massachusetts, hereafter the American Antiquarian Society]
by "A.B." in the *Boston Medical and Surgical Journal:*
"Critical Observations on Dr. Durkee's 'Remarks On Scrofula,'" *BMSJ* (18 December 1839): 297–99.
"Quotations and Remarks on the Blood—No. 1," *BMSJ* (19 February 1840): 24–27.
"Quotations and Remarks on the Blood—No. 2," *BMSJ* (26 February 1840): 43–45.
"Respiratory Apparatus—Mr. Bronson, &c.," *BMSJ* (26 August 1840): 49–51.
Lectures to Ladies on Anatomy and Physiology. Boston: Saxton & Peirce, 1842.
ed., *Health Journal and Independent Magazine*, 1843.
"Letter to Friend Brisbane from M. S. Gove," *Phalanx* (5 February 1844): 64–65.
by "Mary Orme" in *Godey's Magazine and Lady's Book:*
"Marrying a Genius" (September 1844): 104–7.

"The Artist" (April 1845): 154–56.

"The Evil and the Good" (July 1845): 36–38.

"Mary Pierson" (January 1846): 39–41.

"Minna Harmon; or, The Ideal and the Practical" (December 1848): 335–38.

by "Mary Orme" in the *Broadway Journal:*

"The Gift of Prophecy," *BJ* 2, no. 13 (4 October 1845): 187–88.

Lectures to Women on Anatomy and Physiology. New York: Harper & Brothers, 1846. [reprinted in 1855]

[by "Mary Orme"] *Uncle John; or, "It Is Too Much Trouble."* New York: Harper & Brothers, 1846.

by "Mary Orme" in *U.S. Magazine and Democratic Review:*

"Providence" (poem) 18, no. 92 (February 1846): 141.

"Man and the Earth" (poem) 18, no. 95 (May 1846): 388.

Anonymous in the *American Review:*

"Passages from the Life of a Medical Eclectic," *AR* (April 1846): 374–82.

"Passages from the Life of a Medical Eclectic. No. II," *AR* (May 1846): 469–79.

"Passages from the Life of a Medical Eclectic. No. III," *AR* (July 1846): 53–64.

"Passages from the Life of a Medical Eclectic. No. IV," *AR* (September 1846): 264–75.

Agnes Morris; or, The Heroine of Domestic Life. New York: Harper & Brothers, 1849.

The Two Loves; or, Eros and Anteros. New York: Stringer & Townsend, 1849.

Experience in Water-Cure: A Familiar Exposition of the Principles and Results of Water Treatment, in the Cure of Acute and Chronic Diseases, Illustrated by Numerous Cases in the Practice of the Author; with an Explanation of the Water-Cure Processes, Advice on Diet and Regimen, and Particular Directions to Women in the Treatment of Female Diseases, Water Treatment in Childbirth and the Diseases of Infancy. New York: Fowlers & Wells, 1850.

Water-Cure Journal, and Herald of Reforms (a partial listing):

"Case of Uterine Haemorrhage," *WCJ* (January 1846): 55.

"Mrs. Mary S. Gove," *WCJ* (June 1846): 16.

"Mrs. Gove's Experience in Water Cure," *WCJ* (February 1849): 40–41; (March 1849): 68–70; (April 1849): 103–5; (May 1849): 135–40; (June 1849): 165–68; (July 1849): 7–11; (August 1849): 35–38; (September 1849): 70–73; (October 1849): 98–100; (November 1849): 129–32.

"Errors in Water-Cure," *WCJ* (January 1850): 9–10.

"Observations on Pertussis, or Whooping Cough and Asthma," *WCJ* (February 1850): 37–39.

"Hemorrhoids or Piles," *WCJ* (February 1850): 47.

"A Child Supposed to Be Dead Restored to Life," *WCJ* (February 1850): 55.

"Water-Cure in Childbirth—Again," *WCJ* (April 1850): 117.

"Errors in Water-Cure," *WCJ* (July 1850): 6–7; (October 1850): 156–57.

"Maternity and the Water-Cure of Infants," *WCJ* (March 1851): 57–59.

"The New Costume and Some Other Matters," *WCJ* (August 1851): 30.

"A Lecture on Woman's Dresses," *WCJ* (August 1851): 34–36.

"Woman the Physician," *WCJ* (October 1851): 73–75.

"A Word to Water-Cure People," *WCJ* (January 1852): 8.

"Education: A Letter from Mrs. Gove Nichols," *WCJ* (July 1852): 13–14.

"Letter From Mrs. Gove-Nichols to the Women Who Read the Water-Cure Journal," *WCJ* (September 1852): 67–68.

"Letter from Mrs. Gove Nichols," *WCJ* (November 1852): 112.

"Dress Reform: Letter from Mrs. Gove Nichols," *WCJ* (January 1853): 10–11.

"A Letter from Mrs. Nichols," *WCJ* (February 1853): 35.

[all of the above at the Library of Congress]

The Nicholses published some version of their own periodical from April 1853 through 1856. The original *Nichols' Journal* resembled a newspaper in its format, whereas later issues took the form of small pamphlets. The following bibliography of the *Journal's* many incarnations is taken in large part from John B. Blake, "Mary Gove Nichols, Prophetess of Health," *Proceedings of the American Philosophical Society* 106, no. 3 (June 1962): 229.

Nichols' Journal of Health, Water-Cure, and Human Progress (New York) 1, nos. 1–8 (April–November 1853).

[American Antiquarian Society]

Nichols' Journal: A Weekly Newspaper, Devoted to Health, Intelligence, Freedom, Individual Sovereignty and Social Harmony (New York) 2, nos. 1–31 (7 January–12 August 1854); 3, nos. 1–6 (26 August–30 September 1854). [No later issues of this weekly journal seem to have survived, if indeed they ever existed. The third volume's heading varied slightly, reading "*Health, Intelligence, Freedom, Individuality, Equity, Harmony.*"]

[American Antiquarian Society, with the exception of vol. 2, nos. 23–25 and 29]

Nichols' Monthly (New York) [3] no.[2?] (November 1854): 65–134, plus five unnumbered leaves.

Nichols' Monthly, new ser. 1, nos. [1–4] (June, July, August–September, October–November 1855). The June, August-September, and (probably) July issues were published in New York. The October-November issue was published in Cincinnati.

Nichols' Monthly: A Magazine of Social Science and Progressive Literature (Cincinnati), new ser. 2–3 (1856).

[at Stanford University]

[with T. L. Nichols], *Marriage: Its History, Character, and Results; Its Sanctities, and Its Profanities; Its Science and Its Facts. Demonstrating Its Influence, as a Civilized Institution, on the Happiness of the Individual and the Progress of the Race.* New York, 1854.

Mary Lyndon; or, Revelations of a Life: An Autobiography. New York: Stringer & Townsend, 1855.

[with T. L. Nichols], *Nichols' Medical Miscellanies: A Familiar Guide to the Preservation of Health, and the Hydropathic Home Treatment of the Most Formidable Diseases.* Cincinnati: T. L. Nichols, 1856.

    [Library of Congress]

Sixpenny Magazine:

    "Reminiscences of Edgar Allan Poe" (February 1863).

Anonymous in *All the Year Round:*

    "On the Mississippi: From Cairo to Memphis" (27 August 1864): 58–62.

Uncle Angus. London: Saunders, Otley & Co., 1864.

Vital Law. London: Longmans, Green, & Co., 1869.

Despotism. London: Longmans, Green, & Co., 1869.

Jerry; A Novel of Yankee American Life. London: Sampson Low, Marston Low, & Searle, 1872.

A Woman's Work in Water-Cure and Sanitary Education. London: Nichols & Co., 1874.

"The Clothes Question Considered in Its Relations to Beauty, Comfort, and Health," 1878.

    [British Library, London]

LETTERS OF MARY S. GOVE NICHOLS

Harvard University, Houghton Library:

    to Moses A. Cartland, 1833.

    to John Neal, 8 letters, [1839]–1842.

    to James Russell Lowell, 1843, 1849.

University of Virginia Archives:

    Mary S. Gove Nichols Collection (MSS 9040), Clifton Waller Barrett Library of American Literature, Special Collections Department:

        to Alonzo Lewis, 30 November [1845?]; February 1848; 31 July 1848; undated, c. 1848; 20 November 1849; 2 January 1850; [January 1850]; [February 1850]; 15 February 1850; 13 March [1850]; 2 January 1851; 1 September 1851; 5 December 1855; 15 November [1855]; 2 April 1857; 7 November [1857]; 5 September 1859.

John Henry Ingram's Poe Collection (MSS 38-138), Special Collections Department:

to John Ingram, 24 November 1874; 28 November 1874; 3 February 1875; 4 February 1875; 10 March 1875.

Lynn Historical Society & Museum, Lynn, Massachusetts:

to Alonzo Lewis, 4 May 1849; September 1849; 23 October 1849; undated, ca. 1849.

Massachusetts Historical Society:

Caroline Wells Healey Dall papers,

to Caroline Healey Dall, 24 January 1852.

Mt. Holyoke College Archives and Special Collections:

to Martha Grant, 6 December 1845.

Vassar College Library:

to Paulina Wright Davis, 1870; 29 June 1875; 28 July 1875.

BY THOMAS LOW NICHOLS

The Standard, a weekly, Boston, ca. September 1835–May 1836.

[American Antiquarian Society, vol. 1, nos. 1–2 (1835): 15–16, 31, 34–35; (1836)]

"Address Delivered at Niagara Falls, on the Evening of the 29th of December, 1838," on the anniversary of the burning of the *Caroline*. Buffalo: C. Faxon, 1839.

[Buffalo and Erie County Public Library, Buffalo, New York]

The Buffalonian, 25 December 1837–26 February 1838 as weekly; 5 March 1838–? as triweekly; *Daily Buffalonian*, 1839, Buffalo, New York.

[Buffalo and Erie County Public Library, Buffalo, New York]

My Notions on Matters and Things: Inscribed to the Citizens of Rochester. Rochester: Welles & Hayes, 1840.

[University of Rochester Library, Rochester, New York]

Journal in Jail, Kept During a Four Months' Imprisonment for Libel, in the Jail of Erie County. Buffalo: A. Dinsmore, 1840 (Reprint: New York: Arno Press, 1970).

Ellen Ramsay; or, The Adventures of a Greenhorn, in Town and Country. New York: Nichols's Monthly Series, 1843.

The Lady in Black: A Study of New York Life, Morals, and Manners. New York, 1844.

ed., *The Young Hickory Banner* 1, nos. 1–8 (10 August–28 September 1844). New York: A. Dinsmore.

[American Antiquarian Society]

Raffle for a Wife. New York: Burgess, Stringer, & Co., 1845.

Lecture on Immigration, and the Right of Naturalization. New York: Burgess, Stringer, & Co., 1845.

    [Library of Congress]

Woman, in All Ages and Nations; A Complete and Authentic History of the Manners and Customs, Character and Condition of the Female Sex, in Civilized and Savage Countries, from the Earliest Ages to the Present Time. New York: H. Long & Brother, 1849.

An Introduction to the Water-Cure. A Course Exposition of the Human Constitution, the Conditions of Health; etc. Founded in Nature and Adapted to the Wants of Man. New York: Fowlers & Wells, 1850.

Water-Cure Journal, and Herald of Reforms:

    "A Position Defined, on Reasons for Becoming a Water-Cure Physician," *WCJ* 9, no. 4 (April 1850): 100–103.

    "Practice in Water-Cure," *WCJ* 9, no. 6 (June 1850): 186–88.

    "The Art of Healing: An Inquiry into the Influence of Medical Science upon the Public Health," *WCJ* 10, no. 1 (July 1850): 1–2.

    "American Vegetarian Convention," *WCJ* 10, no. 1 (July 1850): 5–6.

    "American Hydropathic Convention," *WCJ* 10, no. 1 (July 1850): 14–15.

    "Practice in Water-Cure," *WCJ* 10, no. 1 (July 1850): 18–20.

    "Dietetics," *WCJ* 10, no. 3 (September 1850): 89–90.

    "Water-Cure in Consumption," *WCJ* 10, no. 3 (September 1850): 107.

    "Medical Miscellanies. No. 1," *WCJ* 10, no. 4 (October 1850): 135–37.

    "The Curse Removed: A Statement of Facts Respecting the Efficacy of Water-Cure, in the Treatment of Uterine Diseases, and the Removal of the Pains and Perils of Pregnancy and Childbirth," *WCJ* 10, no. 5 (November 1850): 167–73.

    "Vaginal Injections," *WCJ* 10, no. 6 (December 1850): 219.

    "A Few Words on Clothing," *WCJ* 11, no. 2 (February 1851): 25–26.

    "Practice in Water-Cure. Case XX-Asthma," *WCJ* 11, no. 2 (February 1851): 30.

    "Rationalism," *WCJ* 11, no. 2 (February 1851): 43–44.

    "The Home Practice of the Water-Cure," *WCJ* 11, no. 3 (March 1851): 71–72.

    "Practice in Water-Cure," *WCJ* 11, no. 4 (April 1851): 86–87.

    "American Hydropathic Institute," *WCJ* 11, no. 4 (April 1851): 91.

    "Medical Laconics," *WCJ* 11, no. 5 (May 1851): 115–16.

    "The Diseases of Women," *WCJ* 11, no. 5 (May 1851): 122–24.

    "The Staff of Life," *WCJ* 11, no. 6 (June 1851): 148.

    "The War on Pathies," *WCJ* 11, no. 6 (June 1851): 150–51.

    "Medical Education: As It Is, and As It Should Be," *WCJ* 11, no. 7 (July 1851): 10–11.

"Disease of the Heart," *WCJ* 12, no. 3 (September 1851): 62–63.

"The Throat Doctors," *WCJ* 12, no. 3 (September 1851): 64–65.

"Medical Education: The American Hydropathic Institute," *WCJ* 12, no. 3 (September 1851): 65–66.

Discussion of American Hydropathic Institute course of study, *WCJ* 12, no. 5 (November 1851): 114.

"Human Physiology, the True Basis of Reform," *WCJ* 13, no. 1 (January 1852): 1–5.

"Illustrations of Physiology," *WCJ* 13, nos. 2–5 (February-June 1852).

"Reply to Dr. Kittredge," *WCJ* 13, no. 4 (April 1852): 81.

"Our New Epoch—A Personality," *WCJ* 13, no. 5 (May 1852): 100–101.

"Glimpses of Popular Physiology," *WCJ* 14, no. 5 (November 1852): 105–6.

Review of Lazarus, *Love vs. Marriage, WCJ* 14, no. 5 (November 1852): 119.

"The Future Results of Water-Cure," *WCJ* 14, no. 6 (December 1852): 129–30.

American Vegetarian and Health Journal:

"Letter From Dr. T. L. Nichols," *AVHJ* 1, no. 2 (February 1851): 41–43.

"Letter From Dr. Nichols," *AVHJ* 2, no. 3 (March 1852): 38–39.

"Letter From Dr. T. L. Nichols," *AVHJ* 2, no. 5 (May 1852): 72–73.

[National Library of Medicine, Bethesda, Maryland]

Esoteric Anthropology (the Mysteries of Man): A Comprehensive and Confidential Treatise on the Structure, Functions, Passional Attractions, and Perversions, True and False Physical and Social Conditions, and the Most Intimate Relations of Men and Women. New York: Author, 1853 [fourteenth edition: London: W. Foulsham & Co., 1916].

The Nicholses published some version of their own periodical from April 1853 through 1856. For a bibliography of its many incarnations taken in large part from John B. Blake, "Mary Gove Nichols, Prophetess of Health," *Proceedings of the American Philosophical Society* 106, no. 3 (June 1962): 219–34, see above under Mary Sargeant Gove Nichols.

[with Mrs. Mary S. Gove Nichols], *Marriage: Its History, Character, and Results; Its Sanctities, and Its Profanities; Its Science and Its Facts. Demonstrating Its Influence, as a Civilized Institution, on the Happiness of the Individual and the Progress of the Race.* New York, 1854.

Religions of the World. An Impartial History of Religious Creeds, Forms of Worship, Sects, Controversies, and Manifestations, from the Earliest Period to the Present Time. Cincinnati: Valentine Nicholson & Co., 1855.

The Illustrated Manners Book, A Manual of Good Behaviour and Polite Accomplishments. New York: Leland Clay & Co., 1855.

[Library of Congress]

Extra. Nichols' Monthly, ca. 1856.

"Memnonia Institute: A School of Health, Progress, and Harmony." Cincinnati, Ohio, 1856.

    [Antioch College Library, Antiochiana Collection, Yellow Springs, Ohio]

Free Love: A Doctrine of Spiritualism. A Discourse Delivered in Foster Hall, Cincinnati, December 22, 1855. Cincinnati: F. Bly, 1856.

    [Western Reserve Historical Society, Cleveland, Ohio]

[with Mrs. Mary S. Gove Nichols], *Nichols' Medical Miscellanies: A Familiar Guide to the Preservation of Health, and the Hydropathic Home Treatment of the Most Formidable Diseases.* Cincinnati: T. L. Nichols, 1856.

    [Library of Congress]

"Letter to a Married Woman, On the Healthy Regulation and Voluntary Control of the Maternal Function," a pamphlet (1856?) that Thomas Nichols claimed was later incorporated into a book called *Maternity*. (I have found no official bibliographic record of either of these works.)

The Paine Festival. Cincinnati: Valentine Nicholson & Co., 1856.

    [William L. Clements Library of the University of Michigan]

The Work of Reform. Cincinnati: Watkin & Nicholson, 1856.

    [William L. Clements Library of the University of Michigan]

Catholic Telegraph and Advocate:

    "Letter From Dr. Nichols" (19 September 1857): 1.

    "Lectures by Dr. Nichols" (21 November 1857).

    (6, 13, and 20 June 1857); (29 August 1857); and (31 July 1858).

Catholic Mirror, Baltimore:

    article on 13 June 1857.

Lectures on Catholicity and Protestantism. New York: Author, 1859.

Esperanza; My Journey Thither and What I Found There. Cincinnati: Valentine Nicholson, 1860.

    [Research Publications Microfilm, Film #1517, Reel E6]

Father Larkin's Mission in Jonesville: A Tale of the Times. Baltimore: Kelly, Hedian & Piet, 1860.

Circular describing Emmett Mansion. New York, April 1860.

    [University of Notre Dame Archives]

Forty Years of American Life. London: J. Maxwell & Co., 1864 [reprint: New York: Negro Universities Press, 1968].

The Gift of Healing or the Sympathetic Cure. London, n.d.

A Biography of the Brothers Davenport. London: Saunders, Otley, & Co., 1864.

ed., *Supramundane Facts in the Life of Rev. Jesse Babcock Ferguson . . . Including Twenty Years' Observation of Preternatural Phenomena.* London: F. Pitman, 1865.

Human Physiology, the Basis of Sanitary and Social Science. London: Trübner & Co., 1872.

How to Live on a Dime and a-Half a Day. New York: J. S. Redfield, 1872.

How to Live on Six-Pence a Day. London: Longman & Co., 1873.
 [National Library of Medicine, Bethesda, Maryland]

Count Rumford: How He Banished Beggary from Bavaria. London: Herald of Health Office, 1873.

How To Behave: A Manual of Manners and Morals. London: Longmans, Green, & Co., 1873.

A Scamper Across Europe. With Glimpses of Paris, Lyons, Geneva, Turin, Milan, Venice, Vienna and the World's Exhibition, etc. London, 1873.
 [British Library, London]

How to Cook; The Principles and Practice of Scientific, Economic, Hygienic and Aesthetic Gastronomy; With Model Recipes in Every Department of Cookery, Original and Selected. London: Longmans, Green, & Co., 1873.
 [Library of Congress]

ed., *Nichols' Journal of Sanitary and Social Science,* Glasgow, 1873–.
 [British Library, London]

The Laws Of Generation. Showing the Modes and Processes of Vegetable, Animal and Human Reproduction ... Being Part Fourth of Human Physiology the Basis of Sanitary and Social Science. Malvern: T. L. Nichols, 1874.
 [British Library, London]

ed., *The Herald of Health,* London, 1875–.
 [National Library of Medicine, Bethesda, Maryland, and the Library of the British Museum]

Herald of Health, London:
 "How Count Rumford Cured Beggary in Bavaria" (March 1875): 110–14.
 [National Library of Medicine, Bethesda, Maryland, and the British Library, London]

The Herald of Health Almanac. 1876–.
 [British Library, London]

Eating to Live. The Diet Cure: An Essay on the Relations of Food and Drink to Health, Disease, and Cure. London, 1877.
 [British Library, London]

The Beacon Light: Lessons in Physiology for the Young. Glasgow, 1878.
 [British Library, London]

One Half-Mile Square in the Heart of London. (A temperance lecture delivered in Salisbury Hall). London, 1878.
 [British Library, London]

Dr. Nichols' Penny Vegetarian Cookery. Nichols & Co., 1883.

    [British Library, London]

Dyspepsia: Its Nature, Causes, Prevention, and Cure. London: Nichols & Co., 1884.

    [British Library, London]

Marriage in All Ages and Nations: As It Has Been, As It Might Be. Its History, Physiology, Morals, and Laws. London: W. Foulsham & Co., 1886.

Nichols' Health Manual: Being Also a Memorial of the Life and Work of Mrs. Mary S. Gove Nichols. London: T. L. Nichols, 1886 (republished in London by E. W. Allen, 1887).

    [National Library of Medicine, Bethesda, Maryland, and the British Library, London]

Social Life: Its Principles, Relations, and Obligations: A Manual of Morals, and Guide to Good Behaviour. London: Nichols & Co., 1895.

    [Boston Public Library]

LETTERS OF THOMAS LOW NICHOLS

Brown University, John Hay Library, Special Collections:

    to Anthony P. Heinrich, 18 February 1848.

University of Virginia Library:

    Mary S. Gove Nichols Collection (MSS 9040), Clifton Waller Barrett Library of American Literature, Special Collections Department:

    to Alonzo Lewis, 8 May 1854.

John Henry Ingram's Poe Collection (MSS 38-138), Special Collections Department:

    to John Ingram, 3 April 1875.

University of Notre Dame Archives:

    to Anthony Blanc, 3 June 1859, CANO, VI-2-a.

University of Rochester Archives:

    to Thurlow Weed, 21 September 1866.

University of Illinois Archives:

    to Richard Bentley, 19 September 1878.

BIBLIOGRAPHY

NOTE ON SOURCES

Let any woman imagine for a moment a biography of herself based upon those
records she has left, those memories fresh in the minds of surviving friends, those
letters that chanced to be kept, those impressions made, perhaps, on the biographer.... What secrets, what virtues, what passions, what discipline, what quarrels
would, on the subject's death, be lost forever?... We tell ourselves stories of the
past, make fictions or stories of it, and these narrations *become* the past, the only
part of our lives that is not submerged.

CAROLYN HEILBRUN, *Writing a Woman's Life*

Prolific writers, the Nicholses sought an audience in their own time and beyond. The couple produced thirty-eight books, four journals, and two newspapers—not to mention their lectures, their medical columns, and Mary's fiction
and poetry. Much of the Nicholses' prose seems confidently intended for some
future biographer. Both wrote autobiographical and didactic fiction. They were
storytellers—and highly self-conscious seekers of their own plot lines. For this
reason, biography seemed to me the most just way to preserve a memory of this
extraordinary couple. They did not preach abstractions or remote theory; rather,
they encouraged their followers to be aware of the holiness and happiness attainable through moral and healthful choices in each moment of life.

Information about Mary's childhood comes from a variety of primary
sources, including (most descriptively) her own autobiography, *Mary Lyndon;
or, Revelations of a Life. An Autobiography*, written in 1855; her 1850 *Experience in Water-Cure;* the *Nichols' Journal* (1853–56); and a memorial written by
her second husband and published in 1886, entitled *Nichols' Health Manual:
Being Also a Memorial of the Life and Work of Mrs. Mary S. Gove Nichols.* Aspects of Mary's adult life described in these texts do find corroborating evidence
in other sources. There is no reason to discount the descriptions offered of her

youth. However, for the sake of narrative coherence and interest, at a few points I have relied exclusively on *Mary Lyndon* for details that lack outside corroboration; these passages have been flagged in the endnotes. My decision to voice Mary's version of her past experiences rather than to skip over these otherwise undocumented periods in her life may not please all academic readers. After all, Mary did write a great deal of fiction. Historians would prefer to cite unpublished manuscripts—letters and diaries—rather than revised, carefully contemplated retrospective accounts. Yet the story one tells of one's own life may be more useful to understanding the individual than anything else: it is, at worst, the imagined and thus wished-for self. If not entirely trusted as fact, it should at the very least be included for consideration.

In a letter to Moses Cartland written on April 12, 1853, Mary Gove Nichols claimed that *Mary Lyndon* possessed "more truth than poetry" (Houghton Library, Harvard University, cited in Noever, "Passionate Rebel," 231–32). And Thomas Low Nichols also vouched for the text's accuracy: "It is an actual life, even to minute particulars, and to the very conversations, and the literal copying of letters. It is not, therefore, in the least degree a work of imagination or artistic skill. . . . Its great merit is in its being perhaps the only actual copy of a real life, in incident, thought and feeling" (*Nichols' Monthly* [Aug. and Sept. 1855]: 200). Historian Janet Noever notes that in writing *Mary Lyndon* Mary chose to present her half-siblings as full siblings and to ignore her father's prior marriage, which most likely ended with his first wife's death. Noever claims that these are the only details in *Mary Lyndon* that she could document as deviating "from the known facts" ("Passionate Rebel," 29 n. 1).

To ease the way for future Nichols scholars, I have described below some potentially fruitful areas of investigation as well as some of the frustrations encountered in my own work. To begin, it is extremely likely that Mary Gove and Thomas Low Nichols saved more of their correspondence than I have yet found. Even if they did not bring an extensive manuscript collection with them to England (assuming a hasty retreat at the start of the Civil War), it seems unlikely that they would have made no arrangements for the preservation of their papers. In her autobiography, Mary described having a friend pack and send her personal library to her after she had left Hiram, for fear that Hiram might sell the books. She also described her grief at discovering that Hiram had found and burned the collection of letters she had saved from her brother. Mary was not a person to abandon her papers; and indeed, Thomas refers to using her diaries, letters, and other personal documents in compiling the *Nichols' Health Manual.* "Among her correspondence I find letters of . . . John Neal, Horace Greeley, N. P. Willis, W. E. Channing, . . . Thomas Carlyle, John Ruskin, Charles Dickens, Charles Kingsley, Charles Reade, Le Compte de Montalembert, [Rev.] Canon

Warmoll [of Bedford], and many others," he wrote (444), noting as well that she personally knew John Audubon, Theodore Parker, William Ellery Channing, and John Greenleaf Whittier (427). He also quoted Mary's claim in 1880 that "at the lowest estimate, I have written one thousand professional letters a year" (219). I believe there is a rich manuscript trove yet to be found.

One letter from Mary S. Gove to Ralph Waldo Emerson (15 August 1843) is cited in Ralph R. Rusk, ed., *The Letters of Ralph Waldo Emerson in Six Volumes* (New York: Columbia University Press, 1939), 453. However, this letter is not cataloged in the Emerson manuscript collection at Harvard University's Houghton Library. Likewise, general query letters to the following British sites have yielded no records of the Nicholses: *Royal Commission on Historical Manuscripts, National Register of Archives; Hereford and Worcester County Council Record Office;* and *Bedfordshire County Council Record Office.*

Other primary sources that I pursued to no avail included the records of Thomas's early trial in Erie County, New York, and any sacramental records of the Nicholses' conversion to Catholicism and possible renewal of their wedding vows. Original records of Mary's expulsion from the Society of Friends are, however, likely to exist.

In the *Nichols' Health Manual* (426–27), Thomas includes an excerpt from what he describes as a three-page listing in Mary's handwriting of stories she had written for various periodicals, all under pen names (not mentioned) and the prices paid for each. Thomas, who guessed that the list had been written around 1847, did transcribe some of the titles of the stories and their respective publication sites:

"Poor Mrs. Dalton"—Bonner's *Weekly Ledger*
"Never Despair"—Bonner's *Weekly Ledger*
"Violetta"—*Sunday Times*
"The Dead Hand"—Bonner's *Weekly Ledger*
"The Doomed One"—Bonner's *Weekly Ledger*
"The Angel of Mop Alley"—*Sunday Times*
"Madaline's Crow"—Bonner's *Weekly Ledger*
"The Black Horse, Beelzebub"—*Mercury*
"Our Bruno"—Bonner's *Weekly Ledger*
"Alia Braithwhite"—Bonner's *Weekly Ledger*
"Pursuit of a Pretty Woman, or, The Crimson Shawl"—Bonner's *Weekly Ledger*
"Shot!"—Bonner's *Weekly Ledger*
"The Model Maiden"—Bonner's *Weekly Ledger*
"The Little Girl Who Did Not Take Her Own Part"—Bonner's *Weekly Ledger*

"That Woman!"—*Mercury*

"Making Both Ends Meet" and "Violets"—*Mercury*

"Neptune, the Newfoundland"—*Mercury*

"The Old Maid"—Bonner's *Weekly Ledger*

"How We Took in the *Ledger*"—Bonner's *Weekly Ledger*

"Rodden the Gambler"—Bonner's *Weekly Ledger*

"Almost a Horsewhipping"—*Mercury*

"Lost and Saved"—*Mercury*

"The Mystery of Iniquity"—*Mercury*

It should also be noted that although volumes 2 and 3 of the *Nichols'
Monthly* are catalogued in the collections of the Library of the University of
Illinois, the journals themselves were not on the shelves, and librarians'
searches proved to be fruitless. Stanford University may therefore be the only
library with copies of the *Nichols' Monthly* for 1856.

PRIMARY SOURCES

Abbott, Jacob. *Emma; or, The Three Misfortunes of a Belle.* New York: Harper &
    Brothers, 1855.

Abernethy, John. *Lectures on Anatomy, Surgery, and Pathology; including observa-
    tions on the nature and treatment of local diseases.* Boston: B. Perkin Co., 1828.

Alcott, Amos Bronson. *Conversations with Children on the Gospels.* Boston: James
    Munroe & Co., 1836.

Alcott, William Andrus. *The Young Mother; or, Management of Children in Re-
    gard to Health.* Boston: Light & Stearns, 1836.

———. *The Young Wife; or, Duties of Woman in the Marriage Relation.* New
    York: Arno Press, 1972 [orig. 1837].

———. *The House I Live In; or, The Human Body.* Boston: Light & Stearns, 1837.

———. *Vegetable Diet: As Sanctioned by Medical Men, and by Experience in
    All Ages. Including a System of Vegetable Cookery.* New York: Fowlers &
    Wells, 1849.

———. *The Physiology of Marriage.* Boston: Dinsmoor & Co., 1866 [orig. 1856].

———. *Forty Years in the Wilderness of Pills and Powders; or, The Cogitations
    and Confessions of an Aged Physician.* Boston: J. P. Jewett, 1859.

Andrews, Stephen Pearl. *Love, Marriage, and Divorce, and the Sovereignty of the
    Individual. A Discussion Between Henry James, Horace Greeley, and Stephen
    Pearl Andrews.* Weston, Mass.: M & S Press, 1975 [orig. 1853].

*Aristotle's Compleat Masterpiece. In Three Parts; Displaying the Secrets of Na-
    ture in the Generation of Man.* The Booksellers, 1740.

Ashton, James. *The Book of Nature; containing information for young people who think of getting married, on the philosophy of procreation and sexual intercourse; showing how to prevent conception and to avoid child-bearing.* 1860.

Austin, Harriet N. *Baths, and How to Take Them.* Boston: B. L. Emerson, 1861.

Ballou, Ellis. *The Patent Hat: Designed to Promote the Growth of Certain Undeveloped Bumps, and Thereby Increase the Thinking, Reasoning, Acting Power of the Wearer.* New York: Carlton & Phillips, 1855.

Beecher, Catharine E. *Letters to the People on Health and Happiness.* New York: Harper & Brothers, 1855.

Boivin, Marie Anne Victoire Gillain. *A Practical Treatise on the Diseases of the Uterus and Its Appendages.* London: Sherwood, Gilbert, & Piper, 1834.

Brisbane, Albert. *Social Destiny of Man, or Association and Reorganization of Industry.* New York: Greeley & McElrath, 1843.

————. *Theory and Functions of the Human Passions: Followed by an Outline of the Fundamental Principles of Fourier's Theory of Social Science.* Westport, Conn.: Hyperion Press, 1976 [orig. 1856].

Bronson, Charles P. *Abstract of Elocution and Music.* Auburn: H. Oliphant, 1842.

————. *Elocution; or, Mental and Vocal Philosophy.* Louisville, Ky.: Morton & Griswold, 1845.

Brown, Mrs. H. F. M. *The False and True Marriage; The Reason and Results.* Cleveland: E. Cowles & Co., 1859.

Combe, George. *Notes on the United States of North America during a Phrenological Visit in 1838-9-40.* Philadelphia: Carey & Hart, 1841.

Conway, Moncure Daniel. *Autobiography, Memories and Experiences of Moncure Daniel Conway.* 2 vols. Boston and New York: Houghton Mifflin, 1904 [orig. 1860].

Cridge, Alfred. *Epitome of Spirit-Intercourse: A Condensed View of Spiritualism in Its Scriptural, Historical, Actual and Scientific Aspects; Its Relations to Christianity, Insanity, Psychometry and Social Reform. Manifestations in Nova Scotia. Important Communications from the Spirits of Sir John Franklin, and Rev. Wm. Wishart, St. John, N.B. with Evidences of Identity, and Directions for Developing Mediums.* Boston: Bela Marsh, 1854.

Cutter, Calvin. *First Book on Anatomy and Physiology.* Boston: Benjamin B. Mussey & Co., 1848.

Dame Dingle's Series. *Life and Death of Rich Mrs. Duck, A Notorious Glutton.* New York: McLoughlin Bros., 1869.

Davis, Andrew Jackson. *The Harbinger of Health; Containing Medical Prescriptions for the Human Body and Mind.* New York: A. J. Davis & Co., 1861.

Dills, R. S. *History of Greene County, Ohio.* Dayton, Ohio, 1881.

Duffey, Eliza B. *What Women Should Know. A Woman's Book About Women Containing Practical Information for Wives and Mothers.* Philadelphia: J. M. Stoddart, 1873; reprint, New York: Arno Press, 1974.

Dunglison, Robley. *Human Physiology.* Philadelphia: Carey & Lea, 1832.

Eberle, John. *A Treatise of the Materia Medica and Therapeutics.* Philadelphia: J. Grigg, 1830.

Farrar, Eliza W. *The Young Lady's Friend.* New York: Samuel S. & William Wood, 1843 [orig. 1836].

Foote, Edward B. *Science in Story: Sammy Tubbs, the Boy Doctor, and "Sponsie," the Troublesome Monkey.* New York: Murray Hill, 1874.

Fowler, Orson. *Amativeness.* New York: Fowlers & Wells, 1844.

———. *Love and Parentage.* New York: Fowlers & Wells, 1851.

———. *Sexual Science; Including Manhood, Womanhood, and Their Mutual Interrelations; Love, Its Laws, Power, etc. . . . as Taught by Phrenology.* Philadelphia: National Publishing Co., 1870.

Fowler, Orson, and Lorenzo Fowler. *Phrenology. A Practical Guide to Your Head.* New York: Chelsea House Publishers, 1969.

Fuller, Margaret. *Woman in the Nineteenth Century.* New York: W.W. Norton & Co., 1971 [reprint of 1855 ed.; orig. 1845].

Gage, Jared. "Address to the Friends, Officers, and Students of Antioch College," ca. 1856. Pamphlet in Archives of Antioch College Library.

Gleason, Rachel Brooks. *Talks to My Patients; Hints on Getting Well and Keeping Well.* New York: Wood & Holbrook, 1870.

Good, John Mason. *The Study of Medicine.* Boston: Wells & Lilly, 1826.

Goodwin, Parke. *A Popular View of the Doctrines of Charles Fourier, With the Addition of Democracy, Constructive and Pacific.* Philadelphia: Porcupine Press, 1972 [orig. 1844].

Gove, William Henry. *The Gove Book. History and Genealogy of the American Family of Gove and Notes of European Goves.* Salem, Mass.: Sidney Perley, 1922.

Graham, Sylvester. *A Lecture to Young Men on Chastity. Also Intended for the Serious Consideration of Parents and Guardians.* Boston: Charles H. Peirce, 1848 [orig. 1834].

———. *Lectures on the Science of Human Life.* Boston: Marsh, Capen, Lyon, & Webb, 1839.

Gregory, Samuel. *Facts and Important Information for Young Women, on the Subject of Masturbation; With Its Causes, Prevention, and Cure.* Boston: Geo. Gregory, 1845.

———. *Man-Midwifery Exposed and Corrected.* New York: Fowlers & Wells, 1848.

————. *Letter to Ladies, in Favor of Female Physicians for Their Own Sex.* Boston: The [Female Medical Education] Society, 1850.

————. *Female Physicians.* Boston: New England Female Medical College, 1864.

Griswold, Rufus W. *Passages from the Correspondence and Other Papers of Rufus W. Griswold.* Cambridge, Mass.: W. M. Griswold, 1898.

Grosvenor, Benjamin. *Health: An Essay on Its Nature, Value, Uncertainty, Preservation and Best Improvement.* Boston: D. J. Kneeland, 1761.

Hale, Sarah Josepha. *Woman's Record.* New York: Harper Brothers, 1855.

Hamilton. *An Address to the People of Rhode Island.* Providence, R.I.: Knowles & Vose, 1844.

Hollick, Frederick. *The Matron's Manual of Midwifery, and the Diseases of Women During Pregnancy and in Child Bed. Being a Familiar and Practical Treatise, More Especially Intended for the Instruction of Females Themselves, But Adapted Also for Popular Use Among Students and Practitioners of Medicine.* New York: T. W. Strong, 1843.

————. *The Marriage Guide, or Natural History of Generation; A Private Instructor for Married Persons and Those About to Marry Both Male and Female.* New York: T. W. Strong, 1850.

————. *Diseases of Woman, Their Causes and Cure Familiarly Explained; With Practical Hints for Their Prevention, and for the Preservation of Female Health.* New York: Excelsior Publishing House, 1876.

Horsell, William. *Hydropathy for the People: With Plain Observations on Drugs, Diet, Water, Air, and Exercise.* New York: Fowlers & Wells, 1850.

Hunt, Harriot. *Glances and Glimpses; Or, Fifty Years Social, Including Twenty Years Professional Life.* Boston: John P. Jewett & Co., 1856.

Jackson, James Caleb. *Hints on the Reproductive Organs: Their Diseases, Cases, and Cure on Hydropathic Principles.* New York: Fowlers & Wells, 1852.

————. *The Sexual Organism, and Its Healthful Management.* New York: Arno Press, 1974 [orig. 1861].

————. *American Womanhood: Its Peculiarities and Necessities.* Dansville, N.Y.: Austin, Jackson & Co., 1870.

Knowlton, Charles. *Fruits of Philosophy; or, The Private Companion of Young Married People.* 1832.

Lazarus, Marx Edgeworth. *Passional Hygiene and Natural Medicine; Embracing the Harmonies of Man and His Planet.* New York: Fowlers & Wells, 1852.

————. *Love vs. Marriage.* New York: Fowlers & Wells, 1852.

Lewis, Alonzo. *History of Lynn.* Boston: J. H. Eastburn, 1829.

Lewis, Alonzo, and James R. Newhall. *History of Lynn, Essex County, Massachusetts: Including Lynnfield, Saugus, Swampscot, and Nahant.* Boston: John L. Shorey, 1865.

Lewis, Dio. *The Dio Lewis Treasury.* New York: Garfield, 1887.

Little, William. *The History of Weare, New Hampshire 1735–1888.* Lowell, Mass.: S. W. Huse & Co., 1888.

Magendie, François. *An Elementary Treatise on Human Physiology, on The Basis of the Précis Élémentaire de Physiologie.* New York: Harper & Bros., 1844.

Marryat, C. B. *A Diary in America, With Remarks on Its Institutions.* New York: Wm. H. Colyer, 1839.

Martineau, Harriet. *The Martyr Age of the United States.* New York: Arno Press, 1969 [reprint; orig. Boston: Weeks, Jordan & Co., 1839].

The Maternal Physician; A Treatise on the Nurture and Management of Infants, from Birth until Two Years Old. Being the result of sixteen years' experience in the nursery. New York: Arno Press, 1972 [reprint; orig. New York: Isaac Riley, 1811].

Mill, John Stuart. *The Subjection of Women.* Cambridge: M.I.T. Press, 1970 [reprint; orig. London, 1869].

Mott, James. *Observations on the Education of Children; And Hints to Young People on the Duties of Civil Life.* New York: Samuel Wood & Sons, 1816.

Noyes, John Humphrey. *History of American Socialisms.* New York: Hillary House, 1961 [orig. 1870].

———. *Male Continence.* Oneida, N.Y.: Oneida Community Mansion House, 1992 [orig. 1872].

Peabody, Elizabeth Palmer. *Record of a School.* New York, 1835.

Peters, John C. *A Treatise on the Diseases of Married Females. Disorders of Pregnancy, Parturition and Lactation.* New York: William Radde, 1854.

Poe, Edgar Allan. "The Literati of New York," *Godey's Magazine and Lady's Book* 33 (July 1846): 16.

Pulte, J. H. *Woman's Medical Guide; Containing Essays on the Physical, Moral and Educational Development of Females and the Homeopathic Treatment of Their Diseases in All Periods of Life, Together with Directions for the Remedial Use of Water and Gymnastics.* Cincinnati: Moore, Anderson, Wilstach & Keys, 1853.

Report of the Woman's Rights Convention, Held at Seneca Falls, N.Y., July 19th and 20th, 1848. Rochester: John Dick, printer [reprinted by Seneca Falls Historical Society].

Richerand, Anthelme Malthasar Baron. *Elements of Physiology.* Philadelphia: Moore, 1823 [orig. London, 1803].

Robinson, Harriet H. *Loom and Spindle; or, Life Among the Early Mill Girls.* Kailua, Hawaii: Press Pacifica, 1976 [orig. 1898].

Rush, Benjamin. *Medical Inquiries and Observations Upon the Diseases of the Mind.* Philadelphia: J. Grigg, 1827 [orig. 1812].

Seymour, Henry J., [an original Community member]. *The Oneida Community. A Dialogue.* New York: Oneida Community Mansion House, ca. 1893; reprint, 1990.

Shew, Joel, ed. *Hand-Book of Hydropathy; or, A Popular Account of the Treatment and Prevention of Diseases, by Means of Water.* New York: Wiley & Putnam, 1844.

———. *The Water-Cure Manual: A Popular Work, Embracing Descriptions of the Various Modes of Bathing, the Hygienic and Curative Effects of Air, Exercise, Clothing, Occupation, Diet, Water-Drinking, &c.: Together with Descriptions of Diseases, and the Hydropathic Means to Be Employed Therein.* New York: Cady & Burgess, 1848.

———. *Hydropathy; or, The Water Cure: Its Principles, Processes, and Modes of Treatment.* New York: Fowlers & Wells, 1850.

Shew, Marie Louise. *Water-Cure for Ladies: A Popular Work on the Health, Diet, and Regimen of Females and Children, and the Prevention and Cure of Disease; With a Full Account of the Processes of Water-Cure.* Revised by Joel Shew. New York: Wiley & Putnam, 1844.

Slavery and Marriage. A Dialogue. New York: Oneida Community Mansion House, 1994 [orig. 1850].

"Socialistic Theories in Their Medical Aspects." *American Medical Gazette and Journal of Health* (January 1856): 35–42.

Stowe, Harriet Beecher. *Pink and White Tyranny. A Society Novel.* Boston: Roberts Brothers, 1871.

Swedenborg, Emanuel. *The Delights of Wisdom Pertaining to Conjugial Love to Which Is Added the Pleasures of Insanity Pertaining to Scortatory Love.* London: J. S. Hodson, W. Newbery, 1841.

———. *Heaven and Its Wonders, the World of Spirits, and Hell: From Things Heard and Seen.* New York: American Swedenborg Printing & Publishing Society, 1854.

Swisshelm, Jane G. *Letters to Country Girls.* New York: J. C. Riker, 1853.

Taylor, George B. *Claiborne.* New York: Sheldon & Co., 1860.

Tefft, B. F. Letter to Joseph Wall. *The Reformer* (18 January 1840): 27.

Thomas, T. Gaillard. *A Practical Treatise on the Diseases of Women.* Philadelphia: Henry C. Lea, 1872.

Tissot, Samuel A. *A Treatise on the Diseases Produced by Onanism.* New York: Collins & Hannay, 1832.

Townsend, Joseph. *Elements of Therapeutics; or, A Guide to Health; Being Cau-*

tions and Directions in the Treatment of Diseases. Designed Chiefly for the Use of Students. Boston: Etheridge & Bliss, 1807.

Trall, Russell T. *The Hydropathic Encyclopedia; A System of Hydropathy and Hygiene in Eight Parts. Designed as a Guide to Families and Students. And a Text-Book for Physicians.* New York: Fowlers & Wells, 1853 [orig. 1850].

————. *Home Treatment for Sexual Abuses: A Practical Treatise on the Nature and Causes of Excessive and Unnatural Sexual Indulgence, the Diseases and Injuries Resulting Therefrom, with Their Symptoms and Hydropathic Management.* New York: Fowlers & Wells, 1853.

————. *Uterine Diseases and Displacements. A Practical Treatise on the Various Diseases, Malpositions, and Structural Derangements of the Uterus and Its Appendages.* New York: Fowlers & Wells, 1854.

————. *The New Hydropathic Cook-Book; With Recipes for Cooking on Hydropathic Principles.* New York: Fowlers & Wells, 1855.

————. *Sexual Physiology: A Scientific and Popular Exposition of the Fundamental Problems in Sociology.* London: Health Promotion, 1861.

A Vindication of the So-Called Clique. Buffalo, 1839.

Walton, George E. *The Mineral Springs of the United States and Canada, with Analyses and Notes on the Prominent Spas of Europe, and a List of Sea-Side Resorts.* New York: D. Appleton & Co., 1874.

Warrington, Joseph. *The Obstetric Catechism; Containing Two Thousand Three Hundred and Forty-Seven Questions and Answers on Obstetrics Proper.* Philadelphia: J. B. Lippincott, 1860.

Webber, Charles Wilkins. *Yieger's Cabinet. Spiritual Vampirism: The History of Etherial Softdown, and Her Friends of the "New Light."* Philadelphia: Lippincott, Grambo & Co., 1853.

————. *A Letter to the Country and Whig Party, With Regard to the Conduct of the "American Whig Review."* Washington, D.C.: John T. Towers, 1847.

Wesselhœft, Robert. *Report of Over Two Hundred Interesting Cases, Selected from Among Those Who Have Been Under Treatment in Dr. Robert Wesselhœft's Water Cure Establishment.* New York: Edward O. Jenkins, 1853.

Wesselhœft, Robert, with Shew, Berdortha, Shieferdecker, Trall, Nichols, and others. *The Water-Cure in America. Over Three Hundred Cases of Various Diseases Treated with Water.* New York: Fowlers & Wells, 1852.

Whitman, Walt. *Leaves of Grass.* New York: Fowlers & Wells, 1855.

Wilkins, Charles. "The Shot in the Eye. A True Story of Texas Border Life," *U.S. Magazine and Democratic Review* 16, no. 80 (February 1845): 144–56.

Wollstonecraft, Mary. *A Vindication of the Rights of Woman.* New York: Penguin, 1992 [orig. 1792].

The Young Lady's Toilet. Hartford, Conn.: E. B. & E. C. Kellogg, 1842.

NINETEENTH-CENTURY JOURNALS AND NEWSPAPERS

All The Year Round. London.
American Journal of Hydropathy. New York, N.Y.
American Review. New York, N.Y.
American Water-Cure Reporter. New Grafenberg, N.Y.
Athenaeum. London.
Boston Medical and Surgical Journal. Boston, Mass.
Boston Quarterly Review. Boston, Mass.
Broadway Journal. New York, N.Y.
Brother Jonathan. New York, N.Y.
Catholic Telegraph and Advocate. Cincinnati, Ohio.
Crayon. New York, N.Y.
Daily Springfield Nonpareil. Springfield, Ohio.
Democratic Review. Washington, D.C.
Dietetic Reformer and Vegetarian Messenger. London.
Doggett's New York City Directory, 1846–52.
Frazer's Magazine, London.
Freedom's Amulet. Lynn, Mass.
Godey's Magazine and Lady's Book. New York, N.Y.
Graham Journal of Health and Longevity. Boston, Mass.
Green Mountain Spring. Brattleboro, Vt.
Herald of Health. London.
Household Words. London.
Hygienic Teacher and Water-Cure Journal. New York, N.Y.
Lady's Amaranth. Philadelphia, Pa.
Laws of Life. Dansville, N.Y.
Library of Health and Teacher of the Human Constitution. Boston, Mass.
Lily. Seneca Falls, N.Y.
Lynn Record. Lynn, Mass.
Magnetic and Cold Water Guide. Rochester, N.Y.
New England Spiritualist. Boston, Mass.
New Grafenberg Water-Cure Reporter. Utica, N.Y.
New York Arena. New York, N.Y.
New York Aurora. New York, N.Y.
New York Daily Times. New York, N.Y.
New York Daily Tribune. New York, N.Y.
New York Evening Herald. New York, N.Y.
Once a Week. London.
Phalanx, or Journal of Social Science. New York, N.Y.

Reformer. Lynn, Mass.

Temple Bar. London.

Una. Providence, R.I.

United States Magazine and Democratic Review. Washington, D.C.

Water-Cure Journal and Herald of Reforms. New York, N.Y.

Water-Cure World. Brattleboro, Vt.

Xenia Torch-Light. Xenia, Ohio.

MANUSCRIPT COLLECTIONS

American Antiquarian Society [AAS]
  Abby Foster Kelley Papers
  Letter of Anna Breed to Abby Foster Kelley, November 1838
  Letter of William Bassett to Abby Foster Kelley, November 1838
Antioch College Library, Antiochiana Collection [AC]
  Horace and Mary Mann letters
  Notes of the Adelphian Literary Society, November 1856
  Advertising circular for "Memnonia Institute," 1856
  Letter of W. N. Hambleton to the Faculty of Antioch College, 1 March 1856
  Jared Gage, "Address to the Friends, Officers, and Students of Antioch College," 1856
Boston Public Library/Rare Books Dept., Courtesy of the Trustees [BPL]
  Griswold Manuscripts
  Letter of John Neal to Mary Gove Nichols, 30 November 1846
Brown University, John Hay Library [BU]
  Letter of Thomas Low Nichols to Anthony P. Heinrich, 18 February 1848
Harvard University, Houghton Library [HU]
  Letter of Mary Gove Nichols to Moses A. Cartland, 1853
  Letters of Mary Gove Nichols to James R. Lowell, two letters, 1843, 1849
  Letters of Mary Gove Nichols to John Neal, eight letters, 1839?–1842
Lynn Historical Society [LHS]
  Letters of Mary Gove Nichols to Alonzo Lewis, four letters, 1849
Massachusetts Historical Society [MHS]
  Letter of Mary Gove Nichols to Caroline Healey Dall, 24 January 1852. Caroline Healey Wells Dall papers.
  Letter of Horace Mann to Mary Peabody Mann, 22 August 1856. Horace Mann papers.
  Letter of Mary Peabody Mann to Horace Mann, 20 March 1856. Horace Mann papers.
Mount Holyoke College Archives [MHC]

Letter of Mary Gove Nichols to Martha Grant, 1845

University of Notre Dame Archives [UNDA]

Letter of John B. Purcell to Peter Paul Lefevre, 22 February 1857, Archdiocese of Detroit Collection, CDET, III-2-i

Letter of John B. Purcell to Anthony Blanc, 6 March 1847, Archdiocese of New Orleans Collection, CANO, IV-1-l

Letter of Peter R. Kenrick to John B. Purcell, 15 April 1857, Archdiocese of Cincinnati Collection, CACI, II-4-n

Letter of John B. Purcell to Anthony Blanc, 5 December 1857, CANO, VI-1-n

Letter of John B. Purcell to Anthony Blanc, 23 March 1859, CANO, VI-2-a

Letter of Thomas Low Nichols to Anthony Blanc, 3 June 1859, CANO, VI-2-a

Circular advertising the Nicholses' Emmet Mansion, April 1860, CANO, VI-2-c

University of Rochester Archives [UR]

Letter of Thomas Low Nichols to Thurlow Weed, 21 September 1866

University of Virginia Library, Special Collections Department [UVA]

Mary S. Gove Nichols Collection (MSS 9040), Clifton Waller Barrett Library of American Literature:

Letters of Mary Gove Nichols to Alonzo Lewis, sixteen letters, 1848–59

Letter of Thomas Low Nichols to Alonzo Lewis, May 1854

John Henry Ingram's Poe Collection (MSS 38–138):

Letters of Mary Gove Nichols to John Ingram, five letters, 1874–75

Letter of Thomas Low Nichols to John Ingram, April 1875

Vassar College Library, Special Collections [VC]

Letters of Mary Gove Nichols to Paulina W. Davis, three letters, 1870, 1875

SECONDARY SOURCES

Abrahams, Harold J. *The Extinct Medical Schools of Baltimore, Md.* Baltimore, Md.: Maryland Historical Society, 1969.

Adams, Grace, and Edward Hutter. *The Mad Forties.* New York: Harper & Brothers, 1942.

Apple, Rima, ed. *Women, Health, and Medicine in America: A Historical Handbook.* New Brunswick: Rutgers University Press, 1992.

Aspinwall, Bernard. "Social Catholicism and Health: Dr. and Mrs. Thomas Low Nichols in Britain." In *The Church and Healing,* ed. W. J. Sheils. Oxford: Basil Blackwell, 1982.

Bacon, Margaret Hope. *Valiant Friend: The Life of Lucretia Mott.* New York: Walker & Co., 1980.

Barker-Benfield, Ben. "The Spermatic Economy: A Nineteenth-Century View of Sexuality." *Feminist Studies* 1 (1972): 45–74.

Barthel, Diane L. *Amana: From Pietist Sect to American Community.* Lincoln: University of Nebraska Press, 1984.

Bartlett, Elizabeth Ann. *Liberty, Equality, Sorority: The Origins and Interpretation of American Feminist Thought: Frances Wright, Sarah Grimké, and Margaret Fuller.* New York: Carlson Publishing, Inc., 1994.

Basch, Norma. *In the Eyes of the Law: Women, Marriage, and Property in Nineteenth-Century New York.* Ithaca: Cornell University Press, 1982.

Battan, Jesse F. "'The World Made Flesh': Language, Authority, and Sexual Desire in Late Nineteenth-Century America." *Journal of the History of Sexuality* 3, no. 2 (October 1992): 223–44.

Battenfeld, Dorothy Eleanor. "'She hath done what she could.' Three Women in the Popular Health Movement: Harriot Kezia Hunt, Mary Gove Nichols, and Paulina Wright Davis." Master's thesis, George Washington University, 1985.

Baym, Nina. *Woman's Fiction: A Guide to Novels by and about Women in America, 1820–1870.* Ithaca: Cornell University Press, 1978.

Bedell, Madelon. *The Alcotts: Biography of a Family.* New York: Clarkson N. Potter, Inc., 1980.

Beecher, Jonathan. *Charles Fourier: The Visionary and His World.* Berkeley: University of California Press, 1986.

Beecher, Jonathan, and Richard Bienvenu, eds. *The Utopian Vision of Charles Fourier: Selected Texts on Work, Love, and Passionate Attraction.* Columbia: University of Missouri Press, 1983.

Bender, Thomas. *Toward an Urban Vision: Ideas and Institutions in Nineteenth Century America.* Baltimore: Johns Hopkins University Press, 1975.

Blair, Kathy. *The Clubwoman as Feminist: True Womanhood Redefined, 1868–1914.* New York: Holmes & Meier, 1980.

Blake, John B. "Mary Gove Nichols, Prophetess of Health." *Proceedings of the American Philosophical Society* 106, no. 3 (June 1962): 219–34.

Blake, Nelson M. *The Road to Reno: A History of Divorce in the United States.* Westport, Conn.: Greenwood Press, 1977.

Blanchard, Paula. *Margaret Fuller: From Transcendentalism to Revolution.* New York: Addison-Wesley, 1987.

Bonner, Edwin B. *"The Other Branch": London Yearly Meeting and the Hicksites, 1827–1912.* London: Friends Historical Society of Philadelphia, 1975.

Bowers, Q. David. *The Waterford Water Cure: A Numismatic Inquiry.* Wolfeboro, N.H.: Bowers & Merena Publications, 1992.

Brandon, Ruth. *The Spiritualists: The Passion for the Occult in the 19th and 20th Centuries.* New York: Alfred A. Knopf, 1983.

Braude, Ann. *Radical Spirits: Spiritualism and Women's Rights in Nineteenth-Century America.* Boston: Beacon Press, 1989.

Brock, E. J., ed. *Swedenborg and His Influence.* Bryn Athyn, Pa.: Academy of the New Church, 1988.

Brodie, Janet Farrell. *Contraception and Abortion in Nineteenth-Century America.* Ithaca: Cornell University Press, 1994.

Brown, Letitia Woods. *Free Negroes in the District of Columbia, 1790–1846.* New York: Oxford University Press, 1972.

Burby, Liza N. *Elizabeth Blackwell.* New York: Rosen Publication Group, 1996.

Butler, Jon. *Awash in a Sea of Faith: Christianizing the American People.* Cambridge: Harvard University Press, 1990.

Cassedy, James H. *Medicine in America: A Short History.* Baltimore: Johns Hopkins University Press, 1991.

Catechism of the Catholic Church. New York: William H. Sadlier, 1994.

Cayleff, Susan E. *Wash and Be Healed: The Water-Cure Movement and Women's Health.* Philadelphia: Temple University Press, 1987.

————. "Gender, Ideology, and the Water-Cure Movement" In *Other Healers: Unorthodox Medicine in America,* ed. Norman Gevitz. Baltimore: Johns Hopkins University Press, 1988.

Christman, Margaret C. S. *1846: Portrait of the Nation.* Washington, D.C.: Smithsonian Institution Press, 1996.

Cogliano, Francis D. *No King, No Popery: Anti-Catholicism in Revolutionary New England.* Westport, Conn.: Greenwood Press, 1995.

Cohen, Patricia Cline. *The Murder of Helen Jewett: The Life and Death of a Prostitute in Nineteenth-Century New York.* New York: Alfred A. Knopf, 1998.

Cominos, Peter. "Late-Victorian Sexual Respectability and the Social System." *International Review of Social History* 8 (1963).

Conrad, Susan Phinney. *Perish the Thought: Intellectual Women in Romantic America, 1830–1860.* New York: Oxford University Press, 1976.

Cott, Nancy. *The Bonds of Womanhood: "Woman's Sphere" in New England, 1780–1835.* New Haven: Yale University Press, 1977.

————. "Eighteenth-Century Family and Social Life Revealed in Massachusetts Divorce Records." *Journal of Social History* 10 (1976): 20–43.

————, ed. *Root of Bitterness: Documents of the Social History of American Women.* New York: E. P. Dutton & Co., 1972.

Coulter, Harris L. *Homeopathic Science and Modern Medicine: The Physics of Healing with Microdoses.* Berkeley, Calif.: North Atlantic Books, 1980.

Danielson, Susan Steinberg. "Alternative Therapies: Spiritualism and Women's Rights in *Mary Lyndon. or, Revelations of a Life.*" Ph.D. diss., University of Oregon, 1990.

Darnton, Robert. *Mesmerism and the End of the Enlightenment in France.* Cambridge: Harvard University Press, 1968.

Davidson, Cathy N. *Revolution and the Word: The Rise of the Novel in America.* New York: Oxford University Press, 1986.

Delano, Marge Ferguson, and Margery A. duMond. *Utopian Visions.* Alexandria, Va.: Time-Life Books, 1990.

D'Emilio, John, and Estelle B. Freedman. *Intimate Matters: A History of Sexuality in America.* New York: Harper & Row, 1988.

Donegan, Jane B. *"Hydropathic Highway to Health": Women and Water-Cure in Antebellum America.* New York: Greenwood Press, 1986.

Douglas, Ann. *The Feminization of American Culture.* New York: Alfred A. Knopf, 1977.

Douglas, Mary. *Natural Symbols: Explorations in Cosmology.* New York: Vintage Books, 1973.

Epstein, Barbara. *The Politics of Domesticity: Women, Evangelism, and Temperance in Nineteenth-Century America.* Middletown, Conn.: Wesleyan University Press, 1981.

Faler, Paul G. *Mechanics and Manufacturers in the Early Industrial Revolution: Lynn, Mass., 1780–1860.* Albany: State University of New York Press, 1981.

Falk, Peter Hastings, ed. *The Annual Exhibition Record of the Pennsylvania Academy of the Fine Arts 1807–1870.* Madison, Conn.: Sound View Press, 1988.

Fitch, William Edward. *Mineral Waters of the United States and American Spas.* Philadelphia: Lea and Febiger, 1927.

Fogarty, Robert S., ed. *Special Love / Special Sex.* Syracuse: Syracuse University Press, 1994.

Foster, Lawrence. *Women, Family, and Utopia. Communal Experiments of the Shakers, the Oneida Community, and the Mormons.* Syracuse: Syracuse University Press, 1991.

Fourier, Charles. *Design for Utopia: Selected Writings of Charles Fourier.* New York: Schocken Books, 1971.

Franchot, Jenny. *Roads to Rome: The Antebellum Protestant Encounter with Catholicism.* Berkeley: University of California Press, 1994.

Francis, Richard. *Transcendental Utopias: Individual and Community at Brook Farm, Fruitlands, and Walden Pond.* Ithaca: Cornell University Press, 1997.

Freedman, Estelle. "Separatism as Strategy: Female Institution Building and American Feminism, 1870–1930." *Feminist Studies* 5 (Fall 1979): 512–29.

Freeman, Rhoda Golden. *The Free Negro in New York City in the Era Before the Civil War.* New York: Garland Publications, 1994.

Galloway, William A. *The History of Glen Helen.* Columbus, Ohio: F. J. Heer, 1932.

Gevitz, Norman, ed. *Other Healers. Unorthodox Medicine in America.* Baltimore: Johns Hopkins University Press, 1988.

Gleason, Adele A. *In Memoriam 1820–1905, Rachel Brooks Gleason*. A. T. Brown, 1905.

Gleason, Philip. "From Free-Love to Catholicism: Dr. and Mrs. Thomas L. Nichols at Yellow Springs." *Ohio Historical Quarterly* 70, no. 4 (October 1961): 283–307.

Golden, Janet F. *A Social History of Wet Nursing in America: From Breast to Bottle*. New York: Cambridge University Press, 1996.

Goldsmith, Barbara. *Other Powers: The Age of Suffrage, Spiritualism, and the Scandalous Victoria Woodhull*. New York: Alfred A. Knopf, 1998.

Gordon, Linda. *Woman's Body, Woman's Right: Birth Control in America*. New York: Penguin Books, 1974.

Green, Harvey. *Fit for America: Health, Fitness, Sport, and American Society*. Baltimore: Johns Hopkins University Press, 1986.

Guarneri, Carl. *The Utopian Alternative: Fourierism in Nineteenth-Century America*. Ithaca: Cornell University Press, 1991.

Hadley, George Plummer. *History of the Town of Goffstown, 1733–1920*. Concord, N.H.: Rumford Press, 1922.

Halttunen, Karen. *Confidence Men and Painted Women: A Study of Middle-Class Culture in America, 1830–1870*. New Haven: Yale University Press, 1982.

Hartog, Hendrik. *Man and Wife in America. A History*. Cambridge: Harvard University Press, 2000.

Heilbrun, Carolyn. *Writing a Woman's Life*. New York: Ballantine Books, 1988.

Hewitt, Nancy A. *Women's Activism and Social Change. Rochester, New York, 1822–1872*. Ithaca: Cornell University Press, 1984.

Himes, Norman E. *Medical History of Contraception*. Baltimore: Williams & Wilkins Co., 1936.

Hodgson, Alice Doan. *Orford, New Hampshire: A Most Beautiful Village*. Orford, 1978.

Hudspeth, Robert N., ed. *The Letters of Margaret Fuller*. 6 vols. Ithaca: Cornell University Press, 1983–88.

Ingle, Larry H. *Quakers in Conflict: The Hicksite Reformation*. Knoxville: University of Tennessee Press, 1986.

Isenberg, Nancy. *Sex and Citizenship in Antebellum America*. Chapel Hill: University of North Carolina Press, 1998.

Johnson, Paul E., and Sean Wilentz. *The Kingdom of Matthias: A Story of Sex and Salvation in 19th-Century America*. New York: Oxford University Press, 1994.

Kasson, John F. *Rudeness and Civility: Manners in Nineteenth-Century America*. New York: Hill & Wang, 1990.

Kaufman, Martin. *Homeopathy in America: The Rise and Fall of a Medical Heresy*. Baltimore: Johns Hopkins University Press, 1971.

Kelley, Mary. *Private Woman, Public Stage: Literary Domesticity in Nineteenth-Century America.* New York: Oxford University Press, 1984.

Kerber, Linda K. *Women of the Republic: Intellect and Ideology in Revolutionary America.* Chapel Hill: University of North Carolina Press, 1980.

———. *Toward an Intellectual History of Women.* Chapel Hill: University of North Carolina Press, 1997.

Kesten, Seymour. *Utopian Episodes.* Syracuse: Syracuse University Press, 1993.

Klaw, Spencer. *Without Sin. The Life and Death of The Oneida Community.* New York: Penguin Press, 1993.

Kline, Nancy. *Elizabeth Blackwell: A Doctor's Triumph.* Berkeley, Calif.: Conari Press, 1997.

Larkin, Jack. *The Reshaping of Everyday Life, 1790–1840.* New York: Harper-Perennial, 1988.

Leach, William. *True Love and Perfect Union: The Feminist Reform of Sex and Society.* New York: Basic Books, 1980.

Leavitt, Judith Walzer. *Brought to Bed: Childbearing in America, 1750–1950.* New York: Oxford University Press, 1986.

———, ed. *Women and Health in America.* Madison: University of Wisconsin Press, 1984.

Leidy, Lynnette E. "Social Roles and Uterine Position: Nineteenth-Century Therapeutics for Prolapse." Paper delivered at the annual meeting of the American Association of the History of Medicine, Pittsburgh, Pa., May 1995.

Letchworth, Edward H. *The Letchworth Family in England and America.* Buffalo, N.Y., 1940.

Lindenmeyer, Kriste, ed. *Ordinary Women, Extraordinary Lives: Women in American History.* Wilmington, Del.: Scholarly Resources Inc., 2000.

Litwack, Leon F. *North of Slavery: The Negro in the Free States, 1790–1860.* Chicago: University of Chicago Press, 1961.

Lystra, Karen. *Searching the Heart: Women, Men, and Romantic Love in Nineteenth-Century America.* New York: Oxford University Press, 1989.

Magdol, Edward. *The Antislavery Rank and File: A Social Profile of the Abolitionists' Constituency.* New York: Greenwood Press, 1986.

Maines, Rachel P. *The Technology of Orgasm: "Hysteria," the Vibrator, and Women's Sexual Satisfaction.* Baltimore: Johns Hopkins University Press, 1999.

Manuel, Frank E., and Fritzie P. Manuel. *Utopian Thought in the Western World.* Cambridge: Harvard University Press, 1979.

Marcus, Steven. *The Other Victorians: A Study of Sexuality and Pornography in Mid-Nineteenth-Century England.* New York: Basic Books, 1975 [orig. 1966].

Marin, Peter. "An American Yearning: Seeking Cures for Freedom's Terrors." *Harper's* (December 1996): 35–43.

Martin, Emily. *The Woman in the Body: A Cultural Analysis of Reproduction.* Boston: Beacon Press, 1987.

Mason, Michael. *The Making of Victorian Sexual Attitudes.* New York: Oxford University Press, 1994.

Matthews, Jean V. *Toward a New Society: American Thought and Culture 1800–1830.* Boston: Twayne Publishers, 1991.

Mayer, Henry. *All on Fire: William Lloyd Garrison and the Abolition of Slavery.* New York: St. Martin's Griffin, 1998.

McPherson, James M. *Battle Cry of Freedom: The Civil War Era.* New York: Oxford University Press, 1988.

Melder, Keith E. *Beginnings of Sisterhood: The American Women's Rights Movement, 1800–1850.* New York: Schocken Books, 1977.

Miller, Perry. *The Raven and The Whale: Poe, Melville, and the New York Literary Scene.* Baltimore: Johns Hopkins University Press, 1997 [orig. 1956].

Mintz, Steven, and Susan Kellogg. *Domestic Revolutions: A Social History of American Family Life.* New York: Free Press, 1988.

Morantz, Regina Markell. "Making Women Modern: Middle-Class Women and Health Reform in 19th-Century America." In *Women and Health in America,* ed. Judith Walzer Leavitt. Madison: University of Wisconsin Press, 1984.

Myerson, Joel. "Mary Gove Nichols' *Mary Lyndon:* A Forgotten Reform Novel." *American Literature* 58, no. 4 (December 1986): 523–39.

Nissenbaum, Stephen. *Sex, Diet, and Debility in Jacksonian America: Sylvester Graham and Health Reform.* Westport, Conn.: Greenwood Press, 1980.

Noever, Janet Hubly. "Passionate Rebel: The Life of Mary Gove Nichols, 1810–1884." Ph.D. diss., University of Oklahoma, 1983.

Pearson, Lynn F. *The Architectural and Social History of Cooperative Living.* New York: St. Martin's Press, 1988.

Peitzman, Steven J. *A New and Untried Course: Women's Medical College and Medical College of Pennsylvania, 1850–1998.* New Brunswick: Rutgers University Press, 2000.

Pessen, Edward, ed. *The Many-Faceted Jacksonian Era: New Interpretations.* Westport, Conn.: Greenwood Press, 1977.

Price, Robin. "Hydropathy in England, 1840–1870." *Medical History* 25 (July 1981): 269–80.

Rexroth, Kenneth. *Communalism: From its Origins to the Twentieth Century.* New York: Seabury Press, 1974.

Reynolds, David S. *Beneath the American Renaissance: The Subversive Imagination in the Age of Emerson and Melville.* Cambridge: Harvard University Press, 1988.

————. *Walt Whitman's America: A Cultural Biography.* New York: Knopf, 1995.

Richards, Irving T. "Mary Gove Nichols and John Neal." *New England Quarterly* 7 (June 1934): 335–55.

Richardson, Robert, Jr. *Henry Thoreau: A Life of the Mind.* Berkeley: University of California Press, 1986.

————. *Emerson: The Mind on Fire.* Berkeley: University of California Press, 1995.

Ronda, Bruce A., ed. *Letters of Elizabeth Palmer Peabody: American Renaissance Woman.* Middletown, Conn.: Wesleyan University Press, 1984.

Rose, Phyllis. *Parallel Lives: Five Victorian Marriages.* New York: Vintage Books, 1983.

Rosenberg, Charles E. "Catechisms of Health: The Body in the Prebellum Classroom." *Bulletin of the History of Medicine* 69 (Summer 1995): 175–97.

————. *No Other Gods: On Science and American Social Thought.* Baltimore: Johns Hopkins University Press, 1976.

————, ed. *Birth Control and Family Planning in Nineteenth-Century America.* New York: Arno Press, 1974 [orig. 1865].

Rosenberg, Charles E., and Carroll Smith-Rosenberg. "The Female Animal: Medical and Biological Views of Woman and Her Role in Nineteenth-Century America." *Journal of American History* 60 (September 1973): 332–56.

————. *The Secret Vice Exposed! Some Arguments Against Masturbation.* New York: Arno Press, 1974.

Rossi, Alice S., ed. *Essays on Sex Equality: John Stuart Mill and Harriet Taylor Mill.* Chicago: University of Chicago Press, 1970.

Rusk, Ralph L. *The Letters of Ralph Waldo Emerson in Six Volumes.* New York: Columbia University Press, 1939.

Sahli, Nancy Ann. "Elizabeth Blackwell, M.D. 1821–1910." Ph.D. diss., University of Pennsylvania, 1974.

Samoff, Joel. "Yellow Springs, Ohio, 1846–1864, or, The Becoming of a Small Town and the Heritage of a College." Thesis, Antioch College, 1965.

Sears, Clara Endicott. *Bronson Alcott's Fruitlands.* Boston: Houghton Mifflin, 1915.

Sears, Hal D. *The Sex Radicals: Free Love in High Victorian America.* Lawrence: Regents Press of Kansas, 1977.

Seidman, Steven. *Romantic Longings: Love in America, 1830–1980.* New York: Routledge, Chapman & Hall Inc., 1991.

Shanley, Mary Lyndon. *Feminism, Marriage, and the Law in Victorian England.* Princeton: Princeton University Press, 1989.

Shepard, Odell. *Pedlar's Progress: The Life of Bronson Alcott.* Boston: Little, Brown & Co., 1937.

Shryock, Richard H. "Sylvester Graham and the Popular Health Movement, 1830–1870." *Mississippi Valley Historical Review* 18 (September 1931): 172–83.

Silbey, Joel H. *The American Political Nation, 1838–1893.* Stanford: Stanford University Press, 1991.

Sklar, Kathryn Kish. *Catharine Beecher: A Study in American Domesticity.* New York: W.W. Norton, 1976.

Smith-Rosenberg, Carroll. *Disorderly Conduct: Visions of Gender in Victorian America.* New York: Oxford University Press, 1986.

———. "The Female World of Love and Ritual: Relations Between Women in Nineteenth-Century America," *Signs* 1 (1975): 1–29.

———. "Beauty, the Beast, and the Militant Woman: A Case Study in Sex Roles and Social Stress in Jacksonian America." *American Quarterly* 23 (October 1971): 562–84.

Spurlock, John C. *Free Love: Marriage and Middle-Class Radicalism in America, 1825–1860.* New York: New York University Press, 1988.

Stage, Sarah. *Female Complaints: Lydia Pinkham and the Business of Women's Medicine.* New York: W. W. Norton Co., 1979.

Stansell, Christine. *City of Women: Sex and Class in New York, 1789–1860.* Urbana: University of Illinois Press, 1982.

Stanton, Theodore, and Harriot Stanton Blatch, eds. *Elizabeth Cady Stanton as Revealed in Her Letters, Diary, and Reminiscences.* New York: Harper & Brothers, 1922.

Starr, Paul. *The Social Transformation of American Medicine.* New York: Basic Books, 1982.

Stearns, Bertha-Monica. "Two Forgotten New England Reformers." *New England Quarterly* 6 (March 1933): 59–84.

———. "Memnonia: The Launching of a Utopia." *New England Quarterly* 15, no. 2 (June 1942): 280–95.

Stein, Leon, and Annette K. Baxter, eds. *Sex and Equality.* New York: Arno Press, 1974.

Sterkx, H. E. *The Free Negro in Antebellum Louisiana.* Rutherford, N.J.: Fairleigh Dickinson University Press, 1972.

Stern, Madeline B. *The Pantarch: A Biography of Stephen Pearl Andrews.* Austin: University of Texas Press, 1968.

Stilgoe, John R. *Common Landscape of America, 1580–1845.* New Haven: Yale University Press, 1982.

Stoehr, Taylor, ed. *Free Love in America: A Documentary History.* New York: AMS Press, 1979.

Symons, Julian. *Sweet Adelaide.* New York: Harper & Row, 1980.

Tharp, Louise Hall. *Until Victory: Horace Mann and Mary Peabody.* Boston: Little, Brown, & Co., 1953.

Tompkins, Jane. *Sensational Designs: The Cultural Work of American Fiction 1790–1860.* New York: Oxford University Press, 1985.

Trobridge, George. *Swedenborg: Life and Teaching.* New York: Pillar Books, 1976.

Verbrugge, Martha H. *Able-Bodied Womanhood: Personal Health and Social Change in Nineteenth-Century Boston.* New York: Oxford University Press, 1988.

Von Mehren, Joan. *Minerva and the Muse: A Life of Margaret Fuller.* Amherst: University of Massachusetts Press, 1994.

Walters, Ronald G., ed. *Primers for Prudery. Sexual Advice to Victorian America.* Englewood Cliffs, N.J.: Prentice-Hall, 1974.

————. *American Reformers 1815–1860,* rev. ed. New York: Hill & Wang, 1997.

Weiss, Harry B., and Howard R. Kemble. *The Great American Water-Cure Craze: A History of Hydropathy in the United States.* Trenton, N.J.: Past Times Press, 1967.

Whitman, Roger. *The Rise and Fall of a Frontier Entrepreneur: Benjamin Rathbun, "Master Builder and Architect."* Syracuse: Syracuse University Press, 1996.

Whorton, James C. *Crusaders for Fitness: The History of American Health Reformers.* Princeton: Princeton University Press, 1982.

Woodward, Helen Beal. *The Bold Women.* New York: Farrar, Straus, 1953.

Woolfolk, George Ruble. *The Free Negro in Texas, 1800–1860: A Study in Cultural Compromise.* Ann Arbor, Mich.: University Microfilms International, 1976.

Wunderlich, Roger. *Low Living and High Thinking at Modern Times, New York.* Syracuse: Syracuse University Press, 1992.

Young, Marguerite. *Angel in the Forest: A Fairy Tale of Two Utopias.* Normal, Ill.: Dalkey Archive Press, 1994 [orig. 1945].

GENERAL REFERENCE

Chase, Harold, et. al, eds. *Dictionary of American History.* New York: Charles Scribner's Sons, 1976.

Fielding, Mantle. *Mantle Fielding's Dictionary of American Painters, Sculptors, and Engravers.* New York: J. F. Carr, 1965.

Gerdts, William H. *Women Artists of America, 1707–1964.* Newark, N.J.: Newark Museum, 1965.

International Genealogical Index. Church of Jesus Christ of Latter-day Saints, 1994.

James, Edward T., ed. *Notable American Women, 1607–1950.* Cambridge, Mass: Belknap Press, 1971.

Johnson, Allen, ed. *Dictionary of American Biography.* New York: Charles Scribner's Sons, 1964.

Magnusson, Magnus. *Cambridge Biographical Dictionary.* Cambridge: Cambridge University Press, 1990.

Morris, George North. "The Tradition." In *A Century and a Half of American Art.* New York: National Academy of Design, 1975.

National Academy of Design Exhibition Record 1826–1860. New York: New York Historical Society, 1943.

Naylor, Maria, ed. *The National Academy of Design Exhibition Record 1861–1900.* New York: Kennedy Galleries, Inc., 1973.

Sahli, Nancy Ann. *Women and Sexuality in America—A Bibliography.* Boston: G. K. Hall, 1984.